Ethics in
Health Services
Management

Ethics in Health Services Management

Third Edition

Kurt Darr

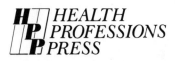

HEALTH
PROFESSIONS
PRESS

Baltimore • Winnipeg • London • Sydney

Health Professions Press, Inc.
Post Office Box 10624
Baltimore, Maryland 21285-0624

Copyright © 1997 by Health Professions Press, Inc.
All rights reserved.

Typeset by PRO-IMAGE Corporation, York, Pennsylvania.
Manufactured in the United States of America by
Thomson-Shore, Inc., Dexter, Michigan.

First printing, January 1997
Second printing, December 1998
Third printing, February 2002
The case study on page 186 is adapted from
CASE STUDIES IN MEDICAL ETHICS by Robert Veatch.
Copyright © 1977 by Robert Veatch.
Reprinted by permission of Harvard University Press.

www.healthpropress.com

Library of Congress Cataloging-in-Publication Data
Darr, Kurt.
    Ethics in health services management / Kurt J. Darr. —3rd ed.
        p. cm.
    Includes bibliographic references and index.
    ISBN 1-878812-36-X
    1. Health services administration—Moral and ethical aspects.
    2. Medical ethics. I. Title.
RA394.D35   1997
174′.2—dc20

                                                        96-26874
                                                        CIP

British Library Cataloguing in Publication Data are available from the British
Library.

Contents

About the Author

Kurt Darr is Professor of Hospital Administration in the Department of Health Services Management and Policy and Professor of Health Care Sciences at The George Washington University. He holds a Doctor of Science from The Johns Hopkins University and a Master of Hospital Administration and a Juris Doctor from the University of Minnesota.

Professor Darr completed his adminstrative residency at Rochester (Minnesota) Methodist Hospital and subsequently worked as an administrative associate at the Mayo Clinic. After being commissioned in the U.S. Navy, he served in administrative and educational assignments at St. Albans Naval Hospital and Bethesda Naval Hospital. He completed postdoctoral fellowships with the Department of Health and Human Services, the World Health Organization, and the Accrediting Commission on Education for Health Services Administration.

Dr. Darr is a Fellow of the American College of Healthcare Executives, a member of the District of Columbia and Minnesota Bars, and serves as an arbitrator and mediator for the American Arbitration Association and the National Health Lawyers Association.

Professor Darr regularly presents seminars on health services ethics, hospital organization and management, quality improvement, and the application of the Deming method in health services.

He is the author and editor of numerous books used in graduate health services administration programs and numerous articles on health services topics.

Preface

In writing the third edition of *Ethics in Health Services Management*, I had the same intent as I had with the first two editions: to assist managers of health services organizations to prevent or solve administrative and biomedical ethical problems and to provide this assistance in a readily usable form. The foci of the book are the methodologies and techniques that assist managers in understanding ethical issues and the analysis and solution of ethical problems when they occur. A collateral focus is to encourage and aid managers in developing and honing a personal ethic.

To facilitate initial reading and subsequent use as a reference, brevity in expression in this volume is a primary criterion. The text informs users about ethical issues and potential problems so that they may be solved knowledgably and effectively, and to this end, cases and vignettes are used extensively. Some are based on events reported in the popular press and professional literature; many are based on the author's personal experience. These cases and vignettes help readers learn how to identify ethical issues and apply the principles examined. Ten cases and vignettes have been added to the third edition, bringing the total number to 66. Enhancements to this edition include greater attention to ethical issues in areas such as managed care. Other issues that appeared in the second edition, such as physician-assisted suicide, are addressed in greater depth in this edition.

No ready answers exist in management problem solving; the same is true in ethical problem solving. "Cookbook" solutions lack feasibility because nuances of fact, setting, and personality vary with each situation. The approach used in this volume is to provide detailed information, examples, and analyses useful in developing the individualized solutions needed by health services organizations and their managers.

Successful managers approach problems in an organized, logical manner. This methodology requires identifying and analyzing the problem, developing alternative means to solve it, and formulating criteria by which to evaluate possible solutions. The implementation plan is critical. Evaluation must be included in the plan; it is preferable that evaluation be built in rather than be added as an afterthought. Evaluation provides the all-important feedback necessary to make the adjustments that enhance results. This methodology is similar to that used in moral reasoning and management problem solving.

Health services organizations have always needed their managers to make ethical decisions (i.e., applied ethics). The development of new technologies, the advent of external pressures from government and community, and the evolution of social mores have combined to cause the decision-making and implementation processes to become critical and to impose harsh penalties on organizations and people who ignore their implications.

Section I describes various moral philosophies and moral principles and examines the ways in which managers approach ethical problems. Section II provides guidelines that assist managers in making ethical decisions. Section III provides an in-depth look at administrative ethical issues found commonly in health services organizations. Section IV examines prominent biomedical ethical issues. Section V analyzes the emerging ethical issues raised by marketing and delivery mechanisms such as managed care and by HIV and AIDS. Also analyzed are the ethical dimensions of resource allocation and the social responsibility of health services organizations.

This is a book that I have long wanted to write. As technology has extended life (and death), as demands for health care and medical services continue to exceed resources, and as economic and competitive pressure buffet health services organizations, their managers will increasingly be leading actors in a complex drama. If this third edition assists them to prevent (if possible), identify, analyze, and solve ethical problems, I will have achieved my goal.

Acknowledgments

This book was conceived as a vehicle to assist health services managers to identify and solve the numerous and complex ethical issues they confront. This goal came to fruition with publication of the first edition in 1987. Publication of the second edition only 4 years later was a response to the pace of change in the health services field. The third edition builds on the achievements of the previous editions.

It would be impossible to prepare three manuscripts and publish three editions without assistance from many individuals and organizations. Those instrumental in preparing the first two editions have my continuing thanks. My late colleague and friend, Robert G. Shouldice, D.B.A., was helpful in preparing the managed care section in the first two editions. I hope he is in a place that allows but does not require reading. Richard F. Southby, Ph.D., Chairman of the Department of Health Services Management and Policy at The George Washington University, has been supportive of and continues to encourage my efforts. F. David Fowler, Dean of The George Washington University School of Business and Public Management, has sought to create an environment that stresses research and writing, and I am grateful for his efforts.

Research and other assistance for this edition was provided by Heidi Gambino, who worked diligently and cheerfully, often under daunting time constraints. She has my appreciation and best wishes for every success in life and her career in the health services field.

At Health Professions Press, Barbara S. Karni offered encouragement and constructive advice as this edition was being researched and written. She has my gratitude. Anita McCabe worked with me patiently. She was consistently helpful and contributed in numerous ways to improving the manuscript and the final result. I thank her.

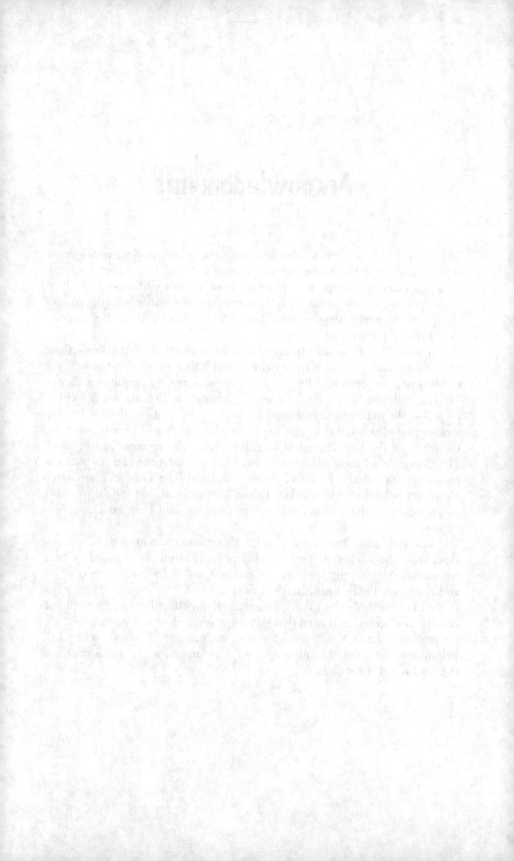

ANNE
As always, lighting the way

Introduction

T wo themes underlie *Ethics in Health Services Management*: the autonomy, primacy, and protection of the patient* and the role of the health
services manager as a moral agent who leads the health services
organization.

This book seeks to help health services managers develop a personal ethic
and gain a basic understanding of administrative and biomedical ethical issues, and suggests a methodology for solving the problems these issues raise.
The emphasis is on normative ethics (*what should be done*). Some attention
is paid to descriptive ethics (*what is actually done*) and metaethics (*study of
ethical systems*) because they assist in understanding normative ethics. Theories of ethical relativism and ethical nihilism are not considered. Ethical
relativism holds that there are no absolutes and that answers to ethical questions are equally right or morally correct, depending on the circumstances and
the culture. Nihilists consider no choice correct. These theories have similarities because neither helps managers meet the needs of patients, staff, and
organizations, nor do these theories assist managers who have the difficult
task of solving ethical problems. Furthermore, relativist and nihilist perspectives are of little value in helping the manager formulate a personal ethic.

For the health services manager, a personal ethic is a moral framework within which the appropriate relationship with employees, patients, organization, and community develops. In this regard, the manager is not,
and cannot be, a morally neutral technocrat. The manager is a moral
agent—someone who morally affects and is morally affected by actions. This
means that decision making by management is not value-free; in a moral
sense, it affects its environment and all touched by it.

---

*For ease of reading, *patient* is used to describe anyone served by a health services
organization.

1

The patient relies on the health services organization and its staff to perform services that are unique in society. Managers' responsibilities to the patients take precedence over their fiduciary responsibilities to their organizations. Protecting the patient is more than providing safe surroundings and competent staff. It is more than accreditation by the Joint Commission on Accreditation of Healthcare Organizations (Joint Commission). It is more than showing a surplus on a financial statement. The manager is the organization's conscience. This duty is exemplified by the organization's willingness, prompted and led by management, to recognize the inherent human dignity of the patient and to do so through effective programs that make this recognition a reality. It means using appropriate consent forms and procedures and aggressively ascertaining that all who have contact with patients are qualified and work for the patient's good. It means not considering the patient an adversary and not deserting the patient should something go wrong during treatment. An organization that has honestly and forthrightly done its best can face the consequences of an error without shame, mitigate the injury, and work out an equitable solution. The loop is closed when the organization, at the impetus of management, determines the cause of the problem and prevents or minimizes the probability of its recurrence, all the while working to continuously improve quality.

Physicians* must respect decisions made by a patient or an appropriate proxy. However, there will be times when the principle of justice requires that a decision process used prospectively includes the criteria of cost–benefit analysis and utilitarianism (*the greatest good for the greatest number*). Even here, the organization recognizes the dignity and worth of people as yet unserved or only partially served.

How does the health services organization develop and implement a "just" policy? How does it strive to treat its patients as equals and to work with them to serve their interests? Implementation of a just policy begins with the organizational philosophy,** which should explicitly state the nature of the relationship between patient and organization. This philosophy should reflect the view that the patient is autonomous and is entitled to be treated with respect and dignity. In a sense, it is based on a contract—an implicit but verifiable understanding between patient and provider, grounded in mutual trust and confidence. It recognizes that whenever possible, patients retain control of their lives.

Once enunciated, the organization's philosophy must be reflected in all derivative mission and vision statements, policies, procedures, and rules, but

---

*For ease of reading, *physician* includes medical doctors and other practitioners of the medical and healing arts licensed to independently treat patients (e.g., dentists, nurse midwives, clinical psychologists, podiatrists, chiropractors).

**Organizational philosophy* is used as a generic concept to include values, core values, shared values, ministry, healing ministry, philosophy, or similar terms used to convey the philosophical framework in which services are delivered.

especially in relationships with patients and community. If not operationalized, the organization will be judged cynical about itself and the persons it serves. This cynicism is easily recognized by staff and will be reflected in the way patients are treated. Although most staff will not succumb to the negative implications of this inconsistency, it will remain an underlying, festering incongruity.

A major participant in developing and maintaining the appropriate relationship is the physician, who is necessarily a primary actor. The roles of physician and organization are complementary, but the organization remains morally (ethically) accountable for the physician's activities.

CONCERN ABOUT ETHICS

Ethics is a word used with increasing frequency in health care. Questions are asked daily about making the ethically right choice. Seemingly straightforward and value-free, management decisions have ethical implications for patients, staff, organization, community, or society. Many decisions that cause ethical dilemmas are the result of the continuing revolutions in biology and technology that began in the 1940s. Fiscal constraints, competition, and new means of delivering services exacerbate existing ethical problems and raise new ones. Beyond these causes is an enhanced level of awareness resulting from the research and writing of ethicists and the work of government commissions on experimentation and bioethics.

Ethical dilemmas occur when decision makers are drawn in two directions by competing courses of action that are based on differing moral frameworks, varying organizational philosophies, conflicting duties or moral principles, or possessing an ill-defined sense of right and wrong. For example, staff members may be asked to follow rules they consider inappropriate or unjust, or two moral principles may conflict with one another. A nurse's duty to preserve life clashes with the patient's wishes not to be kept alive artificially absent a hope of benefit. Another source of ethical dilemma is the existence of two compelling, ethically defensible positions on an issue such as the possible conception of a genetically defective infant. Required genetic screening and counseling for people at risk conflict with individual autonomy. Conclusions vary when decision makers place different weight on various principles, such as the importance of personal liberty or privacy. Ethical decisions are also affected by whether the economic and/or political implications for society are considered. For some issues, one can conclude that reasonable persons could differ as to the ethically "right" result. For the majority of ethical issues, however, one answer emerges as morally superior to the others.

Beyond biomedical ethical problems, some of which become "dilemmas" and receive tremendous attention from the media, there is the important need to identify and solve management problems with ethical dimensions. Administrative ethical problems do not frequently represent competing, eth-

ically defensible choices. Solving these problems is usually a matter of recognition and resolve—doing what is ethically correct.

Are laws and regulations the problem or the solution? Some people perceive that ethical dilemmas exist because laws or regulations external to the
organization fail to guide action clearly. Others perceive that laws force organizations and managers to act in specific ways, thus causing ethical problems. Depending on the issue and facts, both views may be correct. Even
when there are external rules, decision makers must decide when the rules
apply, how they are to be interpreted, and whether they should be obeyed.
In fact, by designating and clarifying rules, there is less middle ground, the
ethical problems are starker, and solving them may be more difficult. Some
people may ignore the rules and apply personal standards. Others will apply
rules dogmatically and choose not to think about the underlying philosophical
or ethical issues that are raised. Conversely, some ethical problems result
because no established external rules assist decision makers. For some issues,
ethical problems have developed more quickly than the ability of the health
services field or society to solve them. For others, there is no consensus as to
what the rules should be.

ETHICS DEFINED

Precisely defining ethics is difficult because it can have several meanings. For
philosophers, ethics is the formal study of morality. Sociologists see ethics as
the mores, customs, and behavior of a culture. For physicians, ethics means
meeting the expectations of profession and society and acting in specified
ways toward patients. Health services managers should consider ethics a special charge and a responsibility to the patient, to the organization and its
staff, to themselves and the profession, and, ultimately but less directly, to
society.

Distinctions often blur, but ethical problems may be divided into administrative and biomedical. Administrative ethical problems involve manager
and profession, organization, patients, and society. Biomedical ethical problems involve individual patients or groups of patients in their relationships
with one another or with providers and organizations. Depending on the issue,
the manager is usually involved less directly in biomedical ethical problems.

Ethical problems are often called *dilemmas* because a word such as this
emphasizes the difficulty of finding the morally correct solution. Ethical problems are often difficult to solve, but few are appropriately labeled *dilemmas*.

SOURCES OF LAW

The relationship between law and ethics (morality) is dynamic. Thus, it is
useful to begin a book about ethics by reviewing briefly the development of
law. Every organized society has a code or system of laws that distinguishes
acceptable behavior from unacceptable behavior and establishes penalties for
transgressors. Law may be defined simply as a system of principles and rules

of human conduct prescribed or recognized by a supreme authority. This definition includes criminal and civil law. Ethics is the study of standards of conduct and moral judgment. For a profession it is the system or code of morals guiding that group.

The moral underpinnings in criminal law are especially clear in reflecting society's sense of right and wrong, or its ethics (morality). In a democratic society laws are said to derive from and reflect the views of justice and fairness held by the majority of the population. This is less true in civil law, which governs relations among individuals and includes contracts and commercial transactions. In civil law the greater emphasis is placed on predictability, stability, and property rights.

Laws in a democracy are thought to reflect the moral values of most people, but substantial minorities may hold contrary views and consider a law or an action of government so unjust that they risk the penalties of breaking it. An historical example is the 1919 Volstead Act, which instituted prohibition by amending the U.S. Constitution. Violation was widespread until the amendment's repeal in 1933. Contemporary examples are draft resistance during the Vietnam war, common disregard of roadway speed limits, and marijuana use.

Some cultures regarded the law as a gift from the gods. Plato's *Republic* postulated the ideal state as one based on rational order and ruled by philosopher-kings. Plato considered written law a regrettable oversimplification that could not take into account the differences and conditions in parties and situations involved in legal disputes. He believed that it was best to have a philosopher apply an unwritten law. His own experience proved this theory impossible, and he accepted a written law administered without regard to the circumstances of the individuals involved.[1,2] This concept of a rule of law, not of men, became established in Anglo American legal tradition. However, because of the absurd results that can occur when civil law is applied without considering the situations of the parties, the concept of unwritten law preferred by Plato was continued but in a limited fashion. Parallel court systems developed in the common law, and actions in civil matters could be brought in either. In some states courts of equity hear cases in which fairness is the primary concern. Most states, however, have combined actions at law and equity into one system.

Because of the link between societal views of right and wrong and the law, morality is reflected in all types of law, whether formal or nonformal. A leading jurisprudent, Edgar Bodenheimer, identifies formal sources of law as constitutions, statutes, executive orders, administrative regulations, ordinances, charters and bylaws of autonomous or semiautonomous bodies, treaties, and judicial precedents. Nonformal sources of law have not received an authoritative, or at least articulated, formulation and embodiment in a formalized legal document. These sources include standards of justice, principles of reason and consideration of the nature of things (*natura rerum*), equity for individuals, public policies, moral convictions, social trends, and customary law.

Bodenheimer's inclusion of the charters and bylaws of autonomous and semiautonomous bodies in the list of formal sources of law has significance for health services management. Such documents include the articles of incorporation and bylaws of the organization. General references to the philosophy and mission may be included in both, but will appear in expanded form in other documents published by the organization. These are key. Medical staff bylaws and rules and regulations also reflect the organization's philosophy and mission and must be consistent with them.

In addition to their importance in reflecting the philosophy and mission, the charter and bylaws are an organization's basic laws. Persons affected by the organization—employees, medical staff, patients—look to them for guidance. Some basic laws, such as the medical staff bylaws, describe in detail the rights and obligations of medical staff. Should a legal controversy develop, courts and other reviewing bodies look to these documents as sources of formal law.

Bodenheimer's definition of formal law is broad enough to include professional codes of ethics. A code can be adequately implemented only when interpreted and enforced. Such activities guide a code's application and related decision making, give it dynamism and life, and ensure the important virtues of consistency and predictability.

RELATIONSHIP BETWEEN ETHICS AND LAW

For professions, ethics is much more than obeying the law. The law is but the minimum standard of morality established by society to guide interactions among individuals and between them and government. The law governing one's relationships includes few positive duties. Only in unique situations is one person obliged to aid another, for example. The law concentrates on prohibitions—the "thou shalt nots." Professions are bound by the law but have a higher calling, one that includes numerous positive duties to patients and society and to one another.

Positive duties are not exclusive to professions. Individuals may believe they have a duty to aid others or to work on their behalf. In many respects this positive duty means practicing the Golden Rule: "Do unto others as you would have them do unto you." This duty is far more demanding than merely refraining from acting so as to interfere with someone else or enacting a law that protects one person from another.

As noted earlier, it is paradoxical that law both prevents and causes ethical problems. Choices must be made whether a public law exists. Absent public law, managers rely on the formal law of the organization (i.e., statements of the organizational philosophy [its ethic] and mission, and managers' personal ethic to guide decision making). The presence of public law may not be determinative in solving a problem. Even when public law is clear, ethical problems may remain. An example is the U.S. Supreme Court decision that a woman has a constitutional right to an abortion during the first trimester of pregnancy. The controversy over the morality (ethics) of abortion is intense.

Statutes, court decisions, and codes of ethics are formal sources of law, but the latter affects only members of a unique group, usually one of voluntary association. Belonging to an association may not be completely voluntary: Colleagues have expectations and demands; employers may consider memberships important in judging qualifications; and better-informed consumers ask questions and express views about an individual's professional associations. At root, however, participating in groups that have codes is voluntary.

Licensure is ubiquitous for clinical personnel. Of health services managers, only nursing facility managers must be licensed. Including ethical standards in the licensing statutes for clinical personnel and managers gives them the force of law. This does not, however, relieve the professional association of the need to regulate members' behavior, even to the point of adopting more stringent guidelines. Groups whose codes are not reflected in statutes or regulations bear a heavier burden. Their codes are only private statements of acceptable behavior; any monitoring must be done by the groups themselves. A profession's obligation to protect society greatly heightens its need to monitor members and is one of the hallmarks of a profession.

In disciplinary proceedings pursuant to a licensing statute, the actions of public regulatory bodies are distinct from those of private groups. If a license is necessary to belong to a group, expulsion may follow delicensure; expulsion occurs only after a separate hearing and review process by the professional group.

The relationship between law and ethics might seem to be one-to-one: Anything lawful is ethical and vice versa. However, this need not be the case. Most important is that the law states the minimum expected from members of society, and contains few, if any, positive duties. Professions expect members to comply with the law, but often add substantially to this standard. The result is that the professional code of ethics may require an action that the law does not. For the professional, then, performing (or not performing) a particular activity may be legal but unethical.

The relationship between law and ethics is shown in Figure 1, a model developed by Henderson. It shows a succession of events leading to corporate decisions being scrutinized by the public and a determination whether they are legal and/or ethical. The judgment is necessarily ex post facto, despite attempts by management to predict consequences of a decision. The model suggests that for many corporate actions it cannot be known with certainty whether the people who finally judge the decision will consider it legal (as determined by law enforcement officials) or ethical (as determined by the profession or the general public). This consideration adds a high degree of

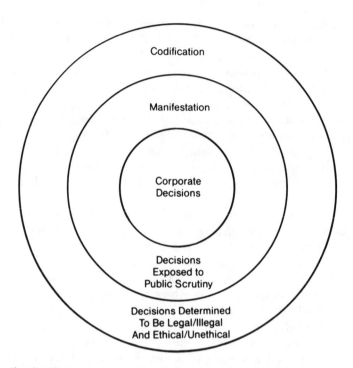

Figure 1. The relationship between law and ethics. (From Henderson, V.E. [1982]. The ethical side of enterprise. *Sloan Management Review, 23,* 37–47. Copyright 1982 by the Sloan Management Review Association. All rights reserved. Reprinted by permission.)

uncertainty to decision making inside and outside health services. It is usually easier to predict whether an action will be deemed legal than to predict whether it will be judged ethical.

The matrix in Figure 2 shows the combinations of legal, illegal, ethical, and unethical. In Quadrant I, managers act legally and ethically.

Quadrant II includes decisions that are ethical but illegal. The American College of Healthcare Executives (ACHE) Code of Ethics defines committing illegal acts as unethical. Given this broad prohibition, it would be virtually impossible for health services managers to justify as ethical an act that is illegal.

Quadrant III includes decisions that are unethical but legal. It incorporates the concept that ethical standards, especially those of a profession, hold the member to a higher standard than does the law. Examples include failing to take reasonable steps to protect the patient from medical malpractice and from manager self-aggrandizement at the expense of patients.

Quadrant IV includes activities that are illegal and unethical. Embezzling falls into this quadrant, as does ignoring local fire safety requirements or filing false Medicare or Medicaid reports.

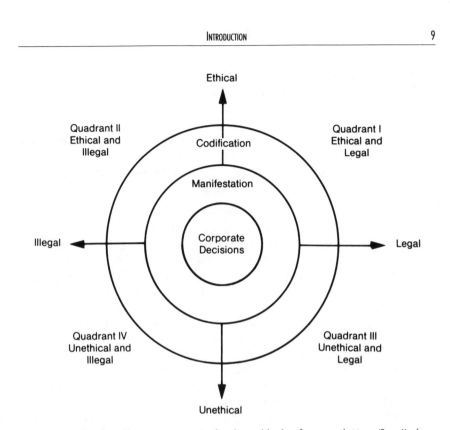

Figure 2.   A matrix of possible outcomes concerning the ethics and legality of corporate decisions. (From Henderson, V.E. [1982]. The ethical side of enterprise. *Sloan Management Review, 23,* 37–47. Copyright 1982 by the Sloan Management Review Association. All rights reserved. Reprinted by permission.)

It is important to stress the dynamic between law and ethics: each affects and is affected by the other. Professional codes and conduct reflect society's perceptions of a profession as well as that profession's self-image. To the extent that the law reflects society's need to protect itself and regulate conduct, licensure laws further clarify what is expected of a profession. Morality reflected in the law evolves but likely lags behind private morality and ethics. In this regard, the law leads some subsets of society but follows others.

CONCLUSION

Gandhi said that noncooperation with evil is as much a duty as is cooperation with good. Edmund Burke said that the only thing necessary for the triumph of evil is that good men do nothing. Both philosophies are germane to health services, especially to its managers. Understanding their ethical obligations and meeting them are essential.

Contemporary demands on health services organizations and managers may seem inconsistent in many ways with the often-idealized statements found in codes of ethics. Managers must recognize their responsibility, however, and strive to transform the ideal into reality. Managers see themselves and are seen by others as moral agents with a critical role in the organization and its efforts to serve, protect, and further the interests of patient and community.

If the findings of a 1984 Gallup poll about corporate ethics are applicable to the health services field, health services managers face an important challenge. The poll showed that 30% of the public believe corporate ethics are slipping; 25% of mid-level executives agree.

> The poll focused on unethical personal behavior in the workplace. Over three quarters of the executives interviewed use company phones to make personal long-distance calls. Almost as many take home office supplies. Thirty-five per cent say that they have somewhat overstated deductions on their tax forms. And 80% have driven while drunk. One financial services executive offered a list of unethical practices that included "bribes, falsifying documents, improper financial statements, bid rigging, and price collusion."
>
> What determines a person's ethics in the workplace? Age, for one thing. In the Gallup poll, younger executives consistently behaved less ethically. Education also influenced responses— negatively. A far higher proportion of college graduates than those without high school diplomas took home office supplies and called in sick when they were not.[3]

The general thrust of the Gallup poll findings is supported by research that found that the typical executive values "self-respect," but is likely to commit financial fraud. The study involved over 400 people, overwhelmingly male, who were asked to play the role of a fictional executive in analyzing hypothetical cases. It was found that 47% of top executives and 40% of controllers were willing to commit fraud by understating a write-down that reduced company profits. A much smaller percentage (14% and 8%, respectively) were willing to make fraudulent decisions in a case regarding anticipated revenue. Graduate students in an MBA program who were part of a pilot of the study were willing to make fraudulent decisions as well: 76% in the write-down case and 40% in the revenue case.[4]

If ethical problems among managers in business are extensive, it is likely that health services are affected by similar problems. The examples of unethical behavior cited above focused on the relationship between manager and organization. What about the manager's relationship with the persons served by the organization or with its staff? Managing health services organizations will always be among the most demanding work in society. No one said it would be easy; few in the field expect kudos for their service. But we raise the pride of profession and self and fulfill our role if we view ourselves as moral agents whose primary duty is to protect patients' interests and further their care. This is the challenge of health services management.

NOTES

1. Edgar Bodenheimer. (1974). *Jurisprudence: The philosophy and method of the law* (p. 6). Cambridge, MA: Harvard University Press.
2. A useful discussion of Plato's political philosophy is found in Jeremy Waldron. (1995). What Plato would allow. In Ian Shapiro & Judith Wagner DeCew, Eds. *Theory and practice: Nomos XXXVII* (pp. 138–178). New York: New York University Press.
3. Hastings Center. (1984, February). In search of the honest executive: A view from the top and the middle. *Hastings Center Report, 14,* 2.
4. Arthur P. Brief, Janet M. Dukerich, Paul R. Brown, & Joan F. Brett. (1996). What's wrong with the Treadway Commission Report? Experimental analyses of the effects of personal values and codes of conduct on fraudulent reporting. *Journal of Business Ethics, 15,* 183–198.

Identifying and
Solving Ethical Problems

C hapters 1 and 2 present important information basic to identifying, understanding, analyzing, and solving administrative and biomedical ethical problems. A generic background and methodology are developed and applied to a
case. The nature and types of ethical problems will evolve, but the framework and
process developed here will have continued usefulness for managers.

Chapter 1 identifies and discusses moral philosophies and derivative principles—a
background that is essential for analyzing and solving administrative and biomedical
ethical problems. They are also essential in developing a personal ethic.

Learning and applying a problem-solving method is part of management education. The problem-solving methodology developed in Chapter 2 builds on that generic
skill, which is modified to accommodate ethical issues. Managers should read the
discussion of moral philosophies and derivative principles with their problem-solving
education and experience, as well as their personal ethic, in mind.

Solving biomedical ethical problems cannot be exclusive to physicians, nor can
administrative ethics be exclusive to managers. Meeting the ethical imperative of an
organization is vital and measures how successfully its mission and objectives are met.
Managers must participate fully if ethical problems are to be solved effectively. Managers who act only as technocrats ignore their responsibilities as moral agents. Applying
ethical principles is too important a task to be left to others.

Considering Moral Philosophies and Principles

What are the sources of ethical guidelines? How do they help us identify and act on the morally correct choice? Philosophers, theologians, and others grapple with such questions. The tradition of ethics in medicine dates from the ancient Greeks. In the 20th century managers and nurses have formally sought to clarify, establish, and sometimes enforce ethical standards. Their codes and activities incorporate philosophies about the ethical relationship of providers to one another, to patients, and to society. For managers, the appropriate relationship with the organization is an added dimension included in their codes.

A natural starting point for discussing ethics and understanding how to resolve ethical problems is to review moral philosophies of major influence in western European culture and thought. Among the most prominent of these philosophies are utilitarian teleology, Kantian deontology, natural law as formulated by Thomas Aquinas, and the work of 20th century American philosopher, John Rawls. Casuistry, virtue ethics, and the ethics of care are distinguished and their contribution to ethical principles is examined.

The principles derived from these moral philosophies provide the framework or moral (ethical) underpinnings for delivery of health services by organizations. These principles will assist managers (and health services providers) in honing a personal ethic. The derivative operative principles are respect for persons, beneficence, nonmaleficence, and justice.

The following case example highlights the moral philosophies and derivative principles.

Baby Boy Doe

In 1970 a male infant born at a major East Coast medical center was diagnosed with mental retardation and duodenal atresia (the absence of a connection between the stomach and intestine). Surgeons determined

15

that although the baby was very small, the atresia was operable, with a high probability of success. The surgery would not alter the baby's mental retardation, but would permit him to take nourishment by mouth and lead a normal life.

The baby's parents decided to forego the surgery—something they had the legal right to do—and over the course of the following 2 weeks the infant was left to die from dehydration and starvation. No basic determination of the extent of mental impairment had been made, nor could it have been, at the time the infant died. Neither hospital personnel nor state family and social services sought to aid the infant.

This case sends a shudder through most people. However, feelings are insufficient. If managers are to be effective in addressing and solving—or, preferably, preventing—such problems, they must identify and understand the issues involved, understand the roles of the staff and the organization, and seek to apply principles of ethical conduct. Following a discussion of moral philosophies and ethical principles, the case of Baby Boy Doe is analyzed.

MORAL PHILOSOPHIES

Utilitarianism

Utilitarians are consequentialists: They evaluate an action in terms of its effect. Synonymous with utilitarians are teleologists (from the Greek, *telos*, meaning end). Utilitarianism has historical connections to hedonism (Epicureanism), which measures morality by the amount of pleasure obtained from an act or a rule as to how to act—greater pleasure is equated with greater morality. This theory was refined by two 19th century philosophers, Jeremy Bentham and John Stuart Mill. The most complete elaboration of utilitarianism was Mill's. Unlike Bentham, Mill sought to distinguish pleasures (the good) on qualitative grounds. Questions about the superiority of certain pleasures, such as listening to a piano concerto, were to be answered by consulting a person of sensitivity and broad experience, even though requiring such judgments diminished the objectivity of utilitarianism.

Mill stressed individual freedom. In *On Liberty* he noted that freedom is requisite to producing happiness, and that this makes it unacceptable for the privacy of any group or individual to be infringed in significant ways.

In selecting the morally correct option utilitarians ignore the means of achieving an end and judge the results of an action by comparing the good brought about by a particular action to the good brought about by alternatives, or the amount of evil avoided. A modified form of utility theory is the basis for the cost–benefit analysis commonly used by economists and managers. "The greatest good for the greatest number," and "the end justifies the means" are statements attributable to utilitarians. However, these statements are only crude gauges of utilitarianism, inappropriately applied without qualification.

Utilitarianism is divided into *act utility* and *rule utility*. Both measure consequences, and the action that brings into being the most good (understood in a nonmoral sense) is deemed the morally correct choice.

Act utilitarians judge each action independently, without reference to preestablished guidelines (rules). They measure the amount of good, or (nonmoral) value brought into being, and the amount of evil, or (nonmoral) disvalue avoided by acting on a particular choice. Each person affected is counted equally, which seems to assign a strong sense of objectivity to this moral philosophy. Because it is episodic, act utilitarianism is incompatible with developing and deriving the ethical principles needed for codes of ethics and a personal ethic. Therefore, it receives no further attention.

Rule utilitarians are also concerned only with consequences, but have prospectively considered various actions and the amount of good or evil brought into being by each. These assessments are used to develop rules (guidelines) for action, because it has been determined that, on average, certain rules produce the most good and least evil. Therefore, these rules determine the morally correct choice. The rules are followed for all similar situations, even if sometimes they are not the best course of action. The rule directs selection of the morally correct choice. Rule utilitarianism assists in developing moral principles for health services management.

Deontology

Deontologists adhere to a formalist moral philosophy (in Greek, *deon* means duty). The foremost proponent of deontology was Immanuel Kant, an 18th century German philosopher. Kant's basic precept was that relations with others must be based on duty. An action is moral if it arises solely from "good will," not from other motives. For Kant, good will is that which is good without qualification. Unlike the utilitarians, deontologists view the end as unimportant, because, in Kant's view, persons have duties to one another as moral agents, duties that take precedence over the consequences of actions. Kantians hold that certain absolute duties are always in force. Among the most important is respect, or the Golden Rule ("Do unto others as you would have them do unto you"). Kant argued that all persons have this duty; respect toward others must always be paid.

Actions that are to be taken under the auspices of this duty must first be tested in a special way, a test Kant termed the *categorical imperative*. The categorical imperative requires that actions under consideration be universalized. In other words, if a principle of action is thought to be appropriate, a determination is made as to whether it can be consistently applied to all persons in all places at all times. No exceptions can be made, nor can allowances be made for special circumstances. If the action under consideration meets this test, it is accepted as a duty. It fails to meet the test if it is contradictory to the overriding principle that all persons must be treated as moral equals and are, therefore, entitled to respect. Truth telling is a prominent example of a duty that meets the categorical imperative.

For the Kantian deontologist, it is logically inconsistent to argue that terminally ill persons should be euthanized because this amounts to the self-contradictory principle that life can be improved by ending it. Similarly, caregivers should not lie to patients to improve the efficiency of health care delivery; such a policy fails the test of the categorical imperative because it treats patients as means rather than as moral equals. The Golden Rule is the best summary of Kant's philosophy. Kantian deontology gives no consideration to results or consequences. This does not mean that managers must be unaware of consequences, but that the consequences of an action are neither included nor weighed in the ethical decision-making process.

Natural Law

Mill defined morally right actions by the happiness or nonmoral value produced. Kant rejected all ethical theories based on desire or inclination. Unlike Mill and Kant, natural law theorists contend that ethics must be based on concern for human good. They also contend that good cannot be defined simply in terms of subjective inclinations. Rather, there is a good for human beings that is objectively desirable, although not reducible to desire.[1] Natural law holds that divine law has inscribed certain potentialities in all things, which constitute the good of those things. In this sense the theory is teleological because it is concerned with ends. Natural law is based on Aristotelian thought as interpreted and synthesized with Christian dogma by St. Thomas Aquinas (1226–1274).[2]

The potentiality of human beings is based on a uniquely human trait, the ability to reason. Natural law bases ethics on the premise that human beings will do what is rational, and that this rationality will cause them to tend to do good and avoid evil. Natural law presumes a natural order in relationships and a predisposition by rational individuals to do or to refrain from doing certain things. Our capability for rational thought enables us to discover what we should do. In that effort we are guided by a partial notion of God's divine plan that is linked to our capacity for rational thought. Because natural law guides what rational human beings do, it serves as a basis for positive law, some of which is reflected in statutes. Our natural inclination directs us to preserve our lives and to do such rational things as avoid danger, act in self-defense, and seek medical attention when needed. Our ability to reason shows that other human beings are like us and therefore entitled to the same respect and dignity we seek. A summary statement of the basic precepts of natural law is "do good and avoid evil." Using natural law, theologians have developed moral guidelines about medical services that are described in later chapters.

Rawls's Theory

Moral philosopher John Rawls provides a hybrid theory of ethics that has applications in health services allocation and delivery. His theory uses an elaborate philosophical construct in which persons are in the "original position," behind a veil of ignorance. Such persons are rational and self-interested, but know nothing of their individual talents, intelligence, social and economic situations, and the like. Rawls argues that persons in the original position behind a veil of ignorance will identify certain principles of justice. First, all persons should have equal rights to the most extensive basic liberty compatible with similar liberty for others (the *liberty principle*). Second, social and economic inequalities should be arranged so that they are both reasonably expected to be to everyone's advantage and attached to positions and offices open to all (the *difference principle*).[3] For Rawls, the liberty principle governing political rights is more important and precedes the difference principle, which governs primary goods (distributive rights), including health services.

Rawls argues that hypothetical rational and self-interested persons in the original position will reject utilitarianism and select the concepts of right and justice as precedent to the good. Rawls concludes that rational self-interest dictates that one will act to protect the least well off because anyone could be in that group. He terms this *maximizing the minimum position* (*maximin*).

When applied to primary goods, one of which is health services, Rawlsian moral theory requires egalitarianism. Egalitarianism is defined to mean that rational, self-interested persons may limit the health services available to people in certain categories, such as particular diseases or age groups, or limit services provided in certain situations. It is also rational and self-interested for persons in the original position not to make every good or service available to everyone at all times.

Rawls's theory permits disproportionate distribution of primary goods to certain groups, but only if doing so benefits the least advantaged. This is part of the difference principle and justifies elite social and economic status for persons such as physicians and health services managers if their efforts ultimately benefit the least advantaged in society.

Casuistry, Virtue Ethics, and Ethics of Care

Casuistry   Many historical definitions of casuistry are not flattering. They include a moral philosophy that uses sophistry and encourages rationalizations for desired ethical results, uses evasive reasoning, and is quibbling. Despite these unflattering definitions and a centuries-long hiatus from the use of casuistry, advocates of this method see it as a pragmatic approach to understanding and solving problems of modern biomedical ethics. Casuistry can be defined as a kind of case-based reasoning in historical context. A claimed strength is that it avoids excessive reliance on principles and rules, which it is argued provide only partial answers and often fall short of comprehensive guidance for decision makers.

A significant effort to rehabilitate casuistry has been undertaken by Jonsen and Toulmin,[4] who argue that

> Casuistry redresses the excessive emphasis placed on universal rules and invariant principles by moral philosophers. . . . Instead we shall take seriously certain features of moral discourse that

recent moral philosophers have too little appreciated: the concrete circumstances of actual cases, and the specific maxims that people invoke in facing actual moral dilemmas. If we start by considering similarities and differences between particular types of cases on a practical level, we open up an alternative approach to ethical theory that is wholly consistent with our moral practice.

At its foundation casuistry is similar to the law in which court cases and the precedents they establish guide decision makers. Beauchamp and Walters[5] state that

> In case law, the normative judgments of a majority of judges become authoritative, and . . . are the primary normative judgments for later judges who assess other cases. Cases in ethics are similar: Normative judgments emerge through majoritarian consensus in society and in institutions because careful attention has been paid to the details of particular problem cases. That consensus then becomes authoritative and is extended to relevantly similar cases.

In fact, this process occurs in organizations as ethics committees, for example, develop a body of experience with ethical issues of various types.

Clinical medicine is case focused as, increasingly, is management education. This development has made it natural to employ a case approach in health services. Traditionally, ethics problem solving in health services has applied moral principles to cases—from the general to the specific, or deductive reasoning. Classical casuists, however, used a kind of inductive reasoning—from the specific to the general. They began by stating a paradigm case with a strong maxim (e.g., "thou shalt not kill") set in its most obvious relevance to circumstances (e.g., a vicious attack on a defenseless person). Subsequent cases added circumstances that made the relevance of the maxim more difficult to understand (e.g., if defense is possible, is it moral?) Classical casuists progressed from being deontologists to teleologists and back again, as suited the case, and adhered to no explicit moral theory.[6] Jonsen[7] argues that modern casuists can profitably copy the classical casuists's reliance on paradigm cases, reference to broad consensus, and acceptance of probable certitude (defined as assent to a proposition, but acknowledging that its opposite might be true). Casuistry has achieved a prominent place in applied administrative and biomedical ethics. Increasing numbers of cases and a body of experience will lead to consensus and greater certainty in identifying morally right decisions.

Virtue Ethics   Western thought about the importance of virtue can be partially traced to Aristotle. Like natural law, virtue ethics is based on theological ethics, but does not focus primarily on obligations or duties. As with casuistry, it is receiving increased attention. Some of this attention results from a perception that traditional rule- or principle-based moral philosophies deal inadequately with the realities of ethical decision making. That is to say, rules take us only so far in solving ethical problems; when there are competing ethical rules or situations to which no rules apply, something more than a coin toss is needed. This is where virtue ethicists claim to have a superior moral philosophy.

Contemporary authors such as Pellegrino and Thomasma[8] argue that ethics has three levels. The first two are observing the laws of the land, and observing moral rights and fulfilling moral duties that go beyond the law. The third and highest level is the practice of virtue.

> Virtue implies a character trait, an internal disposition habitually to seek moral perfection, to live one's life in accord with a moral law, and to attain a balance between noble intention and just action. . . . In almost any view the virtuous person is someone we can trust to act habitually in a good way—courageously, honestly, justly, wisely, and temperately.[9]

Thus virtuous physicians (or managers) are disposed to the right and good that is intrinsic to the practice of their profession and will work for the good of the patient. "Virtue ethics expands the notions of benevolence, beneficence, conscientiousness, compassion, and fidelity well beyond what strict duty might require."[10]

Some virtue ethicists argue that as with any skill or expertise, practice and constant striving to achieve virtuous traits (good works) improves one's ability to be virtuous. Other virtue ethicists argue that accepting in one's heart the forgiveness and reconciliation offered by God (faith) "would lead to a new disposition toward God (trust) and the neighbor (love), much as a physician or patient might be judged to be a different (and better) person following changed dispositions toward those persons with whom . . . (they) are involved." [11]

All people should live virtuous lives, but those in the professions have a special obligation to do so, which is to say that virtuous managers and physicians are not solely virtuous persons practicing a profession. They are expected to work for the patient's good even at the expense of personal sacrifice and legitimate self-interest.[12] Virtuous physicians place the good of their patients above their own and seek that good unless pursuing it imposes injustice upon them or their families, or violates their conscience.[13] Similarly, virtuous managers place the good of the patient (through the organization) above their own.

Ethics of Care Medicine is based on caring, the importance of which is reflected historically and in contemporary biomedical ethics. "Care" focuses on relationships; in clinical practice this means relationships between caregivers and patients. Effective management also depends on relationships between managers and staff and through them to patients. As the ethics of care evolves it may be more applicable to management; at this point, however, it applies almost exclusively to clinical relationships.

The interest beginning in the 1980s in the ethics of care has been attributed to the feminist movement.[14] Its proponents argue that various interpersonal relationships and the obligations and virtues they involve "lack three central features of relations between moral agents as understood by Kantians and contractarians, e.g., Rawls—it is intimate, it is unchosen, and is between unequals."[15] Thus, it emphasizes the attachment of relationships rather than the detachment of rules and duties.

A clear link to virtue ethics exists in that the ethics of care focus on character traits such as compassion and fidelity that are valued in close personal relationships. It has been suggested that the basis for the ethics of care is found in the paradigmatic relationship between mother and child. It is claimed that this paradigm sets it apart from the predominantly male experience, which often uses the economic exchange between buyer and seller as the paradigmatic human relationship, and which it is argued characterizes moral theory, generally.[16]

A leading exponent of the ethics of care, Carol Gilligan,[17] argues that unlike traditional moral theories, the ethics of care is grounded in the assumption that

> Self and other are interdependent, an assumption reflected in a view of action as responsive and, therefore, as arising in relationship rather than the view of action as emanating from within the self and, therefore, "self-governed." Seen as responsive, the self is by definition connected to others, responding to perceptions, interpreting events, and governed by the organizing tendencies of human interaction and human language. Within this framework, detachment, whether from self or from others, is morally problematic, since it breeds moral blindness or indifference—a failure to discern or respond to need. The question of what responses constitute care and what responses lead to hurt draws attention to the fact that one's own terms may differ from those of others. Justice in this context becomes understood as respect for people in their own terms.

Similar to virtue ethics and the renewed interest in casuistry, the ethics of care is a reaction to the rules and systems building of traditional theories. Its proponents argue that the ethics of care more closely reflects the real experiences in clinical medicine and of caregivers who are expected to respond with, for example, warmth, compassion, sympathy, and friendliness, none of which fit well into a system of rules and duties.

Summary   The moral philosophies described in this section span a wide spectrum. Health services managers are likely to be eclectic in selecting those that become part of the organization's philosophy and those that will influence the content of their personal ethic, as well as its reconsideration and evolution. Most important is that managers recognize that a basic understanding of theory is vital.

LINKAGE OF THEORY WITH ACTION

Ethical theories are drawn from abstractions that are often stated broadly. Principles developed from these theories establish a relationship and suggest a course of action. Rules can be derived from the principles; the specific judgments and actions to be applied are the final result. Figure 3 was developed by Beauchamp and Childress to demonstrate the relationship between ethical theories (moral philosophies) and actions implementing decisions.

Ethical theories do not necessarily conflict. Diverse philosophies may reach the same conclusion, albeit through different reasoning, by various constructs, or by focusing divergent criteria (e.g., the rule utilitarian's use of ends versus the Kantian's use of duty). The principles discussed here are considered crucial and should be reflected in the organization's philosophy and the personal ethic of health services managers.

Linking ethical theories and derivative principles permits the development of usable guidelines. To aid in that process, this discussion identifies four principles that provide a context for managing in health services environments: 1) respect for persons, 2) beneficence, 3) nonmaleficence, and 4) justice. Utility is sometimes treated as a distinct principle, but that construct is somewhat artificial and potentially confusing. Here, utility is included as an adjunct to the principle of beneficence.

The theories discussed earlier in the chapter support the conclusion that respect for persons is an important ethical principle. This principle has four elements. The first, *autonomy*, requires that one act toward others in a way that allows them to govern themselves—to choose and pursue courses of

4.   Ethical theories

↑

3.   Principles

↑

2.   Rules

↑

1.   Particular judgments and actions

Figure 3.   Hierarchy of relationships. (From Beauchamp, T.L., & Childress, J.F. [1989]. *Principles of biomedical ethics* [3rd ed., p. 6]. New York: Oxford University Press. Reprinted by permission.)

action. To do so, a person must be rational and uncoerced. Sometimes patients are or become nonautonomous (e.g., the physically or mentally incapacitated). They are owed respect nonetheless, even though special means are required in order to deal with them. Recognizing the patient's autonomy is the reason consent for treatment is obtained, and is a general basis for the way in which an organization views and interacts with patients and staff.

Autonomy is in dynamic tension with paternalism, the concept that one person knows what is best for another. Paternalism is an established tradition in health services. The earliest evidence of it is found in the Hippocratic oath, which directs physicians to act in what they believe to be the patient's best interests. Stressing autonomy does not eliminate paternalism, but paternalism should be limited to certain situations.

The second element of respect for persons is *truth telling*, which requires managers to be honest in all activities. Depending on how absolute a position is taken, this element prohibits "fibs" or "white lies," even if they are told because it is correctly believed that knowing the truth would harm someone. The morality of insisting that patients be told the truth may also be problematic, depending on the circumstances. Some patients would suffer mental and physical harm if told the truth about their illnesses. In doing so, physicians would not meet their obligation of *primum non nocere*, or "first, do no harm." The modern expression of this concept is nonmaleficence, which is discussed later in the chapter.

Confidentiality is the third element of the principle of respect for persons. It requires managers as well as clinicians to keep what they learn about patients confidential. Exceptions to confidentiality are made when the law requires that certain diseases and conditions be reported. For managers, the obligation of confidentiality extends beyond patients. It applies to information about staff, the organization, and the community that becomes known to them in the course of their work.

The fourth element of respect for persons is *fidelity*: doing one's duty or keeping one's word. Sometimes this is called "promise keeping." We treat persons with respect when we do what we are expected to do or what we have promised to do. Fidelity allows managers to meet the principle of respect for persons. Here, too, if exceptions are made, they cannot be made lightly. Breaking a promise must be justified on moral grounds; it must never be done merely for convenience or self-interest.

Like respect for persons, the principle of *beneficence* is supported by most of the moral philosophies described earlier, although utilitarians would require it to meet the consequences test they apply. Beneficence is rooted in Hippocratic tradition and in the history of the caring professions. Beneficence may be defined as acting with charity and kindness. Applied as a principle in health services, it has a similar but broader definition. Beneficence is a positive duty, as distinct from the principle of *nonmaleficence*, which requires refraining from actions that aggravate a problem or cause other negative results. Beneficence and nonmaleficence may be viewed as opposite ends of a continuum.

Beauchamp and Childress[18] divide beneficence into providing benefits and balancing benefits and harms (utility). Conferring benefits is firmly established in medical tradition, and failure to provide them when one is in a position to do so violates the moral agency of both clinician and manager. Balancing benefits against harms provides a philosophical basis for cost–benefit analysis, as well as other considerations of risks balanced against benefits. In this sense it is similar to the principle of utility espoused by the utilitarians. However, here, utility is only one of several considerations and has more limited application.

The positive duty suggested by the principle of beneficence requires organizations and managers to do all they can to aid patients. A lesser duty exists to aid individuals who are potential rather than actual patients. This distinction and its importance varies with the philosophy and mission of the organization and whether it serves a defined population, as would a health maintenance organization. Thus, under a principle of beneficence, the hospital operating an emergency department has no duty to scour the neighborhoods for individuals needing its assistance. However, when they become patients this relationship changes.

The second aspect of beneficence is balancing the benefits and harms that could result from certain actions. This is a natural consequence of a positive duty to act in the patient's best interests. Beyond providing benefits in a positive fashion, one cannot act with kindness and charity when risks outweigh benefits. However it is interpreted, utility cannot be used to justify overriding the interests of individual patients and sacrificing them to the greater good.

The third principle applicable to managing health services organizations is *nonmaleficence*. Like beneficence, it is supported by most of the ethical theories discussed earlier (it must meet the consequences test to claim utilitarianism as a basis). Nonmaleficence means *primum non nocere*. This dictum to physicians is equally applicable to health services managers. Beauchamp and Childress[19] note that although nonmaleficence gives rise to specific moral rules, neither the principle nor the derivative rules can be absolute because it is often appropriate (with the patient's consent) to cause some risk, discomfort, or even harm in order to avoid greater harm or to prevent a worse situation from occurring. Beauchamp and Childress include the natural law concepts of extraordinary and ordinary care and double effect in the principle of nonmaleficence. (These concepts are considered later in this chapter.) Nonmaleficence also leads managers and clinicians to avoid risks, unless potential results justify them.

The fourth principle, *justice*, is especially important for administrative (and clinical) decision making in resource allocation, but applies to areas of management such as human resources policies as well. What is just and how does one know when justice has been achieved? Although all moral philosophies recognize the importance of achieving justice, they define it differently. Rawls defines justice as fairness. Implicit in that definition is that persons get what is due them. But how are fairness and "just desserts" defined? Aristotle's concept of justice, which is reflected in natural law, is that equals are treated equally, unequals unequally. This concept of fairness is used commonly in policy analysis. Equal treatment of equals is reflected in liberty rights (e.g., universal freedom of speech). Unequal treatment of unequal individuals justifies progressive income taxation and redistribution of wealth: People who earn more income should pay taxes at a higher rate. This concept is expressed in health services delivery by expending greater resources on individuals who are sicker and thus in need of more services.

These concepts of justice are helpful, but they do not solve the problems of definition and opinion, which are always troublesome. Macro- and microallocation of resources have received extensive consideration in the literature, but there is little agreement as to operational definitions. Each organization must determine for itself how resources will be allocated. An essential criterion as to whether organizations and their clinicians and managers are acting justly is that they consistently apply clear criteria in decision processes.

MORAL PHILOSOPHY AS A BASIS FOR A PERSONAL ETHIC

This examination of moral philosophies and derivative principles provides a framework for developing a personal ethic and subsequently analyzing ethical problems. Like philosophers, managers are unlikely to agree with all elements of a moral philosophy and make it their own. Most managers are eclectic as they develop and reconsider their personal ethic. In general, however, the principles described here are essential to establishing and maintaining appropriate relationships among patients, managers, and organizations, and should be part of the ethic of health services managers and the value system of the organizations they manage. It should be stressed that the four derivative principles may appropriately carry different weights, depending on the ethical issue being considered. The principle of justice requires, however, that there be a consistent ordering and weighing when the same types of ethical problems are considered.

Application of the Principles

How do the principles summarized in the preceding section and their underlying moral philosophies assist in solving ethical problems in cases such as Baby Boy Doe (see p. 15)? The principle of respect for persons implies certain duties and relationships, including autonomy. Nonautonomous persons, however, must have decisions made for them by a surrogate. The parents of Baby Boy Doe, a nonautonomous person, had to make decisions on behalf of their son. Surrogates cannot exercise unlimited authority, especially when it is uncertain that a decision is in the patient's best interests. If the infant's and parents' interests differ, caregivers (including managers) are duty-bound under the principles of beneficence and nonmaleficence to try to persuade parents to take another course of action. Such an action should have been attempted for Baby Boy Doe.

Extending the principles of beneficence and nonmaleficence, it is acceptable for the organization to seek legal intervention and obtain permission to treat an infant against the parents' wishes. The moral compulsion to do so is especially great when the parents are not acting in the child's best interests, but this moral duty should be exercised only as a last resort. Courts intervene under the theory of *parens patriae* to permit a hospital or social welfare agency to stand *in loco parentis*. Courts take this step reluctantly because of the common law tradition that gives parents control over reproductive and family matters, including decisions about infant children. As noted earlier, although it is an element of beneficence, utility is not an overriding concept that permits trampling on the rights of the person, as happened in the case of Baby Boy Doe.

Intervention has limits. Treating the infant against the parents' wishes but without a court order is inappropriate because it breaks the law. If persons caring for the infant cannot continue to do so because of their personal ethic, they should be permitted to withdraw. The option to remove oneself from a situation that is ethically intolerable should be reflected in the organization's philosophy and policies.

In applying the principle of nonmaleficence, one must consider whether the ethically superior choice would have been to shorten Baby Boy Doe's life through active euthanasia. This consideration raises the question of the moral difference between killing and letting die. Some argue that the identical results make them morally indistinguishable. The analysis cannot end there, however; to do so ignores critical aspects of medical decision making.

When caregivers apply the principle of nonmaleficence they refrain from doing harm, which includes minimizing pain and suffering. Asking caregivers dedicated to preserving life to end it will cause significant role conflict. Furthermore, physicians and nurses in such roles are on a slippery slope that may lead to more exceptions and increasing use of positive acts to shorten lives that are deemed by someone to be not worth living.

The concept of extraordinary care is a part of the principle of nonmaleficence that developed from natural law. *Ordinary care* is treatment provided without excessive expense, pain, or inconvenience and that offers reasonable hope of benefit. Care is *extraordinary* if it is available only in conjunction with excessive expense, pain, or other inconvenience, or if it does not offer any reasonable hope of benefit.[20] With no reasonable hope of benefit, *any* expense, pain, or inconvenience is excessive. Beauchamp and Childress[21] conclude that the "ordinary-extraordinary distinction thus collapses into the balance between benefits and burdens, where the latter category includes immediate detriment, inconvenience, risk of harm, and other costs." For Baby Boy Doe, there was hope of benefit, even though correcting the atresia would not cure his mental retardation. Surgery would have given Baby Boy Doe a normal life for someone with his mental disability. That benefit justifies the use of treatment involving significant expense, pain, and/or inconvenience.

Justice is the final principle to be applied, a principle that was noted earlier to have rather divergent definitions. Rawls defines justice as fairness. Applied to the case of Baby Boy Doe, one could conclude that the result was just. Fairness is arguably compatible with an enlightened self-interest expressed by persons in the original position behind a veil of ignorance—a Rawlsian philosophical construct. Rational persons could decide that no life is preferable to one of significantly diminished quality, even though this arguably limits the liberty principle, which Rawls considers ultimately important.

For a Kantian or an adherent to natural law, the outcome in the Baby Boy Doe case is abhorrent because the infant is being used as a means rather than as an end. Conversely, rule utilitarians would find the result acceptable. Other definitions of justice produce different conclusions. For example, if justice is defined as getting one's just desserts, it is clear that Baby Boy Doe fared badly. Applying an even cruder standard—that individuals equally situated should be treated equally—it is clear that had a similar problem afflicted an adult, the necessary treatment would have been rendered. For Baby Boy Doe, the results of applying the principle of justice are uncertain.

The final regulations about infant care published by the U.S. Department of Health and Human Services (DHHS) in April 1985 focus on beneficence and nonmaleficence. In implementing the Child Abuse Amendments of 1984 ([PL 98-457] amending the Child Abuse Prevention and Treatment Act of 1974), DHHS placed no weight on the parents' traditional right to judge what should be done for impaired infants with life-threatening conditions. The potential problem caused by parents who may not fully understand the implications of the diagnosis and the effects of their decision is obviated by the regulations because medical criteria applied by a knowledgeable, reasonable physician are used. Quality of life criteria cannot be considered. The preliminary regulations to implement the law made specific reference to a case similar to that of Baby Boy Doe, and stated that appropriate medical treatment had to be rendered. The final regulations contain no examples, however. Nevertheless, it is likely that DHHS will view narrowly any decisions to forego treatment of impaired infants with life-threatening conditions. Specifics of the regulations are discussed in Chapter 10.

As with most official efforts to regulate ethical decision making, these regulations are likely to be modified in the future. From an ethical standpoint it is more important to bear in mind the moral considerations that should underlie public policy than to be preoccupied with the semantics of a particular enactment.

Implications for Management

What are the implications of cases such as that of Baby Boy Doe for health services managers? Such events place a heavy burden on caregivers. Whatever the decision, these cases split the staff. The resulting controversy diminishes morale. In addition, criticism may be leveled against management, govern-ance, and medical staff by individuals who question the morality of the de-cision and the organization's role in it. In extreme cases legal action may ensue.

It is crucial that the health services organization implement a view (a philosophy) about matters such as these, and that it is reflected in its policies and procedures. This means the organization has explicitly formulated a course of action—a plan—that it will take when confronted with such prob-lems. Having a philosophy in place permits a deliberate response rather than one that is only reactive, inadequately considered, or governed by rather than governing events. At the very least, the organization must consider these is-sues prospectively and within the constraints of its organizational philosophy.

Paradoxically, prior to the 1984 Child Abuse Amendments, the health services organization could legally do to Baby Boy Doe what the parents could not. Had the parents taken the infant home and allowed it to starve and dehydrate until it died, it is likely that they would have been charged with child neglect or some degree of homicide or manslaughter. However, the organization did not face the same liability. In fact, had it surgically repaired the atresia without parental consent it would have committed battery on the infant for which it could have been sued for civil damages and the staff charged criminally. The latter result is unlikely, but the hospital is legally obligated to obtain consent from the parents or legal guardian for a minor when no emergency exists.

CONCLUSION

This chapter helps the manager develop a personal ethic and stimulates the organization to formulate a philosophy. Few managers will disagree as to the importance of the principles of respect for persons, beneficence, nonmalef-icence, and justice. However, not all managers will embrace unequivocally the principles and underlying moral philosophies discussed here. It is even more unlikely that they will agree about their weighing or priority. Chapter 2 suggests a methodology that managers can use in solving ethical problems.

NOTES

1. Robert Hunt, & John Arras, Eds. (1983). *Issues in modern medicine* (2nd ed., p. 27). Palo Alto, CA: Mayfield Publishing.
2. Edgar Bodenheimer. (1974). *Jurisprudence: The philosophy and method of the law* (Rev. ed., pp. 23–24). Cambridge, MA: Harvard University Press.
3. John Rawls. (1971). *A theory of justice* (p. 60). Cambridge, MA: Belknap Press.
4. Albert R. Jonsen, & Stephen Toulmin. (1988). *The abuse of casuistry: A history of moral reasoning* (p. 13). Berkeley, CA: University of California Press.
5. Tom L. Beauchamp, & LeRoy Walters. (1994). *Contemporary issues in bioethics* (4th ed., p. 21). Belmont, CA: Wadsworth Publishing.

6. Albert R. Jonsen. (1986). Casuistry and clinical ethics. *Theoretical Medicine*, 7, 70.
7. *Ibid.*, p. 71.
8. Edmund D. Pellegrino, & David C. Thomasma. (1988). *For the patient's good: The restoration of beneficence in health care* (p. 121). New York: Oxford University Press.
9. *Ibid.*, p. 116.
10. Edmund D. Pellegrino. (1994). The virtuous physician and the ethics of medicine. In Tom L. Beauchamp & LeRoy Walters, Eds., *Contemporary issues in bioethics* (4th ed., p. 55). Belmont, CA: Wadsworth Publishing.
11. Frederick S. Carney. (1978). Theological ethics. In Warren T. Reich, Ed., *Encyclopedia of bioethics* (Vol. 1, pp. 435–436). New York: Free Press.
12. Pellegrino & Thomasma, p. 121.
13. Pellegrino, p. 53.
14. Beauchamp & Walters, p. 19.
15. Annette C. Baier. (1987). Hume, the women's moral theorist? In Eva Feder Kittay & Diana T. Meyers, Eds., *Women and moral theory* (p. 44). Totowa, NJ: Rowman & Littlefield.
16. Virginia Held. (1987). Feminism and moral theory. In Eva Feder Kittay & Diana T. Meyers, Eds., *Women and moral theory* (p. 111). Totowa, NJ: Rowman & Littlefield.
17. Carol Gilligan. (1987). Moral orientation and moral development. In Eva Feder Kittay & Diana T. Meyers, Eds., *Women and moral theory* (p. 24). Totowa, NJ: Rowman & Littlefield.
18. Tom L. Beauchamp, & James F. Childress. (1989). *Principles of biomedical ethics* (3rd ed., p. 195). New York: Oxford University Press.
19. *Ibid.*, p. 122.
20. Gerald Kelly. (1951, December 12). The duty to preserve life. *Theological Studies*, p. 550.
21. Beauchamp & Childress, p. 153.

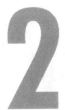

Resolving Ethical Issues

Managers are problem solvers. It is the reason they are hired—organizations without problems do not need managers. Some problems burst on the scene. Something is no doubt amiss when a wildcat strike occurs among the nursing staff or when the local newspaper attacks the organization editorially. Other problems are hard to uncover and often provide no clear evidence or warning. They must be identified and treated early; undetected, they will grow and may threaten the organization's survival (i.e., "a stitch in time saves nine"). Solving them is similar to detection and early treatment of cancer.

Successful managers possess highly developed conceptual and problem identification skills. Preventing (if possible) or identifying and solving ethical problems with the least disruption to the organization is as critical as solving management problems affecting personnel or finances. It is certain that ethical problems have implications for traditional management areas and that traditional management problems have ethical dimensions. It is important to note in using this comparison that the techniques and skills employed in solving ethical problems are essentially the same as those needed to solve the traditional type of management problem. Problem solving is a generic process that applies to both types.

IDENTIFYING ETHICAL PROBLEMS

Often, managers believe that they are inadequately prepared to recognize ethical problems and even less able to solve them. This belief understates the typical manager's credentials. Identifying ethical issues that could become problems is primarily a matter of mind-set, attitude, and application of common sense when reviewing or analyzing a situation. Defining the dimensions of an ethical problem is often less difficult than developing acceptable alter-

31

native solutions and implementing the solution selected. Developing and implementing solutions are more likely to require assistance from within the organization, or even from outside it.

Managers who see their function only as solving problems of staffing, directing, budgeting, controlling, organizing, coordinating, integrating, and planning are more in need of sensitivity to ethical issues than of postgraduate education in philosophy. Methodologies similar to those used to solve traditional management problems can be used to solve ethical problems, whether administrative or biomedical. (This generic process is examined later in the chapter.) However, traditional management issues often overshadow and may even overwhelm ethical dimensions. In addition, ethical dimensions can be subtle, which complicates initial identification and solution.

Using authority delegated by the governing body, managers represent the organization. As considered in Chapter 3, the organization's philosophy provides a general context for the manager's activities and decision making, but does not eliminate the manager's need for a personal ethic. A personal ethic provides individual managers with a framework for action and permits greater refinement of principles, rules, and particular judgments and actions than is likely in the statement of philosophy developed by the typical health services organization. It bears repeating that each human being is a moral agent whose actions have moral consequences. Deleterious conduct cannot be excused simply because someone claims to have been following orders. This is true regardless of the source of the orders. Orders from lawfully constituted authorities, such as courts, pose a special problem. Moral agents who consider such orders unjust or immoral may engage in acts of civil disobedience, but in doing so they must be prepared to bear societally imposed sanctions. The ethical (moral) implications of acts must be considered independently.

Occasionally, there may be conflict between the organization's ethic, as expressed in its philosophy, and the manager's personal ethic. The organization is a bureaucracy and the manager must carefully consider the implications of acquiescing to its values. This follows from the concept of moral agency. Often, it seems easier to "go along to get along" than to risk one's position by speaking out. Professional dissent or whistleblowing are rare, despite evidence that sharp or dishonest practices, criminal behavior, or activities that pose a danger to the public are not uncommon in organizations. Managers must recognize both the distinction between and the integration of an organizational and a personal ethic. They must not perform their daily tasks with little thought about the ethical context or implications of their work.

In terms of the problem-solving methodology described later, the organization's philosophy and the individual's personal ethic are vital. They provide the framework and context in which the manager functions. They enhance sensitization to and identification and solution of ethical problems so that managers can approach these problems as they would traditional management problems.

Another technique that may be useful in identifying ethical problems is the ethics audit.[1] Conducted much like a financial audit, the ethics audit allows the organization to compare actual with desired performance. Small increases in various measures are a warning to managers that ethical problems may exist: patient complaints, incident reports, and legal actions; employee grievances, resignations, terminations, and wrongful discharge complaints; medical staff complaints and resignations; problems with suppliers and other vendors; and adverse publicity. Hofmann[1] recommends three steps in conducting an ethics audit. First, analyze key documents (e.g., vision, mission, and values statements) and their operationalization in policies and procedures, with special attention paid to issues such as uncompensated care, confidentiality, consent, conflicts of interest, and sexual harassment. Second, survey representative board members, managers, physicians, employees, volunteers, and community residents and organizations to determine whether actual performance matches that desired. Third, address deficiencies through education or other appropriate strategies.

Administrative Ethical Issues

Leadership is essential in management. It includes setting goals, establishing direction, and guiding the organization. These activities are more ethics sensitive than are many routine managerial activities. Day-to-day activities seem less tied to values, but even these are based on earlier decisions rooted in ethical principles, whether or not those principles are identified and expressly stated. However management functions are interpreted, human beings cannot escape their role as moral agents. Managers set a tone and establish a context for the organization and staff. They cannot avoid scrutiny of evidence of their personal ethic, or its congruence with the organization's philosophy.

Managers hold positions of trust, which may not be used for personal advantage or aggrandizement, and managers must not raise the slightest hint of wrongdoing by their actions. If one seeks to be an effective leader, these are essential elements of a personal ethic. Actions should be judged by applying the ethical principles developed in Chapter 1. Another effective way to clarify the pragmatic effect of an action is to step back and view what is being done or contemplated as though one were an outsider. One should ask oneself, How would the public and my colleagues see it? This "as seen through the eyes of others" or "light of public scrutiny" standard for judging action is helpful. A cynic's standard is not useful—meeting it is impossible because cynics uncover problems when it is unreasonable to do so. Skepticism is a useful criterion for managers to apply as they seek to understand how their actions might be interpreted. A standard of discovery is unacceptable because the concept of "if you don't get caught, it's okay" negates the need for ethics and substitutes deviousness and deceit.

In a way quite different from a personal ethic or an organization's philosophy, the law is a baseline of what is considered ethical. The Introduction noted that laws provide useful comparisons; however, they guide us only partially because the law is a minimum standard of conduct and no manager can effectively lead by meeting minimum requirements. The manager *qua* leader must set an example that substantially surpasses what is expected of others. Professional codes also guide conduct and provide frames of reference. They have a more demanding level of performance than the law, but should not be seen as incorporating all expectations of ethical performance.

Is it persuasive to argue that where one stands on administrative ethics depends on where one sits? Does the concept of "rank hath its privileges" apply to managing health services? Many senior managers act as to suggest they believe it does. One readily finds situations in which subordinates are reprimanded for behavior unpunished at the upper echelons. Here, it is "do as I say, not as I do"; or "what is sauce for the goose is not sauce for the gander." Few persons fail to distinguish words from actions. This double standard sends staff a clear message of cynicism and inconsistency and greatly diminishes a manager's ability to lead.

Managers can become sensitive to administrative ethical issues in several ways. They should be voracious readers of the popular press and professional literature. Codes of ethics are valuable guides to understanding the concerns of a profession and the parameters of acceptable actions. Asking whether the Golden Rule is being met may suggest that there are ethical problems. Not to be forgotten is intuition and hunch, that sixth sense that something is wrong. Both can be nurtured to alert managers to the presence of ethical problems.

Identifying ethical problems means focusing on the principles of respect for persons, beneficence, nonmaleficence, and justice; asking if the actions contemplated violate them; and determining whether the violation is justified by special circumstances. A questioning mind permits managers to consider the situation further or seek assistance, as appropriate. Identifying administrative ethical problems requires attention to detail and constant vigilance.

Biomedical Ethical Issues

All contemplated and actual interactions with patients present potential sources of ethical problems, which range from paternalism to consent and from truth telling to decisions at the end of life. Managers may feel uncomfortable and out of place working to solve biomedical ethical problems. They should not. *Medicine and the clinician provide key information that assists in making informed ethical decisions, but the decision itself is ethical (moral), not clinical.* The distinction between clinical and ethical aspects of biomedical decision making is critical and is one managers must not forget. Managers will gain confidence with greater experience and exposure to biomedical ethical issues. Their participation is needed because greater medical staff–administration interaction results in a more effective and efficient organization and all biomedical problems have administrative dimensions. Thus the manager's involvement is critical.

Managers do not supersede clinicians, but managers are important to preventing or solving a wide range of biomedical ethical problems, including serving on institutional ethics committees (IECs) and institutional review boards (IRBs) and participating in resource allocation decisions. In addition, managers are key in developing the processes and operationalizing the policies, procedures, and rules that implement the organization's philosophy.

As noted in the section on administrative ethics, managers need not take postgraduate courses in philosophy or ethics to be able to identify the presence of potential problems, although such courses might be helpful. Primarily, learning to identify potential ethical problems requires sensitization, an inquiring mind, and a reasonably well-developed personal ethic. Questions such as "Is this patient being treated as I would wish to be?", "Is the patient protected from unnecessary harm?", and "Does the consent process adequately inform the patient about what is being done?" are useful in identifying biomedical ethical problems. As with all problem solving, asking the right questions may be the most important part of the process.

An important role for managers is stimulating the medical staff and other caregivers to develop the expertise to prevent or deal effectively with biomedical ethical problems. To do so, caregivers must be availed of procedures and rules to follow. Here, the manager's role as a catalyst is much the same as that played in traditional administrative activities. Regrettably, codes of administrative ethics provide little guidance in addressing biomedical ethical issues.

SOLVING PROBLEMS

Unresolved ethical problems exact the same destructive effect on an organization as do problems involving personnel, finance, or the medical staff. Therefore, it is imperative that managers possess a methodology for solving these problems. This poses difficulties, however, because few managers are formally trained in ethics. Ethical issues may seem more subtle than management problems, and because managers tend to be pragmatic, they are less inclined to grapple with nuances. Sometimes ethical problems are combined with and overshadowed by administrative issues. Furthermore, managers may consider ethical issues less important than other problems, perhaps because they do not comprehend their potentially devastating effect. These obstacles are surmountable, however.

In 1910 John Dewey, the American educator and philosopher, wrote in *How We Think* that problem solving comprises three stages: identifying the problem, identifying the alternatives, and determining which alternative is best. Implicitly or explicitly, successful managers use a similar process. The stages of the process include identifying the problem in terms of both the current manifestation (which may be only a symptom) and the underlying cause; developing alternative solutions and the decision criteria to judge them acceptable, unacceptable, or optimal; preparing an implementation plan for the solution selected; and developing a means to evaluate the solution, once implemented.

Philosophers use a similar methodology, *moral reasoning*, to analyze ethical problems. Its components are surprisingly similar to the manager's problem-solving methodology:

- *Analyzing*—separating the overall structure of a problem in a particular case into its major components
- *Weighing*—assessing the strengths and weaknesses of various alternatives that could be used in solving the problem by balancing them against one another
- *Justifying*—providing a compelling and sufficient moral reason that appeals to an established moral principle, such as "always tell the truth" (any such principle must be compatible with the organization's philosophy and the manager's personal ethic)
- *Choosing*—selecting one or more of the available alternatives, preferably on the basis of a position that can be and has been shown to be justified
- *Evaluating*—reexamining the choices and their justifications, identifying unanswered questions, and relating decisions about one particular case to similar cases[2]

Problem solving can be divided into two basic types:

> The specific focus on problem solving is rooted in two broad models, the rational and the heuristic. Problem definition is addressed differently by each. The rational model (sometimes identified with programmed decisions) assumes that one is faced with a specific problem and focuses primarily on a search for the optimal solution.

> Operations research, for example, is primarily a quantitative expression of this approach applied to a wide range of management issues. In the hospital, it includes problems such as work scheduling, e.g., developing a computer program that maximizes the preferred work schedule of a large number of nurses, or a PERT chart used to schedule the construction of a new building. These and similar problem-solving techniques are important for an organization, and help it to establish patterns for problem solving.

> The heuristic model (sometimes identified with nonprogrammed decisions, or a learning model) acknowledges that some problems may be more diffusely defined, poorly structured, and are often not routine. It focuses upon an iterative process of dealing with problem definition, as well as solution. Heuristic general problem-solving techniques have been suggested for training administrators. Heuristic problem-solving approaches which are quantitative and computer-based have been advocated.[3]

The distinction between rational and heuristic models suggests that solving ethical problems is heuristic. First, however, process and substance components must be separated, and ethical problems that recur and have similar features must be distinguished from those that are unique and unlikely to recur. Process components are more amenable to analysis and solution by the rational model than are substance components. Ethical problems that recur and have similar features are also more amenable to using the rational model. Even here, however, implementing the process may uncover unique or subtle problems of substance, such as relative authority of different individuals in the decision-making process. The two problem-solving theories are not mutually exclusive, and the heuristic model often benefits from using a rational model for parts of the analysis. Thus, problem solvers should not choose one model to the exclusion of the other.

Master's degree programs in health services administration and business administration usually teach problem solving. Such methodologies are useful in solving ethical problems, and are similar to the generic problem-solving model in Figure 4. The model is shown in two dimensions, but should be conceptualized with time as the third dimension. In this respect, the model is like a corkscrew: While the process cycles from problem analysis to evaluation of results, the whole activity is moving through time.

In Figure 4 problem analysis begins when the manager objectively or intuitively finds something amiss. Commonly, in solving management problems, it is here that actual results deviate from desired or expected results, or a situation occurs that demands an organizational response. Examples of management situations requiring attention include a rapid decrease or increase in outpatient admissions, increased turnover among staff in a department, more uneaten food returned from patient rooms or the cafeteria to dietary, or an announcement that competing emergicenters are opening or closing. Some of these potential problems are foreseen through analysis of routinely collected data; others are apparent only when the event occurs. Obvious and defined problems are more likely to be amenable to the rational rather than to the heuristic model.

Similarly, the ethical dimensions of some situations are apparent. If a patient is diagnosed as being in a persistent vegetative state (PVS), an ethical problem having both clinical and administrative dimensions exists. An ethical problem is also present when the organization lacks an effective consent process. Under these circumstances heuristic problem solving is not the most effective methodology.

Administrative and biomedical ethical problems are only potentially in need of a solution until the problem solver determines that they must be solved. Sometimes, before planned resolution of the ethical dimensions of a situation can occur, certain events cause the problem to disappear (e.g., the patient in PVS cannot be resuscitated after cardiac arrest). The problem has disappeared, but not because it has been solved.

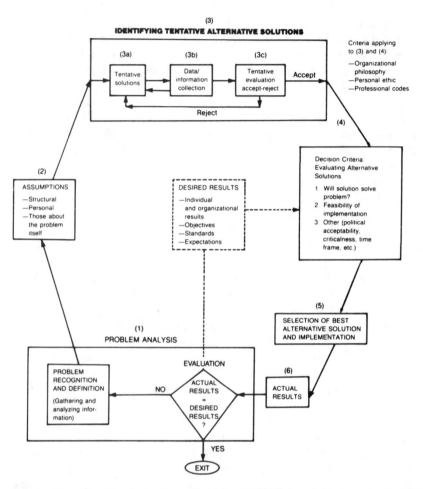

Figure 4.   Schema for solving ethical problems. (Adapted from Rakich, J.S., Longest, B.B., Jr., & Darr, K. [1992]. *Managing health services organizations* [3rd ed., p. 389]. Baltimore: Health Professions Press.)

Berry and Seavey[4] argue that problem definitions "are fundamentally subjective (and) . . . are not objective, concrete realities; they are perceptions of reality." This statement is correct as it bears on perceptions of cause and effect, but must be qualified when applied to certain situations. For example, several mysterious deaths in a nursing facility are a verifiable fact and will be defined by any manager as a problem that needs solving. Perceptions (subjectivity) vary in determining the cause or in identifying the underlying situation (problem) that may be the cause. Views of problems and their solutions are affected by the positions held and responsibilities of the individuals involved. Nursing service is likely to provide a different explanation of the deaths than would management.

Context is far more important in solving problems that are primarily ethical than it is when solving management problems with few ethical dimensions. The context of ethical problems is the organization's philosophy and mission interpreted and applied by a manager who is a moral agent with a personal ethic. Once an ethical problem has been recognized and defined as a problem needing a solution, it must be understood. The information about its extent and character may be available in existing data systems or special efforts may be required. Managers solving ethical problems will experience deficiencies in data similar to those they confront when solving other problems.

Box (2) in Figure 4 asks managers to identify assumptions about the problem, personal implications and views, and the structure within which the problem arises. Staff were undoubtedly affected in the case of Baby Boy Doe, and it is reasonable to assume that in similar cases, staff will become depressed and angry and morale will decline. One may also assume that few staff members will be so upset that they will resign, turn to a union, or refuse to work in the nursery. Assumptions such as these require judgment by managers and may result in a decision to ignore the situation (i.e., not define it as a problem requiring a solution), which is what occurred in the case of Baby Boy Doe. The hospital accepted the parents' directives and determined there was either no problem that required a solution or that the solution was to do nothing. Such a result is dependent on the organization's philosophy and the individual manager's personal ethic. Choosing to do nothing is always an option, if it meets the decision criteria. This may be the best alternative in some situations. However, it must never be the choice by default.

Preliminary review of options occurs in Box (3), in which alternative solutions are identified and assessed. Here, decision makers brainstorm creative solutions. Managers solving administrative or biomedical ethical problems must be mindful of the organization's philosophy as well as their personal ethic. Unless the constraints can be changed, solutions falling outside them must be discarded. Arbitrarily ignoring or applying these constraints creates inconsistencies and discontinuities that eventually cause serious problems for the organization and the manager. Other, more general criteria are also applied in such instances.

Alternative solutions that pass this preliminary screening are subject to detailed assessment. This assessment compares each option against specific decision criteria. Examples of these criteria are shown in Box (4) of Figure 4: time available to solve the problem, real costs of all kinds (e.g., political, financial, reputation), opportunity costs, feasibility of implementation, adequacy of solving the problem, and benefits derived. Applying more specific criteria results in better solutions and outcomes. A primary benefit of greater specificity in the process is that managers are required to review, analyze, and be as precise as possible, both in defining the problem and in considering and selecting the alternative that best solves it. This is a useful exercise because it hones management decision making. A more sophisticated approach is to weight or assign relative values to decision criteria because some are more important than are others.

Prior to and after selecting the alternative, the manager must consider implementation and evaluation. A common failing is that great effort is put into developing a solution and beginning implementation. Then, managers are distracted by other problems and the result is that the solution flounders before it is fully implemented. Implementing the solution should receive as much attention as does selecting it. A means of evaluation must be included in the solution so that difficulties can be identified and timely corrective action taken. Corrective actions are a subset of the problem-solving process and may involve the same or similar steps.

This ethical problem-solving methodology is useful for decision making by one manager, by management as a group, by governing body committees, or by specially established committees, such as institutional ethics committees, infant care review committees, or institutional review boards. It is effective for solving one problem, considering guidelines for a class of problems, or developing a process to bring a similar methodology to bear on solving individual problems or groups of problems. Regardless of the source of decision making, once the process is established and policies (which have gone through a similar problem-solving process) have been formulated and implemented, operating procedures and rules will be established. This means that an issue such as consent has been considered and that the ethically acceptable policies, procedures, and processes have been identified and implemented. Therefore, as a general rule the majority of ethical problems will be prevented. Exceptions and special attention will be necessary when the facts differ sufficiently from the assumptions implicit in the policy and the procedures derived from it.

In this regard it is unnecessary to distinguish administrative from biomedical ethical problems. In terms of general policies and guidelines, both types of problems should be considered prospectively. Resulting policies and procedures will cover the majority of predictable, recurring ethical problems. That is why, for example, a governing body adopts a conflict of interest policy applicable to itself and management staff. Despite the usefulness of general guidelines and specific rules, problems arise in interpreting and applying them and because of unique ethical issues. It bears repeating that the problem-solving model considered earlier is usable on two levels: general policy development and consideration of individual cases.

Although in most ways implementing solutions to administrative or biomedical ethical problems is the same as it is for management problems, some distinctions should be noted. One distinction is that often, ethical issues involve a high level of emotion. Examples are situations that suggest a manager has acted unethically (administrative ethics) or that a patient's view of life and death has been violated or challenged (biomedical ethics). Thus, managers and staff who work to solve ethical problems must exercise greater sensitivity to human factors and must understand that they are not dealing with units of production or ordinary services. Another distinction is that administrative and, especially, biomedical ethical issues often result in significant legal consequences. Although all health services organizations should apply a standard that is much higher than the minimum set by the law, mistakes do occur, and occasionally, there are problems that bring in lawyers. Yet another distinction is that negative public relations consequences may occur inside and outside the organization.

DEVELOPING A PERSONAL ETHIC

Health services managers begin their careers as adults who have, at the very least, developed an implicit personal ethic. In developing that ethic managers have been affected by a host of influences beyond their own introspection, including family and friends, religious principles and teachings, secular education, and the law. It is in this context that adults become managers and that a personal ethic about management emerges. For some managers their personal ethic may be only an intuitive sense of right and wrong, with no identifiable source or explicitly defined code of conduct.

Developing a personal ethic necessitates introspection and self-examination. Questions such as "Who am I?", "How do I view certain actions or activities?", "What do I consider unethical?", and "What is morally right or wrong?" are helpful. Understanding and grappling with questions such as these are critical as managers search for the "right" answer to ethical problems. Both new and experienced health services managers use numerous sources in developing and refining their personal ethic. Chief among these sources are professional codes of ethics, educational socialization, and association and pressure of peers, subordinates, and superiors.

In selecting the principles to be included in a personal ethic managers should apply the criteria of comprehensiveness, consistency, and coherence and ask themselves the following questions: Do the principles apply to the broadest possible range of ethical issues? How useful and applicable are they in solving ethical problems? Do they use the scientific method in terms of exactness, systemization, and predictability? Are the ethical concepts clear and consistent? Are they in conflict with or consistent with other knowledge or life experiences? Are they reasonably adaptable to a changing world? Although the criteria of comprehensiveness, consistency, and coherence are not applied with the rigor employed by a moral philosopher, they should be used when judging, developing, or reconsidering a personal ethic and when analyzing the ethics of others or disputing their reasoning or conclusions.

In addition to the manager's personal ethic, the organization's philosophy is vital to ethical decision making. It is tempting to say that the personal ethic is and ought to remain the most important factor. However, one cannot ignore the realities of bureaucratic life. Some sectarian health services organizations seek to achieve complete congruence between a manager's personal ethic and the organization's ethic by hiring no one above midlevel management who is not an adherent to that faith. The wisdom of such a policy is examined later. Suffice to say that in modern, complex health services organizations a significant and undesirable potential for discontinuity exists between the philosophy of the organization and that of its managers. The extent to which these philosophies *must* be identical, or even congruent, is unclear, however. It is likely that the organization's philosophy will have a greater impact on development of the personal ethic of a younger, less experienced manager. Like others, managers become "set in their ways."

CONCLUSION

In solving problems successful managers implicitly or explicitly use a methodology similar to that outlined in Figure 4. Effectively solving ethical problems requires the same attention and a similar approach. Managers cannot ignore ethical problems and they must be prepared to participate in solving them. This does not mean that health services managers supersede physicians or other clinical staff where biomedical ethics are involved. It does mean that in an effort to operationalize the principles developed in Chapter 1, managers must participate effectively in solving ethical problems of all types. It is the nature of the job that managers serve as team leaders and catalysts. Serving as the organization's conscience is consistent with the manager's role as moral agent in a position of ethical leadership. In terms of administrative ethics, the manager's role is preeminent.

Successful managers have a well-developed personal ethic and a clear understanding of their own views on administrative and biomedical ethical issues. This ethic has been defined by drawing from a wide variety of sources. A personal ethic cannot be chiseled in stone and it can be expected to evolve over time. Although one's basic view of the world is likely to remain relatively stable, experience, maturation, and technological developments do affect one's personal ethic.

NOTES

1. Paul B. Hofmann. (1995, November/December). Performing an ethics audit. *Healthcare Executive, 10*(2), 47.
2. Frank Harron, John Burnside, & Tom Beauchamp. (1983). *Health and human values* (p. 4). New Haven, CT: Yale University Press.
3. David E. Berry, & John W. Seavey. (1984, March/April). Reiteration of problem definition in health services administration. *Hospital & Health Services Administration, 29*(2), 58.
4. *Ibid.*, 59.

II

Guidelines in
Making Ethical Decisions

A significant problem with applied administrative and biomedical ethics is that
many written and unwritten factors influence a manager's behavior. These factors are the by-product of family background, religious orientation and training,
professional affiliations and allegiances, and a too-often ill-defined personal code of
moral conduct—an amalgam of intellect, experience, education, and relationships. A
manager with this mind-set may often provide vague, perhaps contradictory guidance.
When an ill-defined personal code of conduct is combined with a generally high level
of tolerance for varying views, the result is that many managers believe ethical problems have no real answers, only difficult or impossible moral choices. In addition,
events often begin to control, rather than being controlled by managers, who find
themselves being shaped rather than shaping.

An attribute of professions, including health services management, is that its
members engage in activities with a large element of service to humanity. This raises
for managers and the profession generally the problem of the demarcation between
private and professional lives. If the manager's private conduct breaches the profession's code of ethics, the profession may take disciplinary action.

In addition to the dynamic tension between a manager's private and professional
life is that between a manager's personal ethic and the organization's philosophy and
mission. Philosophy and mission are the organization's basic law and guide development and implementation of policies, procedures, and rules. An important question
is "Must the manager's philosophy be identical to the organization's?"

Chapters 3 and 4 suggest development and content of an organizational philosophy and examine its importance in the delivery of services. Codes of ethics and their
role in guiding health services managers and in helping them develop a personal ethic

are examined. The dynamic between the organization's philosophy and the manager's code is analyzed.

Assistance for managers and organizations in solving ethical problems is identified in Chapter 5. Specialized committees that focus on different types of ethical problems and other means of obtaining assistance are suggested. As a moral agent, the manager is a primary actor in efforts to prevent or identify and solve ethical problems.

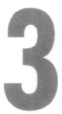

Developing Organizational Philosophy and Mission Statements

Managers confront a variety of moral and symbolic issues in health services organizations. The focus in this chapter is the need for the organization to identify and adopt values and principles—a philosophy. It is within the context of this philosophy that a vision and a mission are developed. The vision statement is the goals the organization seeks to achieve. The mission statement describes its specific activities. Defining the philosophy prospectively resolves conflicts among competing values. The sequence of philosophy–vision–mission is the theoretical ideal. The reality is that more likely the mission is defined first or that it evolves from historical activity in the context of an implicit, rather than explicit, philosophy. The concept of "visioning" in health services organizations developed in the 1980s. This chapter describes the importance of identifying the moral values and principles that govern vision and mission statements and the necessity of reflecting these values across the organization.

Mission (and vision) is necessarily limited by and is a function of the physical location, size, resources, and other aspects of the internal and external environments of the organization. Most of these factors can be affected, but usually only over time. A significant change in these factors necessitates a review of the organization's mission. Many elements in the mission directly relate to the moral values and principles identified by the organization's managers. A nongovernmental acute care hospital may choose not to perform abortions. This decision is derived from a determination that such a service is compatible (or incompatible) with its moral values and principles, as formulated and interpreted by its governing body. A service such as abortion raises other questions, the answers to which must be consistent with the organization's stand on abortion. For example, is performing abortions compatible with legally required efforts to provide medically indicated treatment to live aborted fetuses? Some organizations avoid these questions and the attendant ethical implications by simply adhering to the law. Thus, legality and morality are equated. This action may solve the problem only partially, however, because the law is poorly developed in a number of areas in which administrative and biomedical ethical problems arise.

Because a governing body develops and adopts a statement of philosophy that reflects certain moral values and principles is no indication that the staff agrees. Staff in organizations typically pay little attention to such matters and staff in the field of health services are no exception. Many staff members may not know the organization's philosophy, despite reasonable efforts to communicate it. Even if the philosophy is understood, many members make no commitment to it. When little attention is paid to the organization's stated moral values and principles, it is not surprising that even less attention is paid to what the organization should have said but did not. For these staff members the organization is but a place to work. They do their jobs and are unconcerned about what the board of directors and senior management say is the context for or the goals of service delivery. Absent a significant discontinuity—when even sabotage is possible—staff rarely overtly challenge what is being done. If a challenge is made, results tend to be negative rather than positive in outcome and effect.

Consideration must be given to how much more effective the organization could be were it built on a system of shared values and goals. Adequately communicated to and accepted by staff, a resource-supported goal as simple as "getting the caring back into curing" could reap rewards for the organization through improved efficiency and patient care and relations. Heading staff in the same direction—a direction that is known in advance and recognized as important in the organization—will positively affect staff attitude, productivity, and effectiveness.

DEVELOPING AN ORGANIZATIONAL PHILOSOPHY

The starting point for an organization to solve ethical problems is its philosophy. The statement of philosophy identifies values and principles reflecting the moral right and wrong for the organization, thus distinguishing the acceptable from the unacceptable. It is helpful if the philosophy statement is sufficiently precise that performance in achieving it can be measured. At minimum, the statement of philosophy must be consistent with the law.

The philosophy statement is different from the mission statement and should be developed separately. The philosophy statement provides a context for the mission statement; the mission statement is subordinate to it. Nonetheless, some organizations include references to values in their mission statements. A mission statement that "the corporation owns and operates hospitals to provide care for the sick and injured" provides no information about the moral context of the care. A mission statement that "the hospital provides care for the sick and injured in the context of humanitarian principles" is imprecise, but provides a clearer value or moral context than does the first.

Anecdotal evidence suggests that many health services organizations have not developed a specific, written philosophy. Nonetheless, a de facto or operational philosophy is identifiable because the aggregate effect of decisions and actions taken by the governing body and management have implicit, if ill-defined, philosophical bases. Results of management actions may be contradictory or inconsistent, and this suggests another negative aspect of not prospectively determining a comprehensive philosophy. This problem is reflected in a lack of continuity that may lead to incompatible policies, procedures, and rules. The effect is diminished efficiency.

The theme of identified and shared values is a major thrust of the widely acclaimed book, *In Search of Excellence*, by Thomas J. Peters and Robert H. Waterman. The authors quote Thomas J. Watson, Jr.,[1] former president of IBM: "the basic philosophy of an organization has far more to do with its achievements than do technological or economic resources, organizational structure, innovation and timing." The context of Watson's statement is the focus on consumer service that was so important in creating IBM's reputation and financial success. If *consumer* and *service* are so important to IBM, which has many of the characteristics of a product organization, consider how much more important they are in health services delivery. These emphases are even more noteworthy as health services organizations increasingly face competitive challenges. The centrality of shared values is shown in Figure 5, the 7-S Framework, developed by the consulting firm of McKinsey and Company.

In the book *Corporate Cultures: The Rites and Rituals of Corporate Life*, Deal and Kennedy[2] identified the characteristics shared by successful companies, as follows:

- They stand for something—that is, they have a clear and explicit philosophy about how they aim to conduct their business.
- Management pays a great deal of attention to shaping and fine-tuning these values to conform to the economic and business environment of the company and to communicating them to the organization.
- These values are known and shared by all the people who work for the company—from the production worker right through to the ranks of senior management.

Building on this concept of the importance of shared values or philosophy, Deal and Kennedy[3] describe the following important elements of a culture: 1) shared values and beliefs about success in the environment, 2) heroes who epitomize those values and beliefs, 3) rituals that prescribe how all critical activities are to be carried out, 4) ceremonies that celebrate successes of the culture, and 5) stories and storytellers that keep the mythology of the culture alive.

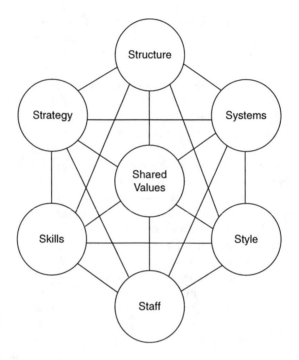

Figure 5.   The McKinsey 7-S Framework. (From McKinsey & Company, Inc. Reprinted with permission.)

In a 1985 explication of corporate cultures Kennedy[4] wrote the following:

> Culture isn't a single thing. It's not a budget; it's not a plan; it's
> not the shape of a building. It is an integrated pattern of all
> the things that go on in an organization on a day-to-day basis.
> Each company has its own unique culture, values, and standards
> communicated internally by style, dress, expectations, and
> assumptions.
>   New people in the workplace find out what is expected of
> them because their peers take them aside and say, "Look, don't
> wear jeans here. Come in to work on time, or you do this or that."
> They lay out some of the unwritten rules of behavior that are
> required for entrance into your workplace. That's how culture
> transmits itself to each new generation of persons. They don't
> come in and invent a whole new style of organization. They come
> in and learn from those around them what's going on in the or-
> ganization and how they are expected to behave.

The barriers to establishing strong corporate cultures in any organization
are a particular problem in health services organizations. Barriers important
to hospitals include the following:[5]

- Hospitals must serve diverse medical needs of heterogeneous populations.
- The number of external variables (forces outside the organization which affect it) is much greater for hospitals than it is in ordinary business enterprise.
- Hospital outcomes are difficult to define and to measure.
- It is difficult to nurture the keen proprietary sense of individual endeavors among leadership and management staff at all levels.
- Hospital board members are not active participants in its culture.
- Hospital physicians are a subculture, and peer acceptance and recognition, participation in professional activities, and stature based on professional contribution and expertise are more important than the rewards of belonging to a particular hospital.
- Elaborate peer reward systems in nursing are complicated by a deep search for professional identity.
- Increasingly, support staff and especially allied medical personnel tend to have a professional identification independent of the hospital.
- Another special subculture in hospitals is the administrators who are caught between the role of facilitating the delivery of medical care and that of running a cost-effective "business," and as a result often isolate themselves from other subcultures.

Beyond these factors, and implicit in them, is the need for managers to view their relationships with patients in a consistent fashion. Paying "lip service" to the organization's avowed goal of patient care, but in fact stressing economic or other nonpatient considerations, is a contradiction that will not be lost on staff, who will respond to real rather than platitudinous incentives.

Management must know and understand the culture and values in its organization. Just as important, management must know how the culture and values mesh with or diverge from those the organization wishes to develop. The organization can mold a culture, but it can move neither faster than nor in directions that are opposed or misunderstood by persons in the organization. This congruence is critical. The organization's philosophy and derivative vision and mission statements are the primary points of reference for its corporate culture and subordinated activities. All efforts to develop excellence are a function of these statements.

A logic is evident in the link between cultural strength and performance. The first piece of logic is that of goal alignment—a strong culture tends to cause staff to march to the same drummer. Second, a strong culture aids in performance by creating an unusual level of motivation among staff—shared values and behaviors make staff feel good about working for an organization; the resulting commitment or loyalty makes them strive harder. Third, a strong culture aids in performance because it provides needed structure and controls without relying on a bureaucracy, which can diminish motivation and innovation.[6]

Closely linked to the concept of organizational philosophy and corporate culture is management's view of the organization's staff. McGregor's Theories

X and Y, Maslow's hierarchy of needs, and the 14 points enumerated by W. Edwards Deming echo the importance of management's view of its employees, which is likely to be similar to how patients are viewed by a health services organization. Dysfunction is rife in an organization that treats employees as adversaries or as a means to an end and distrusts them, while urging staff to treat patients with dignity and respect. Employees observe the hypocrisy and respond negatively. Peters and Waterman[7] sound this theme, quoting Thomas J. Watson, Jr.: "IBM's philosophy is largely contained in three simple beliefs. I want to begin with what I think is the most important: our respect for the individual. This is a simple concept, but in IBM it occupies a major portion of management time."

Content of a Philosophy Statement

Organizational Content The values and principles in the organizational philosophy are broad; the vision statement is developed within this context, as is the mission statement. The philosophy statement provides the context and operative values—it gives delivery of health services a life, a meaning—and recognizes that these values are unique and represent more than delivering a product or rendering a service. Policies, procedures, and rules are derived from the mission statement and make the organization operational. Sibley Memorial Hospital, a nonsectarian hospital, describes its organizational philosophy by listing its values, as follows:[8]

> Our values provide guidelines and parameters for the decisions that we make as we work to improve our processes and respond to our patient's and other customer's needs.
>
> - Personalized and compassionate service
> - Excellence and continually improving quality
> - Teamwork
> - Job satisfaction
> - Professionalism
> - Using resources wisely and providing value
> - Innovation
> - Trust and respect
> - Up-to-date technology
> - A clean, attractive, quiet, and safe environment
> - Honesty, integrity, flexibility, and selflessness

Before its merger into Catholic Health Initiatives (CHI), the Franciscan Health System listed its beliefs in human life, wholism, shared ministry, and peacemaking as the basis for its organizational philosophy.[9] A member hospital, St. Mary Medical Center, has written a derivative mission statement to provide "within the limits of our resources, compassionate and quality holistic care to all in our community, within which we especially cherish the poor."[10]

PHILOSOPHY AND MISSION STATEMENTS

Appendix A includes the values, vision, and mission of Sibley Memorial Hospital and the mission statement of St. Mary Medical Center.

Moral considerations important to the organization must be addressed in the statement of philosophy. These considerations may include the organization's position on specific biomedical ethical issues. If, for example, its view of the sanctity of life prohibits the performance of certain procedures, this should be stated. The organization's view of its relationship with patients, staff (including physicians who are not employees), community, and other institutions should be described. The statement should be sufficiently detailed that performance measures can be developed and applied.

Consistent with the moral philosophies and derivative principles discussed earlier, the organization's philosophy must emphasize the importance of ensuring respect for persons and of benefiting patients and protecting them from untoward results. It is also desirable that justice be addressed by the philosophy statement. These principles are inherent in the independent relationship between the organization and the patient, and are not superseded by the relationship between the physician and the patient. Through its philosophy the organization also implicitly or explicitly states its accountability to the public, regardless of whether it is publicly or privately owned.

Relationship with Patients   It is difficult to imagine a health services organization that does not identify its role vis-à-vis patients in the context of respect for persons, beneficence, nonmaleficence, and justice. These principles stress providing medical services to the patient with respect and in a manner that enhances human dignity. Staff members must know their responsibilities and duties toward patients in this regard. Patients are the reason the organization exists, and all efforts are directed at meeting patient needs by delivering high-quality services safely.

Williams and Donnelly emphasize this relationship in *Medical Care Quality and the Public Trust*.[11] They argue that accountability to the patient takes precedence over other duties of the governing body or relationships between the governing body and other individuals or entities, including physicians. The authors assert that this accountability is such that if medical malpractice has harmed a patient who is unaware of that harm, the hospital has a duty to inform the patient. This advice is not as radical as it seems and a few organizations act in this manner. Although they agree with accountability intellectually, most governing bodies and managers will react to it negatively, primarily because the legal system is seen as demanding an adversarial approach.

The economic hazards in implementing such a philosophy are significant, especially in organizations with a voluntary medical staff. If the organization becomes supportive of patients at the expense of physicians, it risks alienating its economic livelihood. At the least it will have apathetic or angry physicians. A possible answer to this dilemma is to make physicians part of the corporate culture, thus making the organizational philosophy part of their perspective.

Hence, physicians will see substandard clinical treatment as endangering the culture and will work with the organization on the patient's behalf.

The view expressed by Williams and Donnelly is consistent with the high degree of trust the public has traditionally placed in health services organizations, and is an appropriate measure of the duty the organizations should meet in turn. The public has every right to expect that the organization and its managers will treat them with respect and dignity and will seek to right any wrongs. For many, this will mean very different treatment.

Relationship with Staff Like patients, employed and nonemployed (usually physicians) staff are entitled to be treated with respect and fidelity (loyalty). Staff are the organization's most important asset and determine the way that services are delivered. Like patients, staff must not be treated as a means to an end. The ethical aspects of these relations are most apparent in the organization's policies. Examples include reasonable and equitable evaluation standards known in advance and fairly applied; forthright efforts to eliminate capriciousness, arbitrariness, and prejudice in hiring, firing, and promotion; application of due process and access to grievances; and determination of the attributes and capabilities required for each position and matching staff with them.[12] These considerations of ethics in employee relations also make good management sense.

Employees are in an unequal bargaining position with the organization and supervisors: The employment relationship limits their freedom of action. Consequently, for example, a manager who borrows money from employees behaves unethically. This jeopardizes management's credibility, but more important, it reflects a lack of respect for employees, who are being used as a means to an end. Employees are also used as a means to an end if they must undertake high-risk activities without adequate training or supplies and equipment (e.g., treatment of people with highly infectious diseases). This example is a rare instance, in which the duty of beneficence toward the patient is superseded by a duty of loyalty to staff, a decision also supported by a utilitarian calculus.

Physicians are the economic life blood of most health services organizations and are there at the organizations' sufferance, either as employees or independent contractors. In either relationship, the presence of these high-profile professionals complicates the organization's interactions with patients and other staff. If, for example, quality of care issues arise, the organization must meet its obligations to protect patients and further their interests by intervening in the physician–patient relationship. The political problems that are likely to arise for governance and management, exacerbated by the economic dimensions, mean intervention occurs reluctantly and less often than it should occur.

Employees and medical staff should participate in developing the organization's philosophy and vision and mission statements. Increased congruence between the philosophies of organization and staff benefits all involved; most important, it benefits patients. Rapport between the organization and its staff is essential to developing a strong corporate culture.

Relationship with the Community In some geographic areas community (service area) and patients or potential patients are synonymous. The organization's philosophy should specify its relationship to the community: What is its obligation to provide free or less-than-cost care to Medicaid patients or the medically indigent? What is its obligation to provide controversial services such as abortion? Prospectively answering questions such as these causes the organization to consider important issues about itself and its role. This probing assists in honing an organizational philosophy and provides an opportunity for introspection and staff involvement in establishing and strengthening a corporate culture.

Relationship with Other Institutions Revising the organizational philosophy is difficult but necessary as the external environment changes. The organization must deal forthrightly and honestly with other entities, even actual or potential competitors. This ethic fits with effective competition—it simply means the organization competes honestly, with no hint of fraud or deception. In the past there were few incentives for health services organizations to cooperate, but significant changes in the delivery of health services and economic pressures will force them into networks or systems. Large differences in moral philosophies inhibit cooperative efforts, a problem that may be insurmountable when sectarian and nonsectarian organizations contemplate a merger or joint efforts.

DEVELOPING A MISSION STATEMENT

Vision statements are aspirational and inspirational. As such, they sketch out what the organization would like to become. They set a direction for the organization and broadly state its role and activities.

Mission statements are the applied portions of the vision statement. They operationalize the means by which the vision is to be accomplished. The mission statement may originate in the articles of incorporation, the documents filed to establish the health services organization as a legal entity. The statement of objectives or the purposes for which the corporation is formed are useful in developing a mission statement. That the mission statement needs to be consistent with and reflect the organization's philosophy has been amply described herein. A simple mission statement is that a community hospital association will do the following:

- Establish, operate, and maintain a hospital
- Engage in educational activities related to treating the sick and injured
- Engage in health promotion and disease prevention activities
- Promote and perform scientific research related to treating the sick and injured

- Engage in other activities designed to promote the general health of the community

More elaborate are the objectives (mission statement) of Sterling County Hospital,[13] in which elements of an organizational philosophy are included, as follows:

- To recognize man's unique composition of body and soul and man's basic right to life. Sterling County's concept of total care, therefore, embraces the physical, emotional, spiritual, social, and economic needs of each patient.
- To affirm that the primary objective of our health services is to relieve suffering and to promote and restore health in a Christian manner that demands competence, mercy, and respect
- To generate and cultivate a source of allied health manpower by orienting and supporting personnel development in the areas of individual skills, knowledge, and attitudes
- To participate in the development of health services that are relevant to the total community needs by meaningful area-wide and regional planning and in a partnership for health concept

These mission statements show what the two organizations seek to accomplish. An important distinction is that the first statement has no value context, nor is there any attempt to link its activities to a larger value system. The second statement has a philosophical context.

Organizations state their missions in different ways. A well-known children's hospital states that it will provide health services to any child, regardless of ability to pay. This mission statement incorporates the philosophy that treating the child is the primary concern; economics are secondary. Sectarian health services organizations cite their religious creeds; nonsectarian organizations typically link their activities to humanitarian motives. Sterling County Hospital is unique in that it is a publicly owned facility with a religious reference in its mission statement. Appendix A includes sample organizational philosophies and vision and mission statements.

RECONSIDERING THE ORGANIZATION'S PHILOSOPHY

A competitive environment will significantly affect the way many health services organizations born of eleemosynary (charitable) motives view themselves. Competition and reports of large profits will change how others, especially patients and communities, view them. Aggressive competition is at variance with the philosophy and historical mission of many organizations that serve the sick and injured and do so from a sense of duty and charity, rather than from a desire to establish new product lines, increase their market share, or maximize net income over expense. The organization that does not possess the stamina, resources, or mind-set to reconsider its philosophy and mission may become uneconomic and cease to exist. The following case is illustrative.

An Acceptable New Image?

Sebastian Hospital was founded by a Christian congregation in 1891. Its philosophy and mission statement include a strong commitment to care for the sick and injured regardless of ability to pay. This mission posed no problems during its first 90 years. Even after the hospital was purchased by the community in 1950, it continued to function in the same fashion. Sebastian successfully weathered a controversy about abortions in 1973. The compromise limited where in the hospital abortions would be performed and where staff would be assigned.

Increasing cost pressures during the 1970s and diagnosis-related groups (DRGs) in the early 1980s caused substantial financial problems. A switch to all-payer prospective payment, which would prohibit cost shifting, was imminent. In addition, there was pressure for corporate reorganization. Planning consultants first recommended enterprises such as a physician office building, parking facilities, and a motel. Some of these suggestions were complementary to the primary mission. The trustees saw others as only tangential. Another new type of enterprise was proposed: a joint venture with members of the medical staff.

The administrator was concerned that the almost 100-year-old focus of the hospital would change dramatically. It was one thing to manage a facility competently, but quite another to be razzle-dazzle entrepreneurs. Would the caring reputation that Sebastian had achieved so successfully disappear in a blaze of marketing efforts and joint ventures? The administrator wondered whether Sebastian was hopelessly out of step with its environment.

This case illustrates the dilemma confronting many not-for-profit community hospitals. The same or similar problems affect most organizations in the sense that they must continue to adapt to what seem to be revolutionary environmental changes. Interinstitutional competition is less problematic when a community uses one of each type of institutional provider. Even in such a case, however, organizations are beginning to offer competing services. For example, hospitals increasingly find that they are competing with members of their medical staff. Hospitals will lose substantial revenue when highly remunerative ancillary and diagnostic services are performed on the outside. Such tensions will diminish the ability of not-for-profit organizations to carry out their historic mission.

Initially viewed with disdain by managers because it conjured up images of individuals with questionable morals selling unneeded services of little value, marketing has become an accepted, even necessary, part of health services delivery. Preference is still to focus on health promotion and disease and accident prevention and treatment, but marketing is the buzzword; organizations that fail to heed it risk surviving.

Competition is not at variance with a charitable mission. The context has changed, the stakes have increased, but managers should view such changes as a challenge—an opportunity to do what they have been doing even more effectively. Successful corporate restructuring and effective marketing allow the organization to develop revenue streams that enable it to provide charitable services.

A more insidious problem, one that is fraught with conflicts of interest, occurs in certain joint ventures between health services organizations, such as hospitals, and their medical staffs. Physicians who earn income by referring patients to providers in which they have an ownership interest or a profit-sharing arrangement have a conflict of interest. Several states have either prohibited physician referral to such facilities or have mandated disclosure to patients. Organized medicine took note of such conflicts of interest in 1985.[14] Since then, laws have set limits on physician self-referral involving federal program beneficiaries.

A different philosophical dilemma faced St. Joseph Hospital, which was established in 1870 and owned by various orders of Catholic sisters. In 1971 it was sold to the Creighton Regional Health Care Corporation, a not-for-profit corporation with a lay board of directors, which operated St. Joseph as a Catholic teaching hospital for Creighton University. In 1984 a contract was signed with American Medical International (AMI), a for-profit hospital system, under which AMI would acquire St. Joseph Hospital and operate it as a full-service Catholic teaching hospital. Based on this transfer of ownership, the Catholic Health Association (CHA) terminated St. Joseph's membership because "the Hospital is not operated, supervised, or controlled by or in conjunction with the Roman Catholic Church in the United States."[15] The controversy surrounding the decision suggested that other important but unstated reasons were questions about the morality of the profit motive in health services and that other AMI hospitals performed abortions. Those challenging CHA's action argued that the profit motive was compatible with St. Joseph's mission and that the bondholders of St. Joseph's debt were paid several millions of dollars in interest, an action, it was argued, indistinguishable from that of paying dividends to stockholders.

What is important in this case is that CHA took action when it determined that a member hospital was no longer compatible with its philosophy and mission. Regardless of how one judges CHA, the point is that its decision was based on a specific philosophy—a crucial underpinning for any organization.

UNDERSTANDING PATIENT BILLS OF RIGHTS

Patient bills of rights provide guidance about the appropriate ethical relationship between the patient and the organization and its employees. Titles vary, but bills of rights have been published by organizations including the American Hospital Association (AHA), the Joint Commission on Accreditation of Healthcare Organizations (Joint Commission), the U.S. Department of Veterans Affairs (VA), and the American Civil Liberties Union (ACLU). In addition, hospitals and other institutional providers have developed their own statements. All patient bills of rights reflect the law on confidentiality and consent, for example, but no bill is legally binding. Philosophical differences are large, however.

Before 1992 the AHA patient bill of rights[16] was oriented more to institutional than patient needs and contained an element of paternalism, such as the provision that at times patients should not be fully informed of their medical conditions. This paternalism has deep roots in medical ethical tradition dating to the Hippocratic oath, and causes doing good (beneficence) to conflict with enhancing patient autonomy. The AHA's 1992 bill places greater emphasis on patient rights. The institutional bias is muted but continues, and the implementation of several patient rights is limited (e.g., "The patient has the right to make decisions about the plan of care prior to and during the course of treatment and to refuse a recommended treatment or plan of care to the extent permitted by law *and hospital policy*" [emphasis added]). One must conclude from this phrase that hospital policy could force patients to accept care they have declined. The responsibilities of patients in the care process are also addressed.

The ACLU's patient bill of rights[17] was drafted as a model law with the intention that it be enacted by the states. A demanding view of patients' rights distinguishes it philosophically from AHA's bill. The ACLU bill views the patient as an autonomous individual entitled to full involvement in the care process. For example, the bill mandates for each patient a 24-hours-a-day patient rights advocate, who may act on behalf of the patient, and with the patient's consent, assert or protect the rights enumerated in the model bill. Patients also have a right to their medical records, upon their request and on payment of reasonable copying expenses, to receive a complete copy of the records. The ACLU bill details the information to be provided when consent for treatment is obtained. Gone, however, is a suggestion from the previous iteration that patients *have a duty* (emphasis added) to be fully involved in their care. The ACLU bill's stridency in protecting patient rights is unconventional, but its provisions are worth considering.

VA's Code of Patient Concern[18] and the Joint Commission's Standard on Patient Rights[19] lie philosophically between the AHA's and ACLU's patient bills of rights. VA's code recognizes that patients may experience lengthy hospitalizations, and contains provisions on receiving mail, letter writing, and wearing personal apparel. The code also contains sections on patient responsibilities and advance directives. In previous iterations the Joint Commission standard included a section on patients' responsibilities in cooperating with caregivers. In 1996 emphasis was placed on the patient rights that the organization is expected to perfect. Unique sections include ethical issues in research and organ procurement.

Documents such as patient bills of rights set an ethical tone for relationships with patients and serve as a nonformal source of law should a dispute arise. The usefulness of such documents is limited by the organization's willingness to adopt one already available or to develop its own, and more important, to implement the bill of rights by making its contents known to patients and monitoring processes that demonstrate their application.

PLANNING STRATEGICALLY

The organization's philosophy also affects its strategic planning. The philosophy must be articulated if planning objectives are to be consistent as well as set appropriately. The organization's view of its social responsibility should be reflected in its organizational philosophy and vision and mission statements. Once established, the strategic planning process can proceed.

It is widely accepted that an organization's philosophy, vision, and mission state the ideal—ends thought to be unattainable but progress toward that which is believed possible.[20] In this respect, perhaps the most difficult aspect of developing a strategy is determining the balance between social responsibility and economic performance.[21] The perspective that health services organizations are a social enterprise with an economic dimension may no longer apply; however, the obverse may apply. Resolving this dilemma and the paradoxes it raises are increasingly difficult. Although the governing body is primarily responsible for developing a philosophy and vision and mission statements, senior management undertakes the planning process and develops specific operational plans. All participants are responsible for the consistency between the organization's philosophy and its specific procedures and rules.

ACHIEVING CONGRUENCE OF PHILOSOPHIES

Several questions must be asked about the relationship between the manager's personal ethic and the organization's philosophy: To what extent must organizational philosophy and managers' personal ethics mesh? If the organization is to be a community of shared values, must all managers be in full agreement with the philosophy? As a class, are managers sufficiently professional to be effective in an organization when they partially disagree with its values? What degree of congruence is needed? Reading Deal and Kennedy literally suggests that philosophical divergence is to be discouraged; all values must be shared by all employees, including managers.

Some sectarian health services organizations require that managers at midlevel and above be adherents to the religion of the sponsoring group. Apparently, they judge their philosophy and mission as so unique that only coreligionists can effectively manage their organizations. Some moral philosophies are unique, but this requirement seems largely unsupportable. And, if this policy breeds conformity and diminishes innovation, it is also counterproductive.

The organization's interview and preemployment processes should explain its philosophy and determine the applicant's personal ethic about health services delivery. These surveys permit both parties to judge their philosophical congruence, which should occur whether or not the applicant is a coreligionist, because even individuals of the same faith may have divergent views. Similarly, nonsectarian organizations may not want to employ individuals whose ethic constrains them from participating in services such as electro-convulsive therapy. In such cases, this information can and should be known prospectively.

Key is that persons may reach the same conclusions about an organization's activities and its relationship to patients using a moral philosophy that is independent of the organization's religious doctrine. These managers would be effective in achieving the same goals as others in the organization because, as Deal and Kennedy stress, they share the same values, the same philosophy. The measure should be congruence between the organization's philosophy and the results of a manager's decision making, as well as other indications. Someone claiming to be morally neutral is potentially the most inimical to an organization seeking to implement a philosophy and strengthen its corporate culture.

CONCLUSION

This chapter examined the importance of a philosophy, or values, in determining an organization's vision and mission. From them are derived policies and procedures, the stuff from which the abstract and sometimes elusive aspects of an organization are operationalized. Developing a strong corporate culture is the result of shared values. Shared values are crucial in easing discontinuity and achieving corporate effectiveness. However, a school of behavioral science suggests that individuals who disagree must be willing to speak out, and it is problematic if the organization becomes an environment of "group think."

A variety of sources assists in developing an organization's philosophy. These sources include religious affiliation or orientation and humanism or humanitarian motives. Employee and patient bills of rights are also important. Whatever sources an organization uses, the principles of respect for persons, beneficence, nonmaleficence, and justice are essential.

NOTES

1. Thomas J. Peters, & Robert H. Waterman, Jr. (1982). *In search of excellence: Lessons from America's best-run companies* (p. 15). New York: Harper & Row.
2. Terrence E. Deal, & Allan A. Kennedy. (1982). *Corporate cultures: The rites and rituals of corporate life.* Reading, MA: Addison-Wesley.
3. Deal & Kennedy, p. 22.
4. Allan A. Kennedy. (1985, October). Corporate values/corporate culture. In *Excellence in management: Lessons learned from other industries.* Report from a special conference for the American College of Hospital Administrators Fellows, 5–7.
5. Terrence E. Deal, Allan A. Kennedy, & Arthur H. Spiegel, III. (1983, January/February). How to create an outstanding hospital culture. *Hospital Forum, 27,* 21–28, 33–34.
6. John P. Kotter, & James L. Heskett. (1992). *Corporate culture and performance* (p. 18). New York: The Free Press.
7. Peters & Waterman, pp. 15–16.
8. Mission, Vision, and Values Statement of Sibley Memorial Hospital, Washington, DC, 1992.
9. Philosophy of the Franciscan Health System, 1990.
10. Mission Statement of St. Mary Medical Center, Langhorne, PA, 1996.

11. Kenneth J. Williams, & Paul R. Donnelly. (1982). *Medical care quality and the public trust*. Chicago: Pluribus Press.
12. Bonnie J. Gray, & Robert K. Landrum. (1983, July–September). Difficulties with being ethical. *Business, 33*, 28–33.
13. Ed D. Roach, & Bobby G. Bizzell. (1990). Sterling County Hospital. In Jonathon S. Rakich, Beaufort B. Longest, Jr., & Kurt Darr (Eds.). *Cases in health services management* (2nd ed., p. 144). Baltimore: Health Professions Press.
14. Editorial. (1985, September). Dealing with conflicts of interest. *New England Journal of Medicine, 313*, 749–751.
15. Richard L. O'Brien, & Michael J. Haller. (1985, July). Investor-owned or nonprofit? *New England Journal of Medicine, 313*, 198–201. (As of January 1, 1996 St. Joseph Hospital was owned by Tenet Health System, a for-profit corporation. Thus, the issue for the Catholic Health Association remains the same.)
16. American Hospital Association. (1992). A patient's bill of rights. Chicago: Author.
17. George J. Annas. (1989). *The rights of patients: The basic ACLU guide to patient rights* (2nd ed., Appendix B, pp. 283–291). Carbondale and Edwardsville, IL: Southern Illinois University Press.
18. U.S. Department of Veterans Affairs. (1993). *Information booklet on patients' rights and responsibilities*. Washington, DC: U.S. Government Printing Office.
19. Joint Commission on Accreditation of Healthcare Organizations. (1996). Patient rights. In *Accreditation manual for hospitals* (Vol. 1, pp. 38–44). Oakbrook Terrace, IL: Author.
20. R. L. Ackoff. (1981). *Creating the corporate future*. New York: John Wiley & Sons.
21. James Webber. (1982, April 1). Planning. *Hospitals, 56*, 69–70.

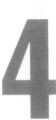

Codes of Ethics in Health Services

Many factors influence human behavior and interaction. Among the most basic factors are those arising from the individual's legal relationships with society—the increasingly pervasive laws, ordinances, regulations, and court decisions. Other formal sources of law, such as the bylaws of a corporation, apply only to it. The link between formal sources of law and ethics was described in the Introduction. In addition, there are nonformal sources of law, such as standards of justice, public policies, moral convictions, customary laws, and notions of individual equity. Both formal and nonformal sources of law are used by health services organizations. Codes of ethics adopted by professional associations are important because they state goals, guide affiliates, and serve as a reference point to discipline those who deviate from the norm.

In 1978 the U.S. Congress created the Office of Government Ethics (OGE) to review the activities of certain executive branch officials in order to determine whether they were in conflict with the officials' public duties. The law provides for financial disclosure by individuals in certain positions; restriction on activities after they leave government service; restrictions on accepting gifts from outside sources; and restrictions on outside earned income, honoraria, and outside employment. Financial interests too remote or inconsequential to affect the integrity of services are exempt. OGE's main source of information is the annual individual financial disclosure statement. Similarly, states provide ethical and legal guidance for their employees.[1]

A 1984 survey by Common Cause of 50 officials designated by federal agencies as "ethics officers" found that only a few spent more than 15% of their time on ethics-related matters. The report was generally critical of ethics enforcement and noted that the most frequently ignored regulations were those limiting contact between employees and the agencies in which they had worked.[2]

Self-regulation has been a hallmark of the learned professions, historically law, medicine, and the clergy. Their ethics are reflected in bar discipline, principles of medical ethics, and ecclesiastic law. As law, medicine, and other, newer professions sought regulation (protection) through legislation or as regulation was forced on them, many of their ethical principles were incorporated into statutes or regulations or, for attorneys, court-adopted disciplinary guidelines.

Groups seeking professional status will put in place a code of ethics. Codes are common in health services, and most managerial and technical groups employ them. Their language is usually general and performance standards are typically so vague as to make fair enforcement impossible. In the latter regard, attorneys are a notable exception. A wag would say that this is as it should be because attorneys seem plagued by ethics problems. Attorneys are officers of the court and have a positive duty to report information that raises substantial questions about another attorney's honesty, trustworthiness, or fitness. Their principles of ethics have judicial sanction, because the highest court in the state usually adopts (with few modifications) the Code of Professional Responsibility of the American Bar Association (a private association) as its rules of professional conduct. This court usually appoints a board of professional responsibility to enforce the rules and to review and investigate complaints, which are heard by a special panel of judges. Adverse action by this panel results in penalties ranging from admonition or probation to suspension or revocation of the attorney's license. The bar association is important because it develops the code of conduct that reflects the profession's ethics.

It is clear, however, that even with reasonably stringent enforcement, a code of ethics can only guide the behavior and decisions of individuals who want to do the right thing but need help determining what that is. Individuals trying to "get away with something" are always on the fringe of a profession, and principles of ethical conduct (and legal requirements) only encourage them to work to avoid being caught. Even absent a code, some actions inevitably raise questions of character, as in the following case example.

Mr. B

Mr. B sought a job as a health services consultant. He contacted two firms and was interviewed by both. One offered him a position. Mr. B verbally accepted the offer, even though it meant moving his family. Several days later, as a courtesy, he called the second firm to tell them he had taken a position. The managing partner said, "Gee, that's really too bad. I was going to offer you a job in your area and pay you $5,000 more than you got from the other firm."

Mr. B faces an ethical problem. No written agreement exists, yet he verbally accepted the first offer—he gave his word. Were Mr. B to call the first firm and explain what happened, they would likely release him. After all, who wants a disgruntled employee? This action does not affect his ethical obligation to take the job he accepted, however. Having made the commitment, Mr. B is morally bound to meet it.

CODES FOR MANAGERS

In addition to what is considered minimally acceptable, codes also state the goals of the profession. These goals may not be achievable. The profession must work toward them, however, because considerable progress is often possible. These aspects of codes of ethics are similar to the philosophy and vision statements developed by the organization.

Research involving business students suggests that ethics can be taught and learned, but that over time (4 years, in one study) lack of reinforcement causes graduates to be no better prepared than before they took an ethics course.[3] The implication for health services managers is that continuing education in ethics is essential.

Code for Health Services Managers

The most prominent health services management group is the American College of Healthcare Executives (ACHE), known prior to mid-1985 as the American College of Hospital Administrators (ACHA). In 1996 ACHE had over 30,000 affiliates. The ACHE (ACHA) has had their Code of Ethics since 1939, 6 years after its founding. Initially, it was linked to the code of ethics for hospitals developed by the American Hospital Association (AHA). Ensuing iterations made the ACHE's code distinct, and it has also become more explicit than the AHA's code.

The ACHE code underwent a major revision in 1987. Significant changes included recognizing health services managers as moral agents who must consider the ethical implications of their decisions and who are charged with a positive duty to report circumstances under which affiliates have violated the code. The latter provision is vital to build esprit de corps among ACHE affiliates and make the code a living document that is clearly applicable to management practice. Increased emphasis is placed on conflicts of interest, and resource allocation and the manager's responsibility for ethical behavior in advertising are specifically mentioned. Beyond these items, the code sets out an affiliate's responsibilities to the profession, patients or others served, the organization, and employees. The 1995 Code of Ethics is reproduced in Appendix B.

Historically, the code paid no attention to biomedical ethical issues. Except for a statement on autonomy and self-determination, this deficit continued in the 1995 version. Little attention was paid to an independent duty owed by managers to patients. The ACHE code has not attempted to define the limits of loyalty (fidelity) to the organization and the point at which that loyalty is superseded by a duty to the patient. This facet is vital to the manager's role as a moral agent.

Disciplinary actions against affiliates under the code are highly structured and emphasize due process. The committee on ethics receives complaints about unethical conduct. The respondent (the affiliate) is informed of the allegations and the committee refers the matter to the regent best able to investigate the alleged infraction. The regent investigates and reports to the committee, making a recommendation. The committee then reviews the report and makes a recommendation to the board of governors. If the respondent appeals, the chairman of the board of governors appoints an ad hoc committee of three fellows to hear the matter and send a report, with recommendations, to the board of governors. The respondent may appear before the ad hoc committee. After that hearing the committee reports to the board of governors, making recommendations. The board of governors makes the final decision.

This lengthy grievance procedure meets a criterion of fairness. It is consistent with the trend to apply legal requirements of procedural and substantive due process to private associations. Respondents can seek judicial review of these decisions, but courts are reluctant to intervene in the actions of private associations.

Expulsion is the maximum disciplinary action allowed by ACHE. Because affiliation is not linked to licensure, expulsion is significant only if colleagues and potential employers consider it important. If they do, the former affiliate's employment and career opportunities are limited. Future employers will be interested as to the reason for the discipline. A policy question the ACHE must address is what use should be made of such information when affiliation in a professional association is voluntary?

When questioned about the pre-1987 code of ethics, ACHE affiliates indicated that it was important to them. They thought the code should be more comprehensive and more specific in guiding decisions on ethical problems. Also, increased emphasis on enforcement and reporting disposition of cases to affiliates, without naming the individual involved, was thought to be necessary. Affiliates also wanted to learn more about ethical problems.[4] A living code has great utility to affiliates as they confront ethical issues and work to solve them.

Code for Nursing Home Administrators

The American College of Health Care Administrators (ACHCA) has adopted a code of ethics for affiliates who are primarily managers of long-term care facilities. The 1994 code is reproduced in Appendix B.

Affiliates are obliged to meet four "expectations," which are divided into prescriptions and proscriptions. These expectations state that affiliates shall 1) hold paramount the welfare of persons for whom care is provided; 2) maintain high standards of professional competence; 3) strive, in all matters relating to their professional functions, to maintain a professional posture that places paramount the interests of the facility and its residents; and 4) honor their responsibilities to the public, their profession, and relationships with colleagues and members of related professions. Examples of the issues receiving specific attention include quality of services; confidentiality of patient information; continuing education; conflicts of interest; promulgation of knowledge, support of research, and sharing of expertise; and provision of information to the standards and ethics committee of actual or potential code violations. The latter requirement suggests a disciplinary dimension, but no enforcement or appeals processes are included. The preamble to the code states that the ultimate responsibility for applying standards and ethics falls to the individual. The ACHCA code pays even less attention to biomedical ethical issues than does the ACHE code—an important lapse for both groups.

CODES FOR CAREGIVERS

Codes for Physicians

Ethics in medicine date from the 18th century B.C. and the Code of Hammurabi, which established a payment schedule for treatments by physicians and veterinarians. Harsh punishments were prescribed if a patient was harmed: A physician could lose his hands if the patient's eye or life was lost as a result of treatment.

A quite-different code developed from the teaching and work of Hippocrates (circa 460–370 B.C.). The Code of Hammurabi was imposed by a ruler, but the Hippocratic philosophy governing relationships among physicians and between physicians and patients was developed by Greek physicians, one of whom could have been Hippocrates, for their own use. The Hippocratic oath has never received public sanction or force of law. It established standards of conduct, some of which are found in state licensing and regulation of physicians.

The Hippocratic oath contains a long, largely obsolete, section describing expected relationships between physicians and their teachers and students. Other provisions no longer universally applied include restrictions on performing surgery, assisting in abortion, and applying dietetic measures in healing. Prohibitions on assisting in suicide and refraining from sexual misconduct with patients and others in the household, and broad restrictions on confidentiality of information learned during medical treatment are found in current medical codes, specifically or by implication.

The American Medical Association (AMA) was founded in 1847. Its first code of medical ethics was based on the work of Thomas Percival, the English physician, philosopher, and writer. The AMA's code has been revised several times. The most recent (as of this writing) edition of the Principles of Medical Ethics was adopted in 1980 and is reproduced in Appendix B. The previous, more proscriptive edition was adopted in 1957, which prohibited advertising and proscribed voluntary association with practitioners who have no scientific basis for treatment. In addition, the code contained a strong element of paternalism—physicians were expected to act in ways that they considered to be in the patient's best interests.

The most significant change in 1980 was philosophical and affects the relationship between physician and patient. The paternalism of the 1957 edition is gone, and although the 1980 principles do not expect a covenant or contract between patient and physician, the profession seems to be moving in that direction. Veatch[5] observed, "It is the first document in the history of professional medical ethics in which a group of physicians is willing to use the language of responsibilities and rights," rather than that of benefits and harms.

AMA members have a positive duty to "strive to expose those physicians deficient in character or competence, or who engage in fraud or deception."[6] The philosophical tone set by the directiveness and specificity of this statement is unique among codes for caregivers. Critics argue that this duty has been widely ignored. The AMA's Council on Ethical and Judicial Affairs assists members in interpreting the principles by publishing opinions on issues such as experimentation, genetic engineering, abortion, and terminal illness. These opinions usefully supplement the principles. The council's 1990 statement, "Fundamental Elements of the Patient–Physician Relationship," complements the AMA principles by focusing on the rights of patients. It is reproduced in Appendix B.

Code for Nurses

The Code for Nurses promulgated by the American Nurses' Association (ANA) was first adopted in 1950. The 1985 version is the most current as of this writing and is reproduced in Appendix B. The preamble states that clients are primary decision makers in matters of their own health, treatment, and well-being, and that "the goal of nursing actions is to support the client's responsibility and self-determination to the greatest extent possible."[7] This philosophy contains no hint of paternalism.

The preamble includes a list of principles similar to those discussed in Chapter 2 that should govern interactions with clients. The introduction to the code states that the code "serves to inform both the nurse and society of the profession's expectations and requirements in ethical matters."[8] Many of the code's 11 provisions are specific. An interpretive statement follows each. One provision is similar to the AMA's requirement to counter or expose certain practice: "the nurse acts to safeguard the client and the public when health care and safety are affected by the incompetent, unethical, or illegal practice of any person."[9]

CODES FOR INSTITUTIONS

Hospitals

The American Hospital Association (AHA) is the most important trade association for hospitals. It adopted revised guidelines for ethical conduct in 1992. These guidelines are divided into community role, patient care, and organizational conduct. Members are expected to improve community health status and deliver high-quality, comprehensive services efficiently. The importance of coordinating with other health services organizations is emphasized. Some provisions are specific: the need for informed consent; confidentiality; and mechanisms to resolve conflicting values and ethical dilemmas among patients and families, medical staff, employees, the organization, and the community. Members should try to accommodate the religious and social beliefs and customs of patients whenever possible. The guidelines identify the expectations regarding employee policies and practices and the accommodation of religious and moral values held by employees and medical staff. Conflicts of interest are defined. No disciplinary or grievance procedures are included.

Nursing Facilities

The American Health Care Association (AHCA) is the national association that serves long-term care facilities, primarily nursing facilities. It has not promulgated a code of ethics. Members are expected to abide by a recommended patient bill of rights, which specifies the need to balance rights and enumerates them for patients in nursing facilities. These rights stress fair treatment, information, communication, choice, and privacy and minimize the dehumanizing aspects of institutional care. Some states require nursing facilities receiving Medicaid funds to follow a patient bill of rights that is based on that of the AHCA.

The American Association of Homes and Services for the Aging (AAHSA) is the national association that represents not-for-profit or government-sponsored organizations that provide housing, health, community, and related services to meet the needs of older adults. AAHSA's ethics are reflected in the "Membership Credo," which was adopted in 1991. Its credo identifies a set of values and a set of beliefs. The values include accountability, benevolence, compassion, competency, integrity, renewal, social responsibility, and stewardship. The beliefs focus on the relationships AAHSA members establish with the people they serve, governing boards, staff, volunteers, communities, government, and other organizations. Each value and belief is followed by short descriptive statements. The credo includes no reporting or disciplinary process.

PHILOSOPHICAL BASES FOR CODES OF ETHICS

Codes of ethics for the health professions blend various moral philosophies and ethical theories. To varying extents, the principles of respect for individuals, beneficence, nonmaleficence, and justice are found in all codes.

The ACHE and ACHCA codes blend consequentialism (teleology) deontology, and virtue ethics, but emphasize the latter two. Respect for persons and beneficence predominate. The section on conflict of interest in the ACHE code, for example, assumes a "right action." Except for the clause that "a conflict of interest may be only a matter of degree," the action, not its results (consequences), determine moral rightness or wrongness. Similarly, the statements on confidential information are based in deontology and virtue ethics, not in consequences. As noted, the duty to report violations was added to the ACHE code in 1987: "An affiliate of the College who has reasonable grounds to believe another affiliate has violated this Code has a duty to communicate such facts to the Committee on Ethics." [10] The 1989 ACHCA code contains a similar provision.

The preamble of the 1980 AMA principles provides the context of its amended view of physician duty and respect for patients: "A physician must recognize responsibility not only to patients, but also to society, to other health professionals, and to self." [11] This philosophy is absent in the Hippocratic oath and the 1957 AMA principles, which emphasized paternalism with no suggestion of balancing the patient's interests against society's. This change carries important implications for resource allocation by suggesting that physicians must consider the societal effects of individual treatment costs. This admonition is based on the principle of justice rather than on beneficence, which focuses on patients and adds a dimension of utilitarianism—to consider the greatest good for the greatest number.

The ANA Code for Nurses is grounded in deontology. Within this philosophical context, respect for individuals and beneficence undergird the relationship with clients.

APPLICATIONS OF CODES OF ETHICS

Enforcement

Codes of ethics assume greater meaning when they are enforced. Unenforced, they are platitudes intended for public consumption, with marginal usefulness to the profession. Enforceable codes are precise and include interpretations of their provisions. Absent sufficient detail to guide affiliates, enforcement results in arbitrary decision making and denial of due process. As noted, private associations are not usually held to constitutional requirements of due process, but it is nonetheless fair (just) that they meet such a standard. This theme should underlie the association's relationships with affiliates. Enforcement with feedback to affiliates provides additional knowledge and understanding for the profession and makes the code a living document. This crucial attribute uses casuistry in building a body of cases and experience.

Codes are typically enforced through a grievance procedure. The ACHE code emphasizes due process and is eminently fair to the grievant. Appeals are heard privately; no information is communicated to affiliates not directly involved. Even when the unethical behavior is the subject of a criminal proceeding and conviction, the ACHE does not identify the affiliate.

When health services professionals are licensed, disciplinary actions are usually a matter of public record. Reports of disciplinary actions against physicians and other caregivers appear occasionally in the press. Among health services managers, only nursing home administrators are licensed—the result of historical problems in nursing facilities. Scandals elsewhere in the field of health services could lead to demands for licensure of other managers, which is much less desirable than self-regulation. This scenario reinforces the importance of voluntary efforts and the need to enforce usable, living (interpreted) codes of ethics.

It is important that professions provide feedback about their codes to affiliates. This information includes interpretation, application, and enforcement. General education that apprises affiliates of code provisions and changes is also needed. Efforts to make health services administrative or institutional codes living documents that are useful in guiding decisions have been inadequate, however. Health services administrators, especially those less experienced, want to learn about their association's code of ethics.[12] Encouraging and responding to this interest remain important, unmet challenges to the profession.

Separation of Private and Public Actions

Managers of health services organizations are public figures and the public's interest in them and their organizations is reflected by their prominence in the community. A manager's public role is greater in small communities, in which the organization, especially an acute care hospital, is economically, politically, and socially significant. This means health services managers are community leaders ex officio. They are in a fishbowl whether or not they desire it. Managers of major health services organizations in urban areas are also community leaders. Health services managers must be prepared to accept this trust and use the public's confidence to improve the community's health. However, such a role demands exceptional performance in all respects.

Community leaders are entitled to some claim of privacy, but greater prominence invariably diminishes privacy. Younger, less experienced managers have difficulty understanding that such persons are unable to escape public scrutiny. They want to guard their privacy jealously, and most younger managers consider what happens in their personal lives irrelevant to managerial performance. Would that this were so, but their role in the organization and the public's expectations do not permit them this luxury.

Three elements affect the dynamic between public and private lives: 1) the corrupt moral standard that the right or wrong of an action is unimportant, the question is whether one is caught; 2) the organization's culture and the community standard of behavior and morality; and 3) administrative effectiveness. "It's okay if you don't get caught" or "It's okay, everybody's doing it" are unacceptable bromides for health services managers. The following simple examples highlight the effect of such views. Most individuals would be embarrassed to be seen photocopying personal papers at their place of employment, or to have their superiors note personal long-distance phone calls made at the organization's expense. Wasted time, personal use of office equipment, and personal phone calls will not result in disciplinary action by a professional association, nor in most cases by the organization. Such actions must be regulated by the individual's personal ethic. Members of the profession must consider that small infractions are governed by the principles developed in Chapter 1, as well as by their personal ethic.

The organization's philosophy and the community standard of morality are important because they affect managers' views of what is acceptable, thus tempering the manager's personal ethic. The microcommunity that is the organization develops a corporate culture whose mores and standards are unique, demanding, and ignored at one's peril.

It Just Isn't Done!

Several university faculty were invited to have lunch with 20 middle- and senior-level managers of a data processing firm. The group was enthusiastic and highly motivated, and most members were younger than age 40. Lunch was a break in a long day of seminars and meetings. When the waiter asked for drink orders, no one from the firm ordered an alcoholic beverage. Instead, they ordered milk or soda. One of the faculty remarked about this unusual behavior and was told there was an unwritten company policy that no member of the staff should have a drink and go back to work.

Regardless whether this policy seems straitlaced, it is different from the "two-martini lunch" once considered the norm in business. Yet this "rule" reflected the group's self-view (culture), and substantial peer pressure would likely be directed at anyone who behaved differently. On both a macro- and a microlevel, this is the type of peer pressure health services managers exercise for the good of patient and profession.

Administrative effectiveness is a question for the manager's supervisor, who determines whether problems have fatally flawed the ability to lead. Managers with badly tarnished reputations lose their effectiveness. The manager who is ridiculed, whose character deficit is blatant and widely known, or for whom respect is eroded or gone must be dismissed.

It may seem unfair that managers are held to a higher standard than the larger community. Employees and the public expect more of leaders than of followers. The health services management profession correctly expects its members to avoid the temptations and problems affecting those outside it.

An example of private behavior considered unacceptable in a health services manager is driving while intoxicated (DWI). Regardless of the view held by professional associations, governing bodies are intolerant of managers charged with DWI, even though such behavior for a housekeeper would go unnoticed. Problems such as DWI run counter to the organization's view of the manager qua leader and its philosophy, which will be unwritten for problems such as alcohol and drug abuse, illicit sexual activity, and spouse abuse. Illegal activities are unethical per se. They are not explicitly prohibited because they are so obviously unacceptable.

A further reason such behavior is unacceptable is that the governing body has no wish to be embarrassed by an errant manager. An organization faced with scandal will separate itself from the source. This reaction reflects the instinct for organizational survival as well as indignation and moral revulsion.

Instilling an awareness of the importance of ethical behavior in others is a challenge.

Is This a Laughing Matter?

One afternoon, Joan Zimmerman, the chief operating officer of a large hospital, encountered two younger members of her management staff conversing in hushed tones. As she approached unnoticed, they burst into laughter. One of the two blushed and turned his eyes downward as Zimmerman greeted them and asked lightheartedly about the source of their amusement. Neither spoke. Sensing there was something she should know, Zimmerman pressed for an answer. The awkward situation was interrupted by Zimmerman's pager, which asked her to call the operator immediately. Later, one of the two managers asked to see Zimmerman. He related an amazing story about the female director of a support department with a high turnover rate. In routine exit interviews conducted by human resources several young male employees said they were leaving because they could no longer endure the sexual harassment by the department's director, who insisted that the young men have sex with her. Employees who refused were given the worst schedules and treated badly in other ways.

Zimmerman was told that the problem had existed for some time and was an open secret in the hospital. She was shocked and distressed that she had not been told.

This case has several dimensions. First, sexual harassment is against the law. Second, sexual harassment breaches the principle of respect for persons. Third, the unfair treatment of staff by the department head breaches the principle of justice.

The immediate problem is to investigate the allegations against the department director and take disciplinary action, if appropriate. Also of concern is that younger managers were amused, not outraged. Their reaction may show immaturity rather than approval; regardless, it is a problem that needs to be solved. Managers lead by actions and words; actions are more important.

Two other issues need attention. The first is that Zimmerman was unaware of the problem. The second issue is the lack of action taken by individuals who knew of the allegations, which, if true, cast a shadow over all managers and the organization. Zimmerman must make clear to all employees that such behavior is intolerable. It breaches the trust that is reposed in managers, breaches their fiduciary duty to the staff and the organization, and is inconsistent with any organizational philosophy worthy of the name.

CONCLUSION

Most codes of ethics provide only general guidelines. Even specific provisions require interpretation and the courage to apply them. Interpretation is crucial, because even great detail cannot address the nuances and intricacies of various situations. A detailed code would be excessively legalistic; applying it would be nightmarish.

Of the professional groups in health services management, the ACHE has developed the most detailed code. This detail makes it useful as a guide to health services managers, whether or not they are ACHE affiliates. The code is, nonetheless, too general to provide standards for performance.

The AMA's Principles of Medical Ethics are useful because its Council on Ethical and Judicial Affairs interprets the principles and their application. Comparing the ACHE and AMA codes shows that the ACHE code has become more explicit and the AMA principles less so as they have evolved.

Codes in the health services field carry only the sanctions available to the professional association, of which expulsion is the maximum disciplinary action. This limitation is unlikely to affect the individual's legal right to engage in the profession.

In addition to the expectations of ethical codes, most clinical groups are regulated by state law. Licensure statutes, or practice acts as they are often called, incorporate ethical principles similar to those of the professional group, and licensing boards are usually composed of individuals from the profession being regulated. This composition gives the group's ethical precepts the force of law; breaching these precepts could lead to license suspension or revocation. It is noteworthy that the proceedings of public regulators are distinct from those of private associations or professional groups. A license is a condition of membership in the professional association, but membership in the association is not required for licensure, an appropriate distinction between private and public action.

For groups such as hospital managers, the lack of licensure increases the significance of self-regulation. The public looks to the profession as a primary force in safeguarding the health services system. Unless self-regulation is effective and maintains the public's confidence, licensing or another form of governmental regulation will result.

Another pragmatic consideration is what contributes to managers' success. A survey of leading hospital chief executive officers showed integrity to be the personality trait rated as most important for success. Integrity was considered to be more important than any skill or other trait or factor.[13] This additional stimulus to be ethical in all aspects of their lives should cause health services managers to be more vigilant about themselves and their colleagues. These are significant reasons for maintaining the public's trust in health services managers and their organizations.

More important than pragmatism to encourage ethical behavior is that it is the right thing to do—it is a principle for life and the profession. The slightest hint of impropriety in personal behavior must be avoided. What a tragedy for the late Hyman G. Rickover, father of the nuclear submarine fleet and a retired U.S. Navy admiral, with an astounding 64 years on active duty, to be forced to admit that he took gifts from defense contractors. Rickover claimed that the gifts were trinkets and that taking them did not affect his judgment. The Secretary of the Navy insisted that the gifts were worth tens of thousands of dollars. Whatever the facts, these revelations badly, and sadly, tarnished a distinguished career. It is just such situations that health services managers must assiduously avoid. Failing this, managers damage the public trust, risk their careers and reputations, and violate the principles of any personal ethic worthy of the name.

NOTES

1. Anita Cava, Jonathan West, & Evan Berman. (1995, Spring). Ethical decision-making in business and government: An analysis of formal and informal strategies. *Spectrum, 68*(2), 34–35.
2. Pete Earley. (1984, November 30). Ethics laws found to be laxly enforced. *The Washington Post*, p. A17.
3. Peter Arlow, & Thomas A. Ulrich. (1983, Spring). Can ethics be taught to business students? *Collegiate Forum*, p. 17.
4. Kurt Darr. (1984, March/April). Administrative ethics and the health services manager. *Hospital & Health Services Administration, 29*, 120–136.
5. Robert M. Veatch. (1980, June). Professional ethics: New principles for physicians? *Hastings Center Report, 10*, 17.
6. American Medical Association. (1980). *Principles of medical ethics*. Chicago: Author.
7. American Nurses Association. (1985). *Code for nurses with interpretive statements* (p. i). Kansas City, MO: Author.
8. *Ibid.*, p. iii.
9. American Medical Association. *Principles of medical ethics*.
10. American College of Healthcare Executives. (1995). *Code of ethics*. Chicago: Author.
11. American Medical Association. *Principles of medical ethics*.
12. Darr, pp. 133–134.
13. Walter J. Wentz, & Terence F. Moore. (1981). Administrative success: Key ingredients. *Hospital & Health Services Administration, Spec. 2*, 85–93.

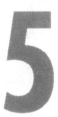

Organizational
Responses to Ethical Problems

Thus far, little has been said about how organizations can be organized to solve administrative and biomedical ethical problems. The starting point in such efforts is the organization's philosophy, which reflects its values and establishes moral direction and a framework for the vision and mission statements. The organization's philosophy is subject to external constraints such as criminal and civil laws and derivative regulations, which set a minimum standard. For example, federal guidelines to protect human subjects are a starting point for the organization's relationship with patients participating in federally funded research.

The personal ethic of the manager, as an employee and a leader, influences the organizational philosophy and is influenced by it. In addition, the manager organizes the organization in order to solve ethical problems. Such problem solving is executed in the context of the organizational philosophy but is affected by the manager's personal ethic, which may be more specific and comprehensive than the organizational philosophy. This dynamic reinforces the importance of the personal ethic.

Since the 1970s health services organizations have established various groups to solve ethical problems; most prominent are institutional ethics committees (IECs) and institutional review boards (IRBs). IECs can provide a broad range of assistance on administrative and biomedical ethical issues. IRBs are specialized IECs that focus on research ethics. They are of more help in preventing and solving problems in biomedical ethics than in administrative ethics.

INSTITUTIONAL ETHICS COMMITTEES

The progenitors to IECs were abortion selection committees, which determined, prior to *Roe v. Wade*, whether a pregnant woman's health or life was at sufficient risk to justify an abortion, and medical morals committees in Catholic hospitals, which assessed certain treatment decisions in light of Church teachings.[1] Later, in the 1960s, committees selected recipients of renal dialysis at a time when there were many more medically suitable patients than machines.

The 1976 court decision regarding Karen Ann Quinlan directed establishment of an "ethics" committee that was to review her prognosis. Such committees confirmed prognoses and helped determine whether to continue life support. In some organizations prognosis committees were called "God squads" because they determined when treatment should be withdrawn and the patient declared dead.

The role of IECs in the 1990s is much broader. An early source of information about them was a national survey completed for the President's Commission for the Study of Ethical Problems in Medicine and Biomedical and Behavioral Research, published in 1983.[2] No hospital with fewer than 200 beds had an IEC. IECs were not ubiquitous in large hospitals, but those with teaching programs most likely had one. The study estimated that there were fewer than 100 IECs in U.S. hospitals. The Quinlan decision encouraged hospitals to establish IECs; in New Jersey, where IECs were most common, 71% were formed because of that case.

Surveys completed in 1983 and 1985 by the National Society of Patient Representatives showed rapid growth of IECs. Of the hospitals responding to the 1983 survey, 26% had IECs; this figure rose to 59% in 1985. The methodology used in the surveys caused disproportionate numbers of large hospitals to respond, thus somewhat skewing the findings. The Babies Doe controversies in the early 1980s caused many hospitals to establish specialized IECs in order to solve the ethical problems of treating profoundly disabled newborns.

The findings of the National Society of Patient Representatives on rapid growth of IECs were consistent with research done by the American Academy of Pediatrics (AAP) reported later in the chapter. The growth in numbers of new IECs slowed in the late 1980s, however.[3] This lack of growth is confirmed by 1993 estimates that nationally about 60% of hospitals have IECs; state and regional ethics networks suggest that 65%–85% is possible.[4] A 1993 survey by the Catholic Health Association found that 92% of its members who responded have an IEC.[5] A Hastings Center report suggests that ethics committees in hospitals have matured and must reconsider their roles to determine whether they should be involved in new ways and in other aspects of organizations.[6] It has been found that IECs are more likely to be involved in issues of appropriateness of technology, a renewed interest in patients' rights, the evolution in relationships among health care providers, and the conflict of social values than they are in case consultation, which seems to have declined.[7]

Delivery of nonacute health services is rapidly moving from hospitals to other types of organizations. The growth in need and use of IECs will be greatest in sites that include nursing facilities, health maintenance organizations (HMOs), and integrated delivery networks. A survey by the American Association of Homes and Services for the Aging found that the numbers of ethics committees among its members had increased from 29% in 1990 to 45% in 1995, and that many others were in the planning stage. The committees review cases and consult, make and review policy recommendations, and educate and advise staff and administration. Of those with committees, 86% found them useful.[8]

IECs in nonacute care organizations are likely to develop along very different lines, consistent with their unique activities and roles. It has been suggested that unlike physicians on IECs in hospitals, physicians on IECs in nursing facilities play a minor role and that administrative staff are much more important. Staff education levels in nursing facilities are lower, which exacerbates cultural and class differences between staff and patients. In addition, because nursing facilities are heavily regulated, it is also likely that considerable focus will fall on legal rather than on ethical issues.[9]

Organization

In this section the author recommends that complex health services organizations, especially acute care hospitals, put in place an ethics committee with at least two subcommittees, each of which addresses different groups of ethical issues. An alternative is to have two ethics committees, one for administrative ethical issues and one for biomedical ethical issues. Specialization is necessary because a committee prepared to address biomedical ethics problems may be inadequately prepared to address administrative ethics problems. Greater specialization may be needed within the broad categories of administrative and biomedical ethics (e.g., an infant care review committee). Committee proliferation or overlap must be avoided, but the various types of ethical problems must be addressed effectively. Because of the need to solve general, organizationwide problems and specific, sometimes very technical, problems, the committee with subcommittees model should be considered.

Veatch[10] has suggested the following models for organizing ethics committees:

1. An *autonomy model*—implements decisions of competent patients whose wishes are known
2. A *social justice model*—grapples with broad issues such as organizational health care policy, resource allocation, and cost effectiveness
3. A *patient benefit model*—makes decisions for patients who are unable to make decisions for themselves

Veatch argues that in many respects, these roles are mutually exclusive because different ethical tasks emphasize different ethical principles. Ethics committees that use an autonomy model are accountable to the patient, whereas ethics committees that use a social justice model must be accountable to the organization (or the community). The first and third Veatch models emphasize biomedical ethical issues. The second model could address administrative as well as biomedical issues, if it were determined desirable to address the two issues in one committee.

Purpose and Role

Since their early, focused beginnings IECs have broadened their activities considerably. Administrative and biomedical IECs undertake generic activities such as policy development, education, case review, and guidance for individuals upon request. Specific activities for administrative IECs could include developing consent procedures, considering the ethics of macroresource allocation, and whistleblowing. Specific activities for biomedical IECs could include developing do-not-resuscitate (DNR) and patient consent policies and advising on withholding or withdrawing life support.

IECs play two roles of general importance. One role is to assist in developing or reconsidering the organizational philosophy and the derivative vision and mission statements. The experience and range of its interdisciplinary membership are likely to produce better reasoned and more thorough results. Education is the second role. The IEC's composition and its members' experience make it a reservoir of knowledge and expertise. These resources should be made available to governing body and staff. Such attributes add a level of sophistication to the organization and improve the quality of clinical and administrative decision making.

Before considering ethical problems the IEC must develop a statement of its ethic, the overall framework for which is the organizational philosophy. The IEC's ethic is not a determination of how to solve each type of problem, but is a statement of general principles that guide deliberations and determine its recommendations. This exercise is essential to the effectiveness of the IEC because it identifies and minimizes differences in members' personal ethics. Only by understanding and enunciating its own ethic can the IEC (for example) appreciate how its values differ from those of a patient, an understanding that is essential if the patient's autonomy is to be respected.

In terms of biomedical ethics, the principal benefits of IECs reported in the President's Commission study include facilitating decision making by clarifying important issues, shaping consistent policies about life support, and providing opportunities for professionals to air disagreements. IECs were found to be ineffective at increasing the ability of patients' families to influence decisions or at educating professionals about issues relevant to life support decisions. The commission found that in the early 1980s IECs focused on solving biomedical ethical problems.

The commission report[11] also made two general observations:

1. Committees that do exist are not involved in large numbers of cases. Existing committees reviewed an average of only one case per year. (This finding remains true in the 1990s.)

2. The composition and function of committees identified in the survey would not allay many of the concerns of patients' rights advocates about patient representation and control. Committees were clearly dominated by physicians and other health professionals. The majority of committees did not allow patients to attend or request meetings, although family members were more often permitted to do so. Yet, chairmen generally regarded their committees as effective.

The latter finding suggests that health services managers should be particularly alert to patient autonomy, a matter affecting several aspects of the organization, especially resource allocation and consent. The evidence that the findings of the President's Commission continue to be true is ample. Important for organizations with culturally diverse clientele, whether patients and families or providers, is that IEC members be sensitized to the views various cultures hold about medical services, but especially about significant events such as death and the process of dying.

Membership

The President's Commission study showed that biomedical IECs were interdisciplinary. Physicians were the most common member of a biomedical IEC, averaging 5.25 members per committee. On average, each committee had at least one representative from the clergy. Other members found on fewer than half of the committees were attorneys, laypersons, social workers, and physicians in graduate education programs (residents). Administrators are included far less often than physicians and served on only about half of the committees. The commission did not find a strong community link, something that governing body members and individuals from the organization's service area could provide. These individuals bring an important perspective to decision making.[12] That managers were underrepresented may reflect limited interest in clinical matters—a problem managers must remedy. It was suggested in the early 1990s that nurses are also underrepresented, in terms of both their number in health services organizations and the number of biomedical ethical problems they encounter.[13]

An administrative IEC will comprise fewer clinical personnel and greater governing body and management personnel. Clinical staff must be included because it is reasonable to conclude that research suggesting that organizations are most effective when they involve clinicians in management decision making also applies to solving administrative ethics problems.

Relationships

The IEC's relationships vary depending on its activity (role). The levels of activity are general and specific. General levels span the organization and can be divided into administrative and biomedical ethics. General levels include

Table 1. Matrix of possible roles for institutional ethics committees

Involvement of committee in decision making	Acceptance and use of advice provided by IEC
Optional	Optional
Optional	Mandatory
Mandatory	Optional
Mandatory	Mandatory

refining the organizational philosophy, developing a conflict of interest policy, or guiding macroallocation decisions. Specific levels are individual cases. An example of a specific level is whether a particular activity is consistent with the organizational philosophy.

The IEC should be proactive in developing and revising the organizational philosophy and in considering the ethical implications of macroresource allocation questions. Similarly, the IEC should take the initiative in reviewing and revising the consent process. However, the committee may choose a more passive role and wait to be consulted in specific instances of conflicts of interest and misuse of confidential information (in the case of an administrative IEC) or in specific clinical matters (in the case of a biomedical IEC).

The President's Commission study suggested that IECs involved in solving biomedical ethics problems are most effective when they wait to be consulted rather than when they interpose themselves. Playing a consultative role means that committees make recommendations, not final decisions.[14] IEC participation in biomedical and administrative decision making may be optional or mandatory. Whether the advice given by an IEC need be followed may be optional or mandatory, as well. Table 1 shows the combinations.

Physicians are unlikely to accept mandatory–mandatory involvement by a biomedical IEC. Furthermore, this type of involvement may not be desirable for most situations, in which the physician is willing to develop alternatives and communicate them to the patient and others concerned. Even if the physician is unwilling to share decision making with an ethics committee, there are benefits to making its analysis and recommendation available.

An important aspect of organizing an IEC is the question of where it should be located administratively. Options include making the IEC a standing committee of the board, the medical staff, or the administration. The fear that the IEC will be dominated by physicians causes some experts to suggest that it be a board or administration committee. Similarly, no committee member should represent only one specific interest or group.[15]

The Administrative Institutional Ethics Committee

The chief executive officer (CEO) of Community Health Plan had been approached by a group from "north of the river." This area of the city was economically depressed and over the previous decade had lost many of its health services delivery organizations and physicians to the suburbs. It seemed to be in a downward spiral, with no end in sight. Decreasing numbers of insured patients meant that organizations were increasingly less able to continue serving the area. The city-owned hospital had made several ill-fated attempts to serve the area "north of the river" with a clinic system, but its efforts had been ridden with scandal. The clinic system was a political football with little credibility in the community.

The representatives from "north of the river" were community leaders, none of whom appeared to have political ambitions. They seemed genuinely willing to do whatever they could to assist in securing high-quality health services for their community. They proposed that Community Health Plan establish and staff three storefront clinics in the area. The community leaders stated that they would find volunteers to remodel the facilities and work in clerical jobs.

The CEO presented the proposed activity to the administrative IEC, which included members of the governing board, managers, and physicians and other caregivers. In making the presentation, the CEO stressed the health plan's historical role in providing services to those in need, its not-for-profit status, and its continuing modest surplus. The members listened patiently, but the minute the CEO was finished, all of them seemed to speak at once. Several members were opposed to the proposal and made the following points about the suggested venture:

1. The area "north of the river" was the city's responsibility. Providing care to the needy was not something a small not-for-profit health plan should attempt.
2. The organization's primary obligation was to enhance benefits for its enrollees and not to become involved in new schemes. New services had been requested by several of their physicians and many plan members.
3. The modest surplus the plan had accumulated over several years could be easily consumed by the proposed venture. The chief financial officer noted that they were expecting an increase in reinsurance premiums in the next quarter.
4. If the plan pulled the city's political chestnuts out of the fire by providing even stopgap assistance, the city would never get its house in order and develop the system needed "north of the river."

Several members spoke in favor of working "north of the river" and made the following points:

1. Helping the "north of the river" community was the right thing to do. The people living there deserved health care services. It was noted that the plan's own start had come about when several physicians in the community had fought the prevailing attitude among their peers about the prepaid practice of medicine.
2. The opposing members were putting dollars ahead of people's health. They must be willing to assist less fortunate people.
3. Plan members would support such an initiative if it were properly explained to them.
4. The positive publicity could further the plan's interests by increasing the number of enrollees.

It seemed to the CEO that this was a no-win situation. The organizational philosophy was not well developed and the proposal was a major step. Should something be done to assist the "north of the river" community? The IEC members had raised valid points that merited further discussion.

This case describes issues arising from decisions about the macroallocation of resources. The problems are even more complex because Community Health Plan is being asked to volunteer assistance and to do so from its own meager surplus. Relevant theories of justice in allocating resources include retribution or compensatory justice (distributing resources so as to make up for past wrongs); just desserts (help would go to those who have not earned it and Community Health Plan's leadership has no right to risk the plan's solvency, which is something the membership paid to achieve); egalitarianism in access to health services and whether it is government's responsibility to provide it to the community "north of the river;" and utility as a prospectively determined element of beneficence.

A significant problem for Community Health Plan is that it did not consider this aspect of its relationship with unique subsets of the community in formulating its organizational philosophy and vision and mission statements. It would do well to develop these prospectively in a comprehensive fashion, rather than address them ad hoc. Resource allocation receives further attention in Chapter 13.

Summary

IECs are useful in many ways. Overall, their effect is likely to be improved clinical and administrative decision making. However, one should not assume that the mere presence of an IEC means that it is successful. As with all undertakings, IECs should be evaluated so that performance can be improved.[16]

IECs present significant potential problems. Organizational concerns, especially legal ramifications and the avoidance of public embarrassment, can easily overwhelm concerns about patient goals.[17] At the extreme, it is suggested that because IECs represent organizations they cannot be objective; thus, when a dispute arises they will take management's side to avoid risk and thus they will fail in their role as patient advocates.[18] Management must ensure that IECs are not subverted in this manner.

INSTITUTIONAL REVIEW BOARDS

Health services managers may think research and experimentation are exclusive to academic medical centers, in which rigorous protection and standards of review are applied. However, many health services organizations engage in research, some types of which may not even be known to nonclinical managers.

Ethical Principles in Research

All codes of research ethics emphasize the subject's voluntary, informed consent. The subject's competence receives less attention. A provision in the Nuremberg Code (1949) states that subjects should be able to halt the experiment if they no longer wish to continue. This proviso places a heavy burden on the subject, who may become incapacitated by the experiment itself or by an unrelated medical problem, or who may be intimidated by the setting or individuals involved. Subjects also usually lack the technical competence to understand when their safety is threatened. This weakness was partially corrected in the Declaration of Helsinki (1964, revised 1975 and 1989), which recommends establishing an independent committee to review and approve the experimental protocol. This is the type of committee required by the U.S. Department of Health and Human Services (DHHS).

All codes and guidelines permit nontherapeutic research and recognize that volunteers for whom the experimental treatment offers no diagnostic or therapeutic advantage are needed for certain research. Clear, utilitarian language is present in all codes (except the American Medical Association [AMA] guidelines, which contain a strong element of paternalism), which compares and balances the risk to the subject (in nontherapeutic research) with the benefit to society. Conversely, emphases on voluntary and informed consent suggest a Kantian philosophy, and reflect the principles of respect for persons and nonmaleficence. This view is found in the DHHS regulations.

A primary problem with research codes other than federal regulations is that they inadequately separate the physician's roles as healer and researcher. Thus, the ethical burden on physicians is heavy because the duality of interests places physician-researchers in a classic conflict of interest situation. What is good for the research subject as a patient may not be good for the experimental design. This problem is exacerbated in nontherapeutic research because the risk to the subject is not balanced by potential benefit. AMA guidelines recognize the dilemma but adopt a paternalistic view of the relationship between physician and patient-subject by expecting the physician to exercise professional skill and judgment to act in the patient's best interests.

Establishment of Institutional Review Boards

In order to protect human subjects health services organizations conducting research should establish IRBs. IRBs are required by many federal agencies when they grant funds or regulate research. In the health services field DHHS and the Food and Drug Administration (FDA) are the most important agencies. Examples of other federal agencies that require IRBs are the Environmental Protection Agency, the National Science Foundation, and the Consumer Product Safety Commission.

Research that involves human subjects and is wholly or partly funded by the DHHS must be reviewed by an IRB with a process that meets DHHS criteria. The FDA regulates the interstate sale of drugs, biologicals, and medical devices and has requirements similar to those of DHHS. Unlike DHHS, however, compliance with the FDA's guidelines, including the use of IRBs, is necessary regardless of the funding source. A few states, especially New York, regulate medical research, but in most cases there is little regulation beyond the DHHS and the FDA.

The FDA does not regulate surgical experimentation. For example, the FDA does not determine whether coronary artery bypass surgery is sufficiently developed to be made generally available or whether radial keratotomy (ophthalmic surgery) can be attempted safely. Neither does the FDA regulate innovative clinical care, which is defined as new uses of existing treatments, drugs, and devices. Innovative care is distinguished from standard clinical activity, and its use requires more than the usual review and consent procedures. Absent government regulation, the organization's managers and clinical staff are essential in monitoring the activities of clinicians who innovate in the use of drugs or treatments or who attempt new types of surgery. A requirement that results be submitted to peer review by publishing them in the professional literature is a type of control, but it is far removed from the research and protects prospective rather than current patients. If current patients are to be protected, such gray, unregulated areas require vigilance by all in the organization. In the final analysis the patient's only recourse may be medical malpractice litigation.

It is not easy for hospitals, most of which have no ongoing research programs, to define experimentation and innovative therapy. Nonetheless, definitions are important, not only because they determine whether there is a need to meet legal requirements or to form an IRB but also because the organization must ensure that its own, presumably more rigorous, procedures for consent and protecting the patient are followed. The following case illustrates the problem.

This is Experimenting?!

An internal auditor conducted an audit of supplies used in biopsies. The data for kidney biopsies revealed significant discrepancies: The use of biopsy packs exceeded the number of procedures by 50%. The auditor was puzzled, but double-checking requisitions and utilization data showed them to be correct. Theft was unlikely.

The auditor made informal inquiries and spoke to technicians in the cytology laboratory. One agreed to speak confidentially about the additional kidney biopsies. The technician told the auditor that one of the nephrology fellows was using a second pack to take additional tissue during kidney biopsies. The tissue was sent to cytology for special studies ordered by the fellow. The technician said the fellow was testing a new theory about treating end-stage renal disease.

Is this research? Taking additional tissue or using part of the specimen in the manner described is experimentation, although the act of obtaining it is not experimental. By trying to prove or disprove a theory, the nephrology fellow is performing research. Even if the patient had given consent for the initial biopsy, no consent was granted to take additional tissue. Taking more tissue or performing a second biopsy puts the patient at additional risk, with no actual or potential diagnostic or therapeutic benefit. The organization and its managers have an absolute duty to prevent unauthorized research, and policies and procedures regarding it should be established. Also, innovative treatments must be closely monitored. In this case, the level of concern increases with the degree of risk. Adequate consent is critical for experimentation and innovative therapy.

Ethical considerations also exist in the economics of this case. The second study adds to laboratory workload. If the charges (or costs) are paid by third-party payers who are told they are part of a patient's diagnosis or treatment, the organization is acting dishonestly toward the payer.

Organizational policies must distinguish unauthorized from authorized experimentation. Obtaining a few extra milliliters of amniotic fluid during amniocentesis causes moderate additional risk. Taking unused urine routinely collected for other purposes or for performing analyses on the placenta poses no risk to the patient, but requires consent nonetheless. Minor or nonexistent risks do not justify ignoring patients' rights and the duties owed to them. DHHS regulations recognize minimal research risk and permit special review procedures.

In the sense that it is defined as attempting new means, methods, and techniques, medicine has always performed research; without it medical knowledge would stagnate. Protecting the human subject remains problematic, however.

Fever All Through the Night

Assistant Administrator Beverley Atchison finished reading the minutes of the utilization review committee. Atchison noted that a lengthy discussion had occurred with regard to the seemingly overlong stay of a pediatric patient. In fact, the attending pediatrician had appeared before the committee to explain the length of stay and her unique treatment regimen.

The case involved a child with a fever of unknown etiology. Routine tests after hospitalization showed no pathology. The physician explained that she had read about fever therapy in the literature and was impressed with its possibilities. Therefore, she decided to determine its appropriateness in cases of fever of unknown etiology. She ordered Tylenol in case the fever went above 102.5°. Otherwise, there was to be no intervention.

The pediatrician stated that the efficaciousness of fever therapy was proven because after 3 days the child had a full recovery. The regimen raised numerous questions among the committee members, however.

This regimen is innovative; it could even be classified as experimental. The case raises two ethical issues: Did the child's parents receive information about the treatment adequate to give informed consent? This question bears directly on how the hospital determines that informed consent has been obtained in such cases. Because the therapy was innovative, special consent and review procedures should have been used. If this therapy is experimental rather than innovative, the second issue is whether the research was therapeutic or nontherapeutic. Experimental treatment that may benefit the subject is therapeutic—the subject is also the patient. Nontherapeutic research involves healthy subjects, or patients with medical problems other than those that might benefit from the experimental treatment. Nontherapeutic research should receive closer attention because the subject will not benefit. Special emphasis should be placed on the quality of consent. Some commentators believe that nondiagnostic and nontherapeutic research on children and on adults who are legally incompetent should be prohibited.[19]

Notable in the fever therapy case is the nursing staff's apparent lack of concern about the unusual orders. Nursing's code of ethics emphasizes protecting the patient and requires the nurse to intervene if the patient is placed at risk unnecessarily. Timely reporting should have been accomplished through the nursing hierarchy.

Membership and Purpose

Both the DHHS and FDA require that an IRB be competent to review research proposals for conformance with the law, standards of professional conduct and practice, and institutional commitment and regulations.[20] IRBs acceptable to DHHS comprise a minimum of five members who have varying backgrounds (at least one must have professional interests that are nonscientific) and who are capable of reviewing research proposals and activities of the type commonly performed by the organization.

The IRB that is acceptable to DHHS must apply the following requirements in reviewing research activities:

- Minimize risk to subjects
- Determine that risks are reasonable relative to anticipated benefits

- Select research subjects equitably
- Obtain and document appropriate consent from research subjects or legally authorized representatives
- Monitor data to ensure safety
- Protect privacy and confidentiality
- Develop special protections when consent is obtained from individuals likely to be vulnerable to coercion or undue influence; this group includes individuals with acute or severe physical or mental illness or individuals who are economically or educationally disadvantaged

In addition, several provisions identify the information needed for informed consent.

The FDA uses the same basic elements of consent as the DHHS but applies special provisions when the subject is in a life-threatening situation that necessitates use of the test article and when the subject cannot provide legally effective consent, when time is insufficient to obtain consent from the participant's legal representative, and when no alternative method of generally recognized therapy that provides an equal or greater likelihood of saving the subject's life is available.

Requirements

Regulations issued in 1981 eliminated the requirement that *any* DHHS funding to an organization required use of DHHS guidelines in all research, regardless of funding source. This marked a significant shift in the role of the federal government in protecting human subjects and in research, generally. The change also enlarges the responsibilities of managers and researchers and necessitates greater reliance on the organization's policies and procedures and on their personal ethic in judging ethical issues. Problems similar to those in the Willowbrook case detailed in subsequent paragraphs may increase state involvement in regulating and reviewing all research.

As a practical matter, organizations with multiple research funding sources, one of which is DHHS, are likely to use the same DHHS-qualified IRB for all formal research. It is easy to slip, however, and managers must be alert to potential ethical problems in formal research programs as well as in isolated innovative therapy or surgical experimentation.

A mix of moral philosophies and values is found in the DHHS regulations. Beneficence and its subsidiary, cost–benefit analysis, determine the benefits of research. Conversely, a Kantian (deontological) perspective and principles of respect for persons and nonmaleficence underlie the requirements for consent, privacy, and confidentiality.

Despite the emphasis on respect for persons and nonmaleficence, nontherapeutic research on children is permitted. A risk–benefit ratio is applied, and no child can be placed in unnecessary jeopardy. Because nontherapeutic research on children is condemned by some prominent commentators and is politically risky, it is rarely undertaken.

Hepatitis for Children with Mental Retardation? [21]

Willowbrook State Hospital was an institution for the care of people with mental retardation located in Staten Island, New York. It housed over 5,000 residents in 1971.

Dr. Saul Krugman was a consultant in pediatrics and infectious diseases. When he began work at Willowbrook in the early 1950s, he discovered that major infectious diseases, including hepatitis, measles, shigellosis, parasitic infections, and respiratory infections, were prevalent. These conditions were like those found at similar facilities elsewhere in the United States. Dr. Krugman and his colleagues undertook a study of these diseases, including research on a measles vaccine and hepatitis.

In 1956 Dr. Krugman and Drs. Joan Giles and Jack Hammond began studies on hepatitis. The final phase of the research (1965–1970) involved 68 children ages 3–10. The researchers injected an infected serum to cause hepatitis in the residents of their research unit. The objective was to gain a better understanding of hepatitis and possibly develop methods of immunizing against it. The research was approved by the Armed Forces Epidemiological Board, one of the funders of the research; the executive faculty and the Committee on Human Experimentation of New York University, where Dr. Krugman held a faculty position; and the New York State Department of Mental Hygiene.

The researchers defended their decision to expose the subjects to strains of hepatitis on the following grounds:

• They were exposed to the same strains that were endemic to the facility.
• They were admitted to a special, well-equipped, and well-staffed unit and were isolated from exposure to other infectious diseases prevalent in the institution. The health risk to subjects was thus lower for those in the experiment than for those in the hospital at large, in which multiple infections occurred.
• They were likely to have a subclinical infection followed by immunity to the particular hepatitis virus.

The researchers emphasized that only children whose parents gave informed consent participated in the experiment.

A storm of adverse publicity arose when the experiment was made public in 1967 by a New York state senator, who charged that children were being used as human guinea pigs. Nevertheless, the research continued. In 1971 the group's work produced spectacular results, when Dr. Krugman and co-workers were able to immunize a small group of children against serum hepatitis (hepatitis B). The preliminary results were hailed as a scientific breakthrough. In defending the research, Dr. Krugman reported that the injections that induced hepatitis in the research group were given only after employing great thought and professional discretion and only with the informed consent of the parents. He stated that the doses were small and that the inoculations usually produced the infections without making the children sick.

In 1975 a federal court ordered that Willowbrook reduce its resident population to 250 people or fewer and that residents be assisted to achieve their fullest potential. Willowbrook was given 6 years to comply. Significant changes, including deinstitutionalization, followed. Progress had been made, but some primary goals remained unmet, and a federal court appointed a special master to supervise the reform program in April 1982. In January 1984 New York Governor Mario Cuomo promised to close the facility, which still housed approximately 1,000 residents. The federal government denied $22 million in Medicaid funds because of a chronic lack of adequate treatment and occupational therapy programs and a finding that food was inadequate for residents on at least one occasion. Living and bathing conditions—not unlike those identified 15 years earlier—were also unsatisfactory. Willowbrook State Hospital closed at the end of 1987 after a federal court approved a final settlement.

Dr. Krugman and his colleagues made a convincing case for undertaking and continuing the research. However, the Willowbrook case illustrates several ethical problems. The consent obtained from parents or surrogates was given under duress—they would almost certainly believe that children who were part of the group purposely infected with hepatitis would fare better than children living among the population at large, in which conditions were much worse. Such considerations make it difficult to apply the principles of beneficence and nonmaleficence.

The general benefit of being included in the special unit is an argument that should receive some credence. The children were somewhat protected from other prevalent diseases and received treatment for the sequelae of hepatitis. In addition, it can be argued that this research is therapeutic; even though the children did not have hepatitis, they were almost certain to become infected. The children in the unit also were likely to be less harmed in other ways than would children living in the general units of Willowbrook, thus meeting the principle of nonmaleficence. The real problem, however, is that the children were being used as a means to an end, despite a potential for great social benefit if the research was successful.

The protocol for the studies had been approved by prominent and appropriate review bodies and the research continued for 16 years (1956–1971). Assuming effective consent from parents or surrogates, federal guidelines would have permitted this nontherapeutic research. At the same time, the organizational philosophy could have applied a more demanding standard, to the point of prohibiting the research. In fact, research that is not clearly therapeutic on children and others unable to give voluntary and competent consent is so fraught with ethical problems that it is rarely, if ever, attempted. Regrettably, this conundrum has resulted in a dearth of certain types of clinical knowledge.

A question of justice in allocating state funds is raised by the horrific conditions at Willowbrook: Is it fair that human beings be treated so? If, however, state appropriations were not increased, the principles of respect for persons, beneficence, and nonmaleficence must be applied within the limits of the situation.

Exempt Research and Expedited Review

The 1981 DHHS regulations identified exempt research and research warranting expedited review as new categories to which different provisions apply. *Exempt research* includes primarily research in the behavioral sciences. It includes certain educational practices and testing, interview procedures and observation, and use of precollected data. Examples of exempt research are research conducted in an established or commonly accepted educational setting involving normal educational practices; use of educational tests, if information from these sources maintains the subjects' anonymity; and observation of public behavior, if certain safeguards are met. *Expedited review* applies special procedures for research that poses no more than a minimal risk and that in which human subjects have very limited involvement. Examples of expedited review include collection of hair and nail clippings in a nondisfiguring manner; collection of deciduous teeth; use of voice recordings; study of existing data, documents, records, and pathological or diagnostic specimens; and moderate exercise by volunteers. These changes greatly facilitate several kinds of research.

Falsification of Research Data

A unique twist to problems in research occurred in the late 1970s and early 1980s.[22] John Darsee, a fellow in cardiology at Emory University and Harvard University and a brilliant physician of unusual talent, perpetrated an amazing fraud. Darsee was found to have falsified large quantities of research data on the genetic and biochemical factors affecting heart disease. Some of these data had been published in leading medical journals. Other data were being used for papers in process. Many of the articles listed prominent physician-researchers as coauthors, some of whom later asserted they had no knowledge they had been listed as coauthors.

Darsee's champions supported him until evidence of his deception proved overwhelming. Darsee's detractors argued that his supporters were too easily charmed by his personality and talents. When researchers and administrators at Emory and Harvard learned of the fraud, they withdrew papers and abstracts that had been submitted for publication. The only step that could be taken regarding articles already published was to urge readers to disregard them. It is claimed that no patients were harmed because of Darsee's clinical work. Although this claim is verifiable by a review of the records at the hospitals involved, much more potential harm lies in the fact that Darsee's list of publications includes over 100 articles and abstracts. Readers unaware of the fraud cannot know which publications contain false data.

The organizations involved acted forthrightly when the problems were uncovered. What happened violated both the ethics of research and proscriptions imposed by funding organizations, such as the National Institutes of Health. The most pointed questions, however, concern the adequacy of surveillance, not only of Darsee but of all physicians in training who engage in research and collect research data. Subsequent self-assessment at Emory Univeristy led to new safeguards in reviewing the work of physicians in training and in monitoring the use of names of teaching staff as coauthors. Research findings are also reviewed much more extensively since the Darsee affair. Despite the safeguards some people argue that "(they) won't prevent the generation of fraudulent data, but under this system someone like Darsee couldn't send out articles at the rate of one a week without raising suspicions." [23]

Summary

Regulations such as those imposed by the DHHS focus responsibility on the organization and its IRB. Irrespective of legal requirements, the organization's managers are charged with independent duties under the principles of respect for persons, beneficence, nonmaleficence, and even justice (e.g., equitable selection of research subjects) in order to protect the patient. Managers must establish and maintain systems and procedures to prevent unauthorized research and to provide the necessary extra protection when innovative treatment is proposed or undertaken. The Darsee affair raises a unique set of potential problems in teaching and research institutions. Most important are staff awareness about the parameters of acceptable practice and the courage to act.

INFANT CARE REVIEW COMMITTEES

Infant care review committees (ICRCs) are another type of specialized IEC. They focus on the biomedical ethical problems of infants with life-threatening conditions. The Child Abuse Amendments of 1984 (PL 98-457) directed DHHS to encourage establishment of ICRCs in health facilities, especially those with tertiary-level neonatal units. The DHHS guidelines identified specific tasks for ICRCs, as follows:

> (1) educate hospital personnel and families of disabled infants with life-threatening conditions; (2) recommend institutional policies and guidelines concerning the withholding of medically indicated treatment from infants with life-threatening conditions; and (3) offer counsel and review in cases involving infants with life-threatening conditions.[24]

The guidelines made it clear that the DHHS considers it prudent to establish an ICRC, but that the organization decides whether to do so. Chapter 10 provides the background for the original Baby Doe regulations and the Child Abuse Amendments.

Certain aspects of the membership and administration recommended in the guidelines are worthy of note. Members should include individuals from varied disciplines and perspectives because a multidisciplinary approach provides the expertise to supply and evaluate pertinent information. The committee should be large enough to represent diverse viewpoints, but not so large as to hinder its effectiveness. Recommended membership includes a practicing physician (e.g., pediatrician, neonatologist, pediatric surgeon), practicing nurse, hospital administrator, social worker, representative of a disability group, lay community member, and a member of the facility's medical staff, who is the chairperson.[25] The recommendation to include a representative of a disability group in the ICRC runs counter to the principle that no specific group should be represented.

The DHHS suggested that the ICRC have adequate staff support, including legal counsel; that the ICRC recommend procedures to ensure that both hospital personnel and patient or resident families are informed of its existence, functions, and 24-hour availability; that the ICRC self-educate about pertinent legal requirements and procedures, including state law requiring reports of known or suspected medical neglect; and that the ICRC maintain records of deliberations and summary descriptions of cases considered and their disposition.[26]

Many groups, including the AMA, the American Hospital Association (AHA), and various medical specialty associations, objected vociferously to the original Baby Doe regulations and led the fight to block implementation. The Child Abuse Amendments and regulations, however, were supported by health services trade associations, which covered the gamut of institutional and personal providers, as well as specialized groups. In fact, the associations were instrumental in developing the law and regulations; their support was reported in the background information provided in the proposed rules issued by the DHHS in late 1984. The new law was enthusiastically backed by the AHA, and hospitals are likely to experience few philosophical problems complying with it.[27]

The form and activities recommended by the DHHS for ICRCs are similar to those reported in a 1984 study of 710 hospitals with special care pediatric units. The American Academy of Pediatrics (AAP) found that of the 426 respondents to the study, 56.5% had ICRCs or IECs. Of hospitals without such a committee, 75% were considering establishing one. The remaining 25% handled ethical problems by other means, including waiting for clarification of legal issues and acting on that information or using a university committee or state board. The committee activity mentioned most frequently was consultation on difficult ethical decisions, followed by advising parents, advising physicians (when consulted), and educating staff. Developing hospital policies was the third most important ICRC function. Committee composition was similar to that found by the President's Commission study of IECs.[28]

The percentage of hospitals with ethics committees reported in the AAP study was much higher than that found in the study undertaken by the President's Commission. The AAP findings were consistent with the findings of the National Society of Patient Representatives discussed earlier. The President's Commission research was undertaken several years before that of the AAP study and differences in findings suggest a significant change in the interim, at least regarding numbers of ICRCs. In fact, the AAP report noted the existence of evidence that many committees had been formed recently (as of 1984). The AAP report found that more administrators were serving on ICRCs than had been found to serve on IECs in the earlier President's Commission study. The greater involvement of managerial staff in biomedical ethical decision making is desirable.

SPECIALIZED PERSONNEL

This section outlines assistance for organizations and their managers and clinical staffs in solving administrative and biomedical ethical problems. Analogues to IECs and specialized committees such as IRBs and ICRCs that can assist managers to identify and solve administrative ethical problems are not as well developed, but can be with patience and perseverance.

Ethics Consultation Service

An ethics consultation service (ECS) is one way health services organizations can provide specialized personnel to advise and assist in solving biomedical ethics problems. Doing so is similar to establishing a clinical service. The ECS is staffed by ethicists with graduate degrees in philosophy, often at the doctoral level, and by clinical personnel who may be physicians or other caregivers. The clinicians have a special interest and/or preparation in ethics and provide a bridge between the ethicist and the clinical staff attending the patient. They also serve as a resource to the ethicists. In this model an ethicist is on call and the clinical member of the ECS is involved as needed. The ECS reports to the hospital IEC, which develops and recommends policy to the governing body. The IEC also serves as a sounding board for problems that develop during ethics consultation. A variant has a primary consultant who is assisted by other members of the ECS. The primary consultants and those assisting them come from various backgrounds, but all have intensive and specialized training in ethics and all participate in case reviews, ethics instruction, and regular meetings of the ECS staff.[29]

Ethicists

A less formal approach than the ECS is common in larger hospitals but should not be limited to them. Often, large hospitals employ full- or part-time ethicists on staff. As in an ECS, these ethicists are often doctorally qualified philosophers who may be faculty members at a university or medical school and who consult with clinical staff on biomedical ethical issues. Organizations needing the assistance of an ethicist can look beyond universities and medical schools and consider anyone with specialized preparation in ethics and its application in health services delivery. In this case, as with the ECS, an ethicist is the clinically oriented, problem-solving extension of an IEC.

DISPUTE RESOLUTION

The American Arbitration Association (AAA) has conducted seminars to train hospice staff to resolve disputes about appropriate patient care more effectively.[30] Resolving disputes is necessary because health care professionals often hold different ethical views about issues and thus reach different conclusions about cases. The objective of improved dispute resolution is to weld a multidisciplinary group into a cohesive and mutually supportive team so that they can resolve their differences and maintain the quality of patient care. Such formal preparation could also assist IECs, ICRCs, and IRBs. It is overly optimistic to assume that the act of establishing an interdisciplinary ethics committee means it will be successful. Specific preparation in dispute resolution should improve its effectiveness.

CONCLUSION

This chapter has examined committees established to address ethical issues. These committees include the general type, which are called here IECs, and IRBs and ICRCs, which are specialized ethics committees. In addition to hospitals, ethics committees can provide assistance in a wide range of health services organizations, including nursing facilities, HMOs, and hospices, all of which experience ethical problems similar to those experienced by hospitals. It is nonhospital settings where the greatest growth is likely. Hospices and nursing facilities, for example, confront ethical issues related to death and dying; HMOs confront ethical issues of resource allocation and physician incentive plans. Ethics committees in all settings will be involved in solving complex ethics issues, some of which (e.g., organizational philosophy) may come under mandatory review.

ECSs and ethicists can be involved on a more discretionary basis to assist in identifying and analyzing the moral obligations, rights, responsibilities, and considerations of justice that bear on a general issue or on the ethical issues in a specific clinical case.[31] They can assist physicians and are more likely to be used than are biomedical ethics committees, which physicians may view as cost ineffective. Beyond considerations of efficiency, it may be more palatable for physicians to consult with a single ethicist than to seek guidance from a committee. Ethicists can serve a similar function for managers by assisting them in identifying and solving administrative ethics problems and working with an administrative IEC.

Economic pressures resulting from cost cutting by third-party payers—especially government—and new competitive pressures are affecting all health services organizations, especially acute care hospitals. Managers may be tempted to use economic justification for decisions that implicitly, or even explicitly, affect quality of care negatively. The conflict between economic interests and quality considerations lies near the surface in most relationships with patients. The technical nature of health services and the average consumer's limited ability to judge results make it imperative that individuals associated with health care delivery expend every effort to further the quality of care and protect the interests of patients.

NOTES

1. Judith Wilson Ross, John W. Glaser, Dorothy Rasinski-Gregory, Joan McIver Gibson, & Corrine Bayley. (1993). *Health care ethics committees: The next generation*. (p. 1). Chicago: American Hospital Publishing.

2. President's Commission for the Study of Ethical Problems in Medicine and Biomedical and Behavioral Research. (1983). *Deciding to forego life-sustaining treatment: Ethical, medical, and legal issues in treatment decisions* (p. 443). Washington, DC: U.S. Government Printing Office.
3. Right-to die: An executive report. (1989, November 20). *Hospitals*, p. 34.
4. Ross et al., p. ix.
5. Joanne Lappetito, & Paula Thompson. (1993, November). Today's ethics committees face varied issues. *Health Progress*, p. 34.
6. Cynthia B. Cohen, Ed. (1990, March/April). Ethics committees. *Hastings Center Report, 20*, 29–34.
7. Lappetito & Thompson, p. 34.
8. American Association of Homes and Services for the Aging. (1995, July). Summary report: Survey on ethics involvement in aging services. Washington, DC: Author.
9. Ross et al., p. 8.
10. Robert M. Veatch. (1983, July). Ethics committees proliferation in hospitals predicted. *Hospitals, 57*(13), 48–49.
11. President's Commission, p. 448.
12. Marilyn M. Mannisto. (1985, April). Orchestrating an ethics committee: Who should be on it, where does it best fit? *Trustee, 38* (no. 4), 18–19.
13. Ross et al., p. 5.
14. Benjamin Freedman. (1981, April). One philosopher's experience on an ethics committee. *Hastings Center Report, 11*, 20–22.
15. Mannisto, pp. 18–19.
16. Linda S. Scheirton. (1993). Measuring hospital ethics committee success. *Cambridge Quarterly of Healthcare Ethics, 2*, 495–504.
17. Mannisto, pp. 17–20.
18. Amy Haddad, & George Annas. (1994, July). George Annas quoted in "Do ethics committees work?" *Trustee, 47*(7), 17.
19. Paul Ramsey. (1970). Research involving children or incompetents. In *The patient as person* (p. 252). New Haven, CT: Yale University Press.
20. President's Commission for the Study of Ethical Problems in Medicine and Biomedical and Behavioral Research. (1981). *Protecting human subjects* (Appendix B). Washington, DC: U.S. Government Printing Office.
21. Articles from several issues of *The New York Times* were used to prepare the Willowbrook material and the background information: January 11, 12, and 13, 1967; March 24, 1971; April 18, 1971; January 11, 1972; May 25, 1981; January 8, 1984; April 19, 1985; and March 3, 1987.
22. *Emory Magazine*. (1983, December). pp. 6–15.
23. *Ibid.*, p. 15.
24. Department of Health and Human Services, Office of Human Development Services. Final Rule, Child Abuse and Neglect Prevention and Treatment Program, 45 *C.F.R.* § 1340 (1985).
25. Department of Health and Human Services, Office of Human Development Services. Services and Treatment for Disabled Infants; Model Guidelines for Health Care Providers to Establish Infant Care Review Committees, 50 *Fed. Reg.* 14893 (1985).
26. *Ibid.*

27. Summary: Survey of infant care review committees. (1984). Paper delivered at the Annual Meeting of the American Academy of Pediatrics, Chicago.

28. Editorial. (1984, December). *Hospitals, 58* (no. 24), 10.

29. John C. Fletcher, Margo L. White, & Philip J. Foubert. (1990). Biomedical ethics and an ethics consultation service at the University of Virginia. *HEC Forum, 2* (no. 2), 89–99.

30. American Arbitration Association. (1984, Summer). *Arbitration Times*, p. 7. New York: Author.

31. John C. Fletcher, Norman Quist, & Albert R. Jonsen. (1989). *Ethics consultation in health care*. Ann Arbor, MI: Health Administration Press.

III

Administrative Ethical Issues

Virtually all administrative problems that arise in managing health services organizations and programs have ethical dimensions. These ethical problems are qualitatively very different from those encountered in the business world.

The business ethics literature burgeoned in the 1980s and courses in business policy and ethics are now common in graduate and undergraduate business programs. Little tradition exists in business of an independent duty or obligation beyond that established by law; the emphasis in business has been and is on profitability and *caveat emptor* (let the buyer beware). The business ethics literature examines concepts such as honesty, integrity, and benevolence; duties employees have to each other and to the organization; and duties organizations have to employees. These aspects are similar to those found in health services. Lacking, however, is the concept of respect for persons, with its emphasis on autonomy, fidelity, and confidentiality. Neither is beneficence a focus in business ethics. The principle of justice is found only at the periphery of business ethics. These differences between business and health services are cited here not to criticize business but to distinguish the two fields of endeavor, whose foci and purposes are, simply put, quite different.

The public's view and that of the health services field have been that we have a higher calling, one going well beyond the bottom line. Codes of ethics assist in defining this calling and the duty of managers. This definition stems from the link with physicians and nurses and the not-for-profit status common in the health services field. For acute care hospitals, the historic link with religious orders and humanistic motivation created a special image. In total, this higher calling resulted in a strong emphasis on the caring as well as on the curing aspects of health services delivery. It reflects society's view that the sick are a unique group, one with special status, that needs protection and is not to be exploited. Despite occasional, harsh negative publicity, especially as to financial management and quality of care, the humanitarian, caring image of health services organizations is largely intact.

The issues of administrative ethics confronting the health services manager run the gamut from conflict of interest to governing body and medical staff relations to duty to the patient. Although they can be subtle and appear in many guises, these problems are identifiable and solvable to alert and conscientious managers.

In this part of the book administrative ethical issues are identified and examined. Many are distinct from the biomedical ethical issues considered in Part IV. Although the differences between administrative and biomedical ethical issues are important, they are often blurred in practice. The best example of these differences is patient consent. A major difference between administrative and biomedical ethical issues is that administrative ethics are likely to affect patients as groups rather than as individuals and will affect the managers' relationships with the organization, peers, profession, and community. Biomedical ethics usually affect patients as individuals or as specific types. Exceptions are issues such as resource allocation, which affect macro- and microallocation. Often, administrative and biomedical ethical problems have an actual or potential effect on one another. The primary focus of each type of problem is usually different, however.

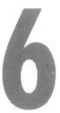

Conflicts of
Interest and Fiduciary Duty

onflict of interest is the most commonly reported administrative ethical problem confronting health services organizations. The American
College of Healthcare Executives (ACHE) Code of Ethics devotes
significant attention to conflict of interest, and trade associations, such as the
American Hospital Association (AHA), have issued policy statements about
it. A conflict of interest exists when duties are owed to two or more persons
or organizations and meeting the duty to one makes it impossible to meet
the duty to another. The classic case occurs when a decision maker (a director
[trustee] or a manager) is also a decision maker for an organization with which
the health services organization does business. The manager cannot meet the
duties owed to each organization—the duties conflict. Conflicts of interest
also arise for clinicians. Conflicts between duties owed to different patients
by the same physician are an important reason, for example, to separate the
organ transplant team from the physician treating the potential donor. Other
conflicts of interest arise when duties owed to the organization by a physician
are in conflict with those owed to patients or colleagues, or when patients
with the same diagnosis and physician but in different payment categories
receive different care in the same organization.

Conflicts of interest are an insidious problem area into which one can
slip, almost without realizing it. The ACHE code notes that the line between
acceptable and unacceptable behavior is sometimes fine. This pragmatic view
recognizes that the relationships of normal business often create a duality of
interests, which may result in conflicts of interests.

The manager's relationships with the organization and interactions with
the health system and other organizations in it can cause conflicts of interest.

In addition to potentially affecting the manager's relationship with the organization, conflicts of interest can affect managers' relationships with the profession and their personal development.

Conflicts of interest can be subtle and can affect all managerial activities. Has the manager who uses a position of influence and authority to gain titles, stature, and income at the expense of the organization or patient care acted ethically? Is the manager who is lax in developing and implementing an effective patient consent policy and process acting ethically? Is it ethical for a manager to review and cleanse negative information from reports to the governing body? Is it ethical for a manager who has reason to believe that quality of care problems may exist in a clinical department to do nothing to prove or disprove their presence? Is it ethical for managers who have serious concerns about their abilities to continue managing? To the complexity of such questions from an ethical perspective must be added the legal implications. Regardless, managers must first be concerned about their independent, positive duty to the patient.

Managers must avoid any hint of wrongdoing, especially the suggestion of divided loyalties. A bad odor emanates from a situation in which a hospital's chief executive officer (CEO) owns stock in a corporation that contracts the hospital's data processing and in which the principal stockholder and CEO is the hospital's comptroller. This odor lingers regardless of the discounted price or other advantages the hospital gains. Outside observers cannot but think that the relationships have hidden aspects that are detrimental to the organization or its patients and that managers are reaping a personal advantage. Attempts to convince the public otherwise probably reinforce the perception of wrongdoing. The only course of action is to avoid arrangements or entanglements that contain any hint of conflicts of interests. The problem is well put by Harlan Cleveland in *The Future Executive:* "If this action is held up to public scrutiny, will I still feel that it is what I should have done, and how I should have done it?" [1]

FIDUCIARY DUTY

Fiduciary is an ethical and legal concept arising from Roman jurisprudence. A fiduciary relationship exists whenever confidence and trust on one side result in superior position and influence on the other. This superiority and influence raise duties of loyalty and responsibility. The definition suggests that numerous fiduciary relationships exist in health services. Governing body members, for example, are fiduciaries. Their duty of loyalty prevents them from using their position for personal gain and they must act only in the organization's best interests. This definition has been interpreted to mean that no secret profits can be made in dealings with the organization and that the governing body member may not accept bribes or compete with the organization. The duty of responsibility requires governing body members to exercise reasonable care, skill, and diligence, as demanded by the circumstances.[2] Members of governing bodies have a duty to avoid errors of omission and errors of commission. Breaching these duties could result in personal liability, whether or not the corporation is organized for profit.

Trusts are common in the health services field. Many not-for-profit health services organizations engaging in charitable activities were established because of a gift or bequest that directed the establishment of a trust; trustees manage the assets of the trust. Examples are trusts to defray the costs of a nursing unit or specific clinical activity in a hospital. Other uses include funding schools of nursing or providing scholarships to educate health services personnel.

The term *trustee* is commonly used to describe governing body members of not-for-profit corporations in the health services field, even though there is no trust and they are not true trustees. Technically, the legally correct term is *director* or *corporate director*. The title *trustee* is preferred in the not-for-profit sector, however; perhaps because governing body members want to be distinguished from governing body members in for-profit organizations, in which *director* is used.

The legal standard for true trustees is much more stringent than is that applied to directors of corporations or to individuals responsible for monies or properties not held in trust. True trustees actually hold title to property or the corpus of the trust and manage it for the beneficiary. True trustees must act in good faith and practice undivided loyalty in administering the trust. All situations and relations that interfere with discharging these duties must be avoided. Breaching these standards results in personal liability. In many jurisdictions the standard of care required of directors of not-for-profit corporations who are not true trustees is higher than that required of other corporate directors. The usual standard for directors who are not true trustees is that they are liable for ordinary negligence, errors in judgment. The minority rule is that to be legally liable directors must have committed an act of gross negligence, usually defined as an intentional failure to perform a manifest duty with reckless disregard of the consequences.

Sibley Hospital

An important court case involving governing body members of a health services organization is *Stern et al. v. Lucy Webb Hayes National Training School of Deaconesses and Missionaries et al.* (1974).[3] The members of the board of Sibley Hospital, a not-for-profit hospital in Washington, D.C., were called "trustees" even though they were not true trustees. David M. Stern brought a class action suit against Sibley Hospital on behalf of his minor son and other patients alleging that patients had overpaid for care because several board members had engaged in mismanagement, nonmanagement, and self-dealing (succumbing to self-interest). The suit alleged that the acts of omission and commission resulted from a conspiracy between those "trustees" and various financial institutions with which several "trustees" were affiliated. The court found no evidence of a conspiracy. In considering the other allegations, however, it determined that:[4]

> The charitable corporation is a relatively new legal entity which does not fit neatly into the established common law categories of corporation and trust . . . the modern trend is to apply corporate rather than trust principles in determining the liability of the directors of a charitable corporation, because their functions are virtually indistinguishable from those of their "pure" corporate counterparts.

This ruling meant that defendant "trustees" were held to a less stringent standard of care.

The court found that the "trustees" had violated their duties as fiduciaries, even when held to the lesser standard. Mismanagement occurred because the "trustees" ignored the investment sections of yearly audits, failed to acquire enough information to vote intelligently on opening new bank accounts, and generally failed to exercise even cursory supervision over hospital funds. Nonmanagement was evidenced by the same failure to exercise supervision and was most starkly demonstrated because although certain "trustees" were repeatedly elected to the investment committee, they did not object when the committee failed to meet in over 10 years. The allegation of self-dealing was substantiated by the following facts: A number of "trustees" were officers of banks in which Sibley Hospital kept hundreds of thousands of dollars in noninterest-bearing checking accounts, interest-bearing accounts paid less than market conditions would have permitted, and one "trustee" advised approval of and voted to approve a contract for investment services with a corporation of which he was president.

The court did not find evidence of personal gain by the "trustees," although in several instances they had been associated with organizations that had benefited from the transactions. That there was no evidence of a conspiracy seems to have had significant impact on the ruling.

The court did not order any "trustees" removed from the board and no personal liability was attached to their wrongdoing. To prevent similar problems in the future, the court ordered the board to adopt a written investment policy, review relevant committees to determine whether hospital assets conformed to the policy, and establish a regular process of disclosure of board members' business affiliations. During the pendency of the case the board adopted the AHA's guidelines on conflicts of interest. This action occurred long after the fact, but was thought to demonstrate the board's good faith.

The conflict of interest statement suggested by the AHA is shown in Figure 6. It reflects the less stringent corporate director standard.

The decision in the Sibley case was handed down in a trial court and therefore has limited legal significance as a precedent. Nevertheless, it is one of the few cases that considers the standard of care for governing body members (directors) of not-for-profit organizations. Fiduciary duty requires governing body members to exercise reasonable care, skill, and diligence; under

Disclosure of Certain Interests of Governing Board Members

WHEREAS, The proper governance of the nation's health care institutions depends on governing board members who give of their time for the benefit of their health communities; and,

WHEREAS, The giving of this service, because of the varied interests and backgrounds of the governing board members, may result in situations involving a dual interest that might be interpreted as conflict of interest; and,

WHEREAS, This service should not be rendered impossible solely by reason of duality of interest or possible conflict of interest; and,

WHEREAS, This service nevertheless carries with it a requirement of loyalty and fidelity to the institution served, it being the responsibility of the members of the board to govern the institution's affairs honestly and economically, exercising their best care, skill, and judgment for the benefit of the institution; and

WHEREAS, The matter of any duality of interest or possible conflict of interest can best be handled through full disclosure of any such interest, together with noninvolvement in any vote wherein the interest is involved:

NOW, THEREFORE, BE IT RESOLVED: That the following policy of duality and conflict of interest is hereby adopted:

1. Any duality of interest or possible conflict of interest on the part of any governing board member should be disclosed to the other members of the board and made a matter of record, either through an annual procedure or when the interest becomes a matter of board action.
2. Any governing board member having a duality of interest or possible conflict of interest on any matter should not vote or use his personal influence on the matter, and he should not be counted in determining the quorum for the meeting, even where permitted by law. The minutes of the meeting should reflect that a disclosure was made, the abstention from voting, and the quorum situation.
3. The foregoing requirements should not be construed as preventing the governing board member from briefly stating his position in the matter, nor from answering pertinent questions of other board members since his knowledge may be of great assistance.

BE IT FURTHER RESOLVED: That this policy be reviewed annually for the information and guidance of governing board members, and that any new member be advised of the policy upon entering on the duties of his office.

Figure 6.   Conflict of interest statement of the American Hospital Association (AHA). (Reprinted with permission of the American Hospital Association, copyright 1990.)

a negligence theory they are liable for acts of commission or omission that violate this standard. *Reasonable care* is the care an ordinary, prudent director would exercise under the same or similar circumstances. The rule enunciated in the Sibley case is that governing body members (directors) of a not-for-profit corporation may be liable for ordinary negligence as well as gross negligence or willful misconduct. This standard is the one usually imposed on a director of a business enterprise.

CEOs and other managers are not fiduciaries in the same sense as directors, but they are held to a similar standard: a duty to exercise reasonable care, skill, and diligence, or the care that an ordinary, prudent manager would exercise in the same or similar circumstances. Many states' laws provide immunity from liability for directors of not-for-profit organizations. Often, however, the statutes contain limitations and exclusions from immunity, loopholes, and vague language, thus providing little real protection for directors and officers against liability.[5]

ETHICAL OBLIGATIONS OF TRUSTEES AND DIRECTORS

Legal standards represent a minimum standard of performance. What are the ethical obligations of trustees and directors? The AHA guidelines in Figure 6 assist governing body members to avoid conflicts of interest. They emphasize disclosure—putting other governing body members on notice about potential or actual conflicts. In the Sibley case it is uncertain that disclosure would have made a difference. The "trustees" must have known about their colleagues' outside affiliations and activities. Adopting the AHA guidelines and knowing their content might have alerted them to the ethical unacceptability of self-dealing and mismanagement. A conflict of interest statement probably would have made no difference as to nonmanagement because the "trustees" did not take seriously their fiduciary duty to invest hospital funds prudently.

Health services managers possess the characteristics of fiduciaries. They are also moral agents, and an important part of their work is assisting the organization, through the governing body, to meet its ethical and legal obligations. Concomitant with this effort, managers have a duty to help the governing body to avoid conflicts of interest and problems of nonmanagement. Managers are the conscience of the organization; they recognize potential administrative and biomedical ethical problems and act to avoid them or minimize their effect.

Hermann Hospital

A scandal uncovered in early 1985 involved activities of both administrators and trustees of the Hermann Hospital, an 800-bed facility, and the Hermann Hospital Estate, a trust established in 1914 to provide charity care to the poor of Houston, Texas. An investigation of the two entities showed evidence of theft, kickbacks, insider stock deals, lavish perquisites and expenditures, and costly trips taken by trust and hospital executives and employees at the trust's expense. Among the allegations were that the former executive director of Hermann Hospital paid money to his mistress for work that was never done and that he received kickbacks from overcharges paid by Hermann Hospital to a company of which he was president. The trust sued the former hospital executive director, asking that he repay $100,000 in kickbacks, $500,000 that he allegedly paid his pregnant mistress, and other funds he allegedly laundered. The suit also alleged that he took improper trips that, with related expenses, cost the hospital $250,000. It also alleged that he used Hermann Hospital's name, credit, and money to create an interior decorating firm for his mistress, most or all of whose income came from the hospital.

The Hermann Hospital Estate's former executive director was alleged to have stolen over $300,000. Allegations against a trust employee stated that a luxury automobile was traded in at less than 20% of its market value for a new automobile paid for by the trust. The undervalued automobile was then purchased by the employee at the grossly understated price. In addition, there was evidence that trustees and employees had entertained lavishly at trust expense, with $10,000 spent by six people on a 4-day weekend in California. Newspaper accounts stated that the Hermann Hospital Estate actually spent less than 3% of its funds on financially disadvantaged patients.

As a result of the investigation, two trustees and eight high-ranking trust and hospital executives resigned. Three individuals connected with the estate, including a trustee, were indicted on criminal charges.[6]

Many of the activities at the Hermann Hospital Estate and Hermann Hospital were unethical because they violated the law. The misconduct involved in this case goes beyond a breach of that minimum standard. The trustees violated their fiduciary duty to protect trust assets by squandering funds that should have been spent treating financially disadvantaged patients. True trustees and directors alike are allowed neither hints of conflicts of interest nor improper benefit from their association with an organization. Similarly, hospital managers must be above reproach in all that they do. They act unethically when there is self-dealing or when organization assets are diverted, whether or not these are indictable actions.

Cedars of Lebanon Hospital

Unlike Sibley, but like Hermann Hospital, circumstances at the Cedars of Lebanon Hospital involved a hospital CEO who engaged in both unethical and criminal behavior. The latter resulted in a prison term for the CEO. As noted, criminal behavior is in itself unethical. In addition to conflict of interest, the case contains instances of self-dealing, bribery, and failure to obey federal laws. The following summary of some of the transactions in which the CEO engaged outlines the problems:

- The CEO owned a consulting firm in the Caribbean with which the hospital contracted for architectural consulting services that were never performed.
- The CEO falsified board minutes to cover the fraudulent contract with his own consulting firm.
- The CEO received over 2,500 shares of stock with a market value of $75,000 in a computer company from which the hospital had purchased a $1.8 million diagnostic computer to be used for multiphasic screening; later underutilization of the equipment caused a loss of over $2,000 per day.
- The CEO bribed public officials to obtain approval for construction and loans for an unnecessary addition to the hospital.

- The CEO attempted to ease the hospital's desperate cash flow situation by not paying federal withholding on employees' salaries.[7]

Several other violations of ethical principles occurred, but these are illustrative. The CEO's activities forced the hospital into receivership; he was convicted and sent to prison. Important in the Cedars of Lebanon case is that the governing body paid grossly insufficient attention to the CEO's activities and did not meet their duties as fiduciaries.

CODES OF ETHICS CONCERNING CONFLICTS OF INTEREST

The ACHE code focuses significant attention on conflict of interest. The particular section of the code begins by stating: "A conflict of interest may be only a matter of degree." [8] This statement suggests that certain behavior, if limited, is unlikely to cause, or is presumed not to cause, a problem. The same behavior exaggerated, however, may result in a conflict. Gratuities are an example in applying this criterion. Few would suggest that a conflict of interest arises when a manager is treated to lunch in the cafeteria by a sales representative. A 2-week, all-expenses-paid vacation suggests something very different. Extravagant gifts or kickbacks can be reasonably assumed to encourage or reward certain behavior. Nevertheless, the appearance of a conflict of interest results by accepting *any* gratuity from those with whom business is done—even to the extent of a small gift or inexpensive lunch.

Earlier in the chapter, conflict of interest was defined as duties and obligations, the meeting of one of which causes derogation of another. In the ACHE code a conflict of interest exists "when the healthcare executive: Acts to benefit directly or indirectly by using authority or inside information, or allows a friend, relative or associate to benefit from such authority or information," or when the health care executive "uses authority or information to make a decision to intentionally affect the organization in an adverse manner." [9]

To minimize the potential for conflicts of interest and to eliminate them once they occur, the ACHE code recommends making all decisions in the best interests of the organization and the people served by it, disclosing conflicts to the appropriate authority, and avoiding conflicts of interests. These guidelines rely on the manager's judgment. Only managers possess the knowledge about personal activities and those of the organization, which helps them determine when there are potential or actual conflicts, when a solution is required, or when certain facts should be brought to the attention of the organization.

The Code of Ethics of the American College of Health Care Administrators (ACHCA) provides some assistance to managers in solving conflicts of interest. ACHCA affiliates shall not "participate in activities that reasonably may be thought to create a conflict of interest or have the potential to have a substantial adverse impact on the facility or its residents." [10] Affiliates are expected to "disclose to the governing body or other authority as may be appropriate, any actual or potential circumstance concerning him or her that might reasonably be thought to create a conflict of interest or have a substantial adverse impact on the facility or its residents." [11]

ACCEPTANCE OF GIFTS

Health services organizations must help staff to avoid conflicts of interest by adopting policies to guide their decision making in the acceptance (or nonacceptance) of gifts. Failing to receive guidance, employees and managers will perform in a manner they believe to be reasonable. This may or may not make them more objective.

Bits and Pieces

John Henry Williams liked his new job in the radiology department of Affiliated Nursing Homes and Rehabilitation Center. He had been appointed acting head when his predecessor, Mary Beth Jacobson, asked for a 6-month maternity leave. John Henry would be responsible for two and one half technicians, an appointments clerk, and $350,000 in equipment. He would have the authority to purchase radiographic supplies, the annual value of which was approximately $110,000. Most supplies were obtained from three vendors, companies from which the Center had bought for years.

As Mary Beth oriented John Henry, she emphasized how much she liked the meetings with sales representatives from the three vendors. Over the years, one had become a close personal friend. She told John Henry that most meetings were held at the nice restaurant near the Center. Some were held in her office and, if so, the reps always brought along "a little something." When John Henry asked what she meant, Mary Beth gave some examples: perfume, a bottle of brandy, and a pen set in a leather case. John Henry remembered thinking that his wife would like the perfume, but he was more interested in the lunches. It would be a chance to get away from the dreary cafeteria as well as his boring sandwich from home. Mary Beth said the lunches were nothing fancy. She estimated the cost to the sales rep to be similar to that of the small gifts—in the $40–$50 range.

John Henry asked Mary Beth whether there was a policy about accepting gifts from vendors. Mary Beth was upset by the question, which implied something might be wrong with what she was doing. She responded curtly that the Center trusted its managers and allowed them discretion in such matters. John Henry then asked if accepting gratuities might suggest to other staff that her decisions were influenced by the pecuniary relationship with the sales reps. Mary Beth's anger flashed: "I know you think that this thing doesn't look right. That isn't fair! I work long hours as a manager and get paid very little extra. It takes effort and time to order and maintain proper inventory. If things go wrong, it's my head in a noose. These gifts make me feel better about my efforts. My work has been exemplary. I'd be happy to talk to anyone who thinks otherwise!!"

This case illustrates a common problem in many health services organizations. Several facts support Mary Beth's position: Taking clients to lunch and providing small gifts is common in business relationships. The organization incurs no direct cost because everything is paid for by the sales representatives, who use their expense accounts. At least one sales representative has become a personal friend. Taken individually, it seems unlikely that Mary Beth's judgment could be influenced by the small amounts of money involved, but a long-term pattern could result in a different interpretation. It must be asked, however, whether other vendors are being ignored because of what might be characterized as "cozy" relationships.

Apparently there was no guidance from organizational policy. Neither the ACHE code nor the ACHCA code addresses the more subtle aspects of conflicts of interest. For example, the ACHE code states that one should "accept no gifts or benefits offered with the express or implied expectation of influencing a management decision." Applying this provision requires that one be able to judge the giver's motivation—a difficult, if not impossible, task. It seems that external evidence, including what is offered and accepted, is needed to judge that a conflict of interest exists.

Decision makers may gain or potentially gain from conflicts of interest in many ways. Often ignored are situations in which the parties understand that the decision maker will be considered favorably for employment or other benefits in the future. A promise or suggestion of future benefit creates potential or actual conflicts of interest and should be included in professional codes of ethics prohibitions. Classic nonhealth sector examples of these circumstances are common. Active duty military personnel interact with contractors and suppliers; on retirement, they accept employment with the same organizations. Former members of Congress and staff of federal agencies find lucrative employment as lobbyists or employees of organizations they formerly affected. Federal law limits how soon such contacts can occur, but advising those who actually make contact is permitted—a tremendous loophole. Former health services executives are employed by consulting firms with which their organizations have done business. Such problems in the health services field are more than theoretical and their likelihood increases as health care becomes more politicized and as large aggregations of health services organizations become common.

Anyone who takes something of value knowing the giver intends to influence the recipient acts unethically. Bribery is obvious: The recipient knows what is being done and what (or who) is being bought. Typically, however, the relationship of giver and recipient is more subtle. What does the pharmacy director do about the proffered lunch from the drug retailer? Does the CEO stop a dietitian from accepting a basket of holiday fruits, nuts, and sweets from the greengrocer? What about a modest gift from the equipment salesperson who was the successful bidder during the renovation program completed 3 years ago? Or 10 years ago? Such transactions suggest potential conflicts of interest. The gift might be given to receive special consideration in the future, or might be payment for past decisions.

Such situations become even more complex because it is difficult to distinguish the conflict-fraught activities of managers and staff from normal interactions. People develop relationships and friendships, whether as buyer and seller or as professional colleagues. As friends or professional colleagues, however, one should expect the buyer to be equally generous in making gifts to the seller.

Health services organizations must establish a policy on gratuities. They have three options. One is to prohibit accepting any gift, regardless of value. This position is that of the American Society for Hospital Materials Management. Its Code of Ethics states: "Decline all gifts or gratuities and do not enter into any transactions that would result in . . . personal benefit." [12] This rule may cause stress for staff who feel awkward declining gifts of trivial value; simplicity and no need to judge are its strengths. This clear, unequivocal rule justifies refusing all gifts, which adds to its usefulness.

The second option is pragmatic but more complex because judgment and occasional difficult decisions are involved. A criterion of reasonableness is applied to the first option, which allows for various circumstances and recognizes that staff have friends and relationships. What must be assiduously avoided, however, is any hint of wrongdoing or conflict of interest in decision making. As noted, this is achieved with difficulty. The test should be what the reasonable person objectively viewing the situation would conclude about the intent of the giver and the gift's effect on the decision maker.

A third option is a hybrid of the first two and is a compromise for organizations that prefer not to enforce an absolute prohibition, but want to minimize conflicts of interest and aid staff with a rule for a reference point. This policy considers all gratuities as gifts to the organization. They are made available for its use by sending them to the materials manager, either for redistribution to staff or other corporate uses. If given to the organization or widely shared with staff, the potential for a personal conflict of interest ceases to exist, even though a conflict between the organization and patient may continue.

Option three is similar to a health services organization that receives gifts from businesses. Suppliers of goods and services commonly make cash or in-kind contributions to not-for-profit organizations. Accepting them is not a conflict of interest. The contribution benefits the organization directly and as a whole, just as would a price cut or a discount. The gift does not benefit one individual, even though the reflected glory of such contributions may enhance the reputations of the individuals managing the organization.

Only a Matter of Degree

Stimson received four Super Bowl tickets in the mail. Attached was a note from the local sales rep for a major equipment manufacturing company, which read: "Thought you might be able to use these." The nursing facility of which Stimson is CEO recently decided to build an addition for a rehabilitation unit. The sales rep's company manufactures equipment that could be used in the unit. Stimson had called the manufacturer several months earlier to discuss equipment that might be available in order to make the specifications for the bidding process more precise.

Stimson is in a difficult situation. Super Bowl tickets are expensive, difficult to obtain, and generally highly prized. However, their intrinsic value is subjective; some recipients would place little value on them. Absent a personal relationship, such as a long-standing friendship, the proffered tickets seem intended to affect the CEO's decision. Important to discussing this conflict is whether Stimson is the sole owner of a for-profit organization. If so, Stimson's interests and the organization's are one—there cannot be an economic conflict of interest. Nevertheless, the owner's financial interests may conflict with the interests of facility residents, a different type of conflict.

APPROVAL OF SELF-DIRECTED EXPENDITURES

More subtle questions of conflict of interest can be self-induced. It seems a safe assumption that health services managers usually identify a personal obligation to put patient interests before their own. How much, then, should be spent to refurbish the CEO's office? What type of automobile should be leased for the CEO? Answers to such questions vary by type of organization and ownership.

Patient or Self?

Anderson is the CEO of Community Hospital, a not-for-profit organization. Anderson has assembled an effective administrative staff. Because Anderson's results have been good year after year, the governing body pays little attention to internal operations and focuses on fund-raising and community relations. Anderson has a large discretionary fund available for any purpose. In the past it has been used for entertainment, gifts, and staff education.

At the urging of several governing body members and managers, Anderson redecorated the administrative suite. Rosewood and leather sofas were ordered, elegant carpet and drapes were installed, a burled oak desk was delivered, and several original oil paintings were selected by the interior decorator. The project cost $50,000.

When the cost was criticized, even by the more financially successful members of the medical staff, Anderson reacted defensively. Anderson's primary argument in justifying the expenditure was that the CEO of a multimillion-dollar enterprise needed the accoutrements of office to be effective. Few critics were placated.

Whether such expenditures are appropriate varies by context and setting. A heavily endowed private hospital, in which the CEO's office is expected to reflect success and sophistication, will view this case differently from a public hospital, in which each nickel is spent reluctantly. Organizations at either extreme, however, could fund worthwhile administrative and clinical projects with $50,000. No one expects a CEO to sit on a lawn chair or use brick and board bookshelves, but the criterion should be good judgment tempered by reason. Again, it is useful to view such actions as would an informed, objective outsider.

CONFLICT OF INTEREST WITHOUT DIRECT PERSONAL GAIN

The case of Miriam Hospital is similar to that of Hermann Hospital.[13] Both cases lie between those of Sibley Hospital and Cedars of Lebanon. This case has an element of conflict of interest; other aspects make it unique.

Miriam Hospital

Before 1980 routine blood tests at Miriam Hospital were performed by a 6-channel analyzer. In 1980 the hospital purchased and put into operation a 12-channel analyzer. Because of a computer programming error, patients continued to be charged for both sets of tests, even though only the 12-channel machine was used.

A year later, Blue Cross raised questions about the unusually high laboratory charges at Miriam as compared with other hospitals. The explanation was that doctors at Miriam simply ordered more laboratory tests. In 1982 a professional standards review organization audit clerk uncovered the double billing. The manager of information systems was ordered by his immediate superior to eliminate the programming error. Shortly thereafter, however, he was told by "top officials" at Miriam to reinstate the programming error.

Later in 1982 a Blue Cross auditor uncovered the same problem and asked for a copy of the program. The manager of data processing was told to erase any evidence in the program that showed that the original error had been reintroduced. Blue Cross received the sanitized program.

A short time later, two data processing personnel were accused of allowing an outside company to use Miriam's computer in contravention of hospital policy. Each was offered the opportunity to resign. Fearing he would be made a scapegoat, one data processor told his story to Blue Cross, who went to the state's attorney general. Six months later, a grand jury brought indictments against the hospital and several senior managers. The charges included obtaining money under false pretenses, conspiracy, and filing false documents. The alleged overbilling totaled almost $2.8 million.

The hospital's and managers' defense was based on their interpretation of the rules under which reimbursement was made. They argued that the rules required hospitals to continue using the same accounting methods for the entire fiscal year, even though there were errors such as those found in this case. An end-of-fiscal-year audit would determine what financial adjustments were needed.

Unlike Cedars of Lebanon and Hermann Hospital, there is no evidence that managers at Miriam gained personally from their action. Miriam Hospital was the only direct beneficiary of the double billing procedure. This explanation does not excuse the action, ethically or legally, but does put it in a different light. Unlike the Sibley Hospital case, these executives did not benefit other organizations to the hospital's detriment. Regardless, to the extent that the double billing improved Miriam's financial situation, the managers enhanced their positions. Thus, they benefited through continued employment, enhanced status and reputation, and, perhaps, proffered financial rewards from the organization. Miriam's financial position was unclear; some sources stated it could not afford to refund the overcharges, even though management stated that doing so posed no problem. Saving a financially troubled organization at personal risk is altruistic and self-sacrificing; however, such efforts also benefit managers. Nevertheless, selfless or self-sacrificing activities cannot take precedence over moral values and ethical codes. The end cannot be used to justify the means.

SYSTEMS CONFLICTS

Health services managers typically serve on boards of health-related organizations. Examples of such organizations include health planning agencies, charities, insurance companies, Blue Cross plans, health maintenance organizations (HMOs), and hospital associations. Increasingly, such service has a great potential for conflicts of interest. The ACHE code advises affiliates to "Inform the appropriate authority and other involved parties of potential or actual conflicts of interest related to appointments or elections to boards or committees inside or outside the healthcare executive's organization." Such information puts the organization on notice and allows it to judge the extent of the potential conflict of interest. If an actual conflict occurs, the manager must withdraw. However, dramatic changes in the health services environment may have rendered these precautions inadequate.

This dilemma begins with the manager's civic duty and professional responsibility to assist the community in meeting its health needs. These efforts are reinforced by codes of ethics and the stimulus of governing bodies. Health services managers should be encouraged to apply their professional expertise to improving community health services, but the potential conflicts of interest are apparent and can be present even if other health services providers are not discussed. If a health services manager is also a Blue Cross director, for example, there are potential conflicts of interest as to rates, programs, and covered services. Furthermore, Blue Cross is becoming a competitor and developing services delivery capability. Even if managers abstain from debating or voting on matters directly affecting their organizations, it is impossible to avoid being privy to corporate thinking and strategies for other activities that in general and specific ways affect the managers' health services organizations. Once known, this knowledge cannot be ignored.

Increased competitiveness in the field of health services makes all information about one's competitors important in order to meet threats to market share or to blunt unfriendly initiatives. In fact, duties of fidelity and loyalty require a manager to preserve or expand the organization's market share. If managers minimize the problem of conflict through disclosure and withdrawal when necessary, they diminish their effectiveness as a director of the organization and potentially violate their fiduciary duty. Furthermore, they risk charges of impropriety simply by participating in other organizations.

How is this problem solved? How does a health services organization obtain important expertise without exposing itself and manager-directors to charges of impropriety and conflicts of interest? One option is to permit service only by individuals from noncompeting organizations. This solution has the disadvantage of potentially excluding individuals with operational experience in that geographic area. However, over time, out-of-area directors will develop expertise. This solution is complicated by the growing number of integrated delivery systems, which replace the traditional, locally based organization with one that is regional or national.

A second option is that health services organizations use full-time directors, individuals who are directors of noncompeting organizations and who are not employed elsewhere. Full-time directors are common in business enterprise but rare in health services, especially in the not-for-profit sector. These individuals are usually paid, an expenditure that should pose no problem for health services organizations, especially the larger ones. Organizations that are unable to bear the cost should consider option three.

The third option uses professionally prepared and experienced individuals not actively managing health services organizations. Examples include retired health services managers and health services administration educators. Physicians and well-informed members of the public could serve effectively. This option possesses most of the advantages of option two. In this case, an economic relationship is desirable because it will produce greater levels of commitment and higher-quality involvement.

Managers working to improve community health services through cooperative efforts face an increasingly competitive environment. This challenge makes some types of cooperation difficult or impossible. Other types, such as sharing services and participating in joint ventures, are stimulated. Survival is a primary corporate goal for health services organizations and new ethical guidelines are needed to address these problems.

CONCLUSION

Avoiding conflicts of interest requires constant vigilance. Managers of government-owned facilities risk fines and criminal charges if they are involved in conflicts of interest. The likelihood of legal penalties is less in the private sector. This does not obviate the ethical problem, however. Disclosure to eliminate or minimize the problem is stressed by the ACHE, ACHCA, and AHA. Disclosure presumes that one recognizes potential conflicts. Failure to recognize conflicts means that managers are well into a conflict situation before they realize it. Conflicts of interest can be subtle and continual questioning and self-analysis are needed to identify them. Their potential and actual effect will increase as competition intensifies.

In addition to disclosure, conflicts of interest may be avoided or eliminated in other ways, including divesting a potentially conflicting outside interest, seeking guidance from the governing body, and not participating in or attempting to influence matters in which conflicts may exist. Such steps eliminate the conflict or put the governing body on notice. Both are important, but it is managers who must remember their inherent moral agency and who must work to minimize or eliminate the risk of conflict of interest once it is present.

Systems conflicts will cause unique problems as well as opportunities in the new competitive environment. To avoid conflicts of interest, managers must be especially alert and may need to withdraw from all involvement in governing and advising competing or potentially competing health services organizations. Nontraditional means will be required to maximize the assistance that individuals experienced in health services can offer, while minimizing the potential for systems conflicts.

NOTES

1. Harlan Cleveland. (1972). *The future executive* (p. 104). New York: Harper & Row.

2. Arthur F. Southwick. (1988). *The law of hospital and health care administration* (2nd ed., pp. 123–126). Ann Arbor, MI: Health Administration Press.
3. Stern et al. v. Lucy Webb Hayes National Training School of Deaconesses and Missionaries et al., 381 F. Supp. 1003 (1974).
4. *Ibid.*, p. 1013.
5. James E. Orlikoff. (1990, January). What every trustee should know about D & O liability. *Trustee, 43*, 8–9.
6. *The Houston Post*, articles dated March 5, 9, 10, 12, 13, 16, and 19, 1985, and *The Washington Post*, article dated March 21, 1985.
7. Summarized from a case study written by the late Milton C. Devolites, Professor Emeritus, Department of Health Services Administration, The George Washington University, Washington, D.C. The case was prepared from various issues of *The Miami Herald* and *The Miami News* published in 1974.
8. American College of Healthcare Executives. (1995). Code of ethics. In *Annual Report & Reference Guide, 1995–1996* (p. 62). Chicago: Author.
9. *Ibid.*
10. American College of Health Care Administrators. (1994). Code of ethics. In *Agenda for Advocacy* (p. 16). Alexandria, VA: Author.
11. *Ibid*, pp. 15–16.
12. American Society for Hospital Materials Management. (1980, October 19). *Code of ethics*. Chicago: Author.
13. *Providence* (Rhode Island) *Journal-Bulletin*, articles dated September 22, 1983; October 2, 5, and 6, 1983; and May 16, 1984.

7

Ethical Issues Regarding Organization and Staff

A wide variety of administrative ethical issues arise as health services managers do their jobs. Issues linked to performance appraisal, for example, are a function of formal relationships. Other issues, such as working with independent practitioners of the medical staff, often result from informal relationships. Managers have an ethical and legal fiduciary relationship with the organization as represented by the governing body. In an ethical sense, managers are fiduciaries for all staff in the organization, and this relationship raises special obligations. Self-dealing was examined briefly in Chapter 6, but is given expanded attention in this chapter.

In the course of their duties health services managers are privy to copious confidential and insider information. Much is sensitive; almost all is proprietary. Administrative information is distinguished from that collected, used, and maintained for patient care. Using and safeguarding both types of confidential information is a major ethical concern in health services organizations, but it receives little attention.

ORGANIZATIONAL CONTEXT OF RELATIONSHIPS

Managers are employed to carry out the organization's mission in the context of its philosophy. The governing body selects and evaluates the chief executive officer (CEO). In turn, the CEO selects and evaluates subordinate managers, perhaps down to the middle management level. Regardless of organizational level, managers are moral agents who are ethically accountable for the effects of actions and inactions on patients, staff, and organization. Their decisions are not excused because they are employees or because they were following orders. The law may hold individuals who are not prime actors or decision makers to a different standard, but managers remain morally accountable for what they do or do not do.

As an employee, the manager has a duty of loyalty to the organization and its staff. In terms of the organization, this duty means that the manager supports the employer's goals and activities and keeps confidential what is learned. Disagreements about policy and its implementation are neither broadcast nor otherwise shared with individuals without a need to know. The duty of loyalty has special importance in light of a common malady, backbiting the employer. Backbiting is not the grumbling or complaining usually considered normal, perhaps even healthy, behavior. Although employees may have a legitimate reason to complain about their treatment (even the best employer does not get it right every time), rabid, negative comments are problematic. Employees who persistently speak ill of their employer act in an unacceptable fashion and should find new employment, voluntarily or involuntarily.

Managers must achieve the difficult balance between loyalty to the organization and fidelity to their personal ethic and professional integrity. Where does the manager draw the line? How far should a manager go in following the crowd or in standing alone? A clear and well-considered personal ethic is needed to answer questions such as these. Professional codes of ethics play a role, but provide only general guidance and are unlikely to be useful in helping a manager decide what to do in specific cases. At the extreme, the limits of loyalty are part of whistleblowing, which is examined in Chapter 8.

As posited earlier, the manager has an independent duty and responsibility to the patient, which, at minimum, means managers protect patients and further their interests. What follows from that is the need for integrity and the courage to speak out and act to transform that responsibility into a reality. What happens, however, when the duty to protect the interests of patients conflicts with the duty of loyalty in achieving part of the organization's mission?

All She Had to Do Was Ask

Richard Weidner experienced angina on mild exercise. His internist referred him to a cardiologist at University Hospital for a cardiac catheterization. After her examination, the cardiologist explained the procedure and obtained Weidner's consent. As the cardiologist turned to leave, Weidner asked her, "You'll be taking care of me, won't you, doc?" "I'll see you in the cardiac cath room," she replied. Weidner was reassured and especially pleased that he had such a long, friendly visit with the cardiologist.

That afternoon, Weidner was lying on the table waiting for the catheterization to begin. He had a clear view of the television monitor, and as the procedure began he saw the catheter moving from his groin toward his heart. At one point he asked a question and was startled when the cardiologist appeared near his head and described what was happening. Weidner asked her who was threading the catheter and was told it was a resident in cardiology.

Later, Weidner was in the recovery area waiting to be discharged. He was quite agitated that a resident had performed the procedure, especially because he thought he had an understanding with the cardiologist. He described what had happened to the nurse and demanded an explanation. The nurse tried to calm him. "You know," she said, "this is a teaching hospital—we train residents so they can perform these procedures to help other people." Weidner was not placated. He said, "Had I been asked, I probably would have agreed to have the resident participate. But they didn't ask me, and I'm damned angry about it. Please tell a manager to see me immediately. I want some answers!"

Weidner was not harmed physically, but he is emotionally distraught. He believes that he was misled and that a promise was broken. Weidner was concerned about who would perform the procedure and sought reassurance from the cardiologist, whom he trusted. Her answer was evasive. She purposefully or negligently misled him and thus breached her obligation to tell the truth. In sum, Weidner was deceived and treated disrespectfully. What happened does not seem to be the result of maliciousness; all involved would likely be distressed to learn that Weidner is angry about his treatment. Weidner's expectations were unmet, however.

What should the manager of cardiology do when Weidner relates his story? Except to reassure and placate, little can be done for Weidner. More important is what should be done to prevent similar problems. The manager of cardiology should be the force for staff education and necessary process changes. The personal ethic of this manager's peers and the organizational philosophy should demand this level of attention to the principle of respect for persons.

To become fully qualified, physicians in residencies need specialized training, which can only be gained by treating patients. Far less acceptable, of course, is the assumption that all patients are willing to participate in medical education. Being used as a means to an end is a crude statement of utilitarianism, and one incompatible with the principle of respect for persons, specifically patient autonomy.

The admissions forms of teaching hospitals disclose their involvement in medical education. Few patients, however, read or understand the implications of that disclosure. Judged by legal standards of informed consent, signing such a form holds little validity. More important than the law, however, is the organization's ethical obligation to inform the patient. Even if the form has been read and understood, minimum ethical conduct demands that patients be informed when teaching activities are to occur and that permission is obtained. Medical education and consent are covered in more detail in Chapter 9.

ORGANIZATIONAL INFORMATION

In addition to patient information, the manager is privy to confidential information about the organization, much of it proprietary. As with patient information, a basic criterion for confidential information is need to know. Examples of confidential organizational information include decisions about capital equipment, staff development, business and marketing strategies, and financial and human resources programs. Equally important, but less commonly included, are general information concerning the staff and organization and specific information such as their strengths, weaknesses, and peculiarities, concerning individual managers or governing body members.

In a competitive environment "loose lips" will result in significant adverse consequences. It is unethical to deliberately or negligently make confidential information available to unauthorized organizations or individuals. This is true whether the manager's organization is put at risk, actually experiences a loss, or the manager making the communication gains personally.

The 1995 American College of Healthcare Executives (ACHE) code directs the health care executive to "respect professional confidences." This wording provides little guidance about confidential information in the organization. Managers, governing body members, and staff must ensure that confidential information is safeguarded. Physicians who are independent contractors usually have limited loyalty to the organization, which in a competitive environment makes sharing proprietary information with them problematic. Increasingly, health services organizations must provide confidential information on an absolute need-to-know basis.

Self-Dealing

Narrowly defined, self-dealing occurs only when a person with access to confidential information uses it for advantages such as monetary gain or self-aggrandizement. Misuse of confidential information that does not involve self-dealing is considered simply a breach of confidentiality. Examples of misusing insider information include the following: a manager, knowing that the organization intends to establish a surgicenter, purchases the property through a straw man and later resells it to the organization for a profit; a manager discloses information about organizational decision making that gives associates an advantage in doing business with the organization; and a manager discloses market strategies (proprietary information) to competitors, with no resulting personal gain. If, in the first example, the manager is decision maker for both the sale and the purchase, that is also a conflict of interest.

What's a Manager to Do?

S.L. Rine joined the management staff of a large health services provider after working as a health services manager for several years. Rine is a member of ACHE and wants to build the best set of credentials in the shortest time. Rine wants to become a CEO.

Rine is responsible for several support departments as well as some clinical areas. Shortly after beginning employment, Rine realized that the organization is very political. Much of what happens at the senior level is the result of personal relationships and obligations.

Maintenance is one of Rine's departments; it is responsible for all of the grounds. Rine learned that grounds crews were being sent to the homes of senior members of the governing body to maintain their lawns, shrubs, and trees. Rine asked the maintenance director to explain and was told that the practice had a long history and should be left alone. When Rine asked the director for a cost estimate of the grounds work being done at the private homes, the director refused, saying that he feared the wrath of the governing body members who were benefiting. Rine pondered what to do.

Soon after talking to the maintenance director, Rine had lunch with the laboratory director. Without discussing specifics, Rine described the problem in maintenance. The laboratory director exclaimed, "That's nothing!," and described how two governing body members were selling reagents and supplies to the laboratory at higher-than-market prices. Rine asked the laboratory director why she had not done anything about the situation. She replied that her predecessor had tried to stop the practice and was fired. Again, Rine pondered what to do.

This case has two dimensions, one involving governing body members, the other involving managers. Governing body members whose yards are maintained by the organization or who sell to the laboratory at inflated prices are explicitly or implicitly using their authority for personal benefit. Selling overpriced reagents and supplies to the laboratory seems more unethical than receiving free grounds maintenance; both improperly divert (steal) organizational resources. In principle the two acts are indistinguishable. Most destructive for the organization's moral health is that the governing body members are setting bad examples, which at best make the staff cynical, and at worst encourage staff to use their authority improperly.

The second dimension is the role of managers. Knowing about improper behavior but not acting (nonfeasance) is no better than committing an unethical act (malfeasance). Codes of administrative ethics are of limited help. Rine and the laboratory manager agree that the behavior is unacceptable. The problem they face is to identify their ethical obligations and act on them.

By confronting the individuals involved Rine will achieve little more than embarrassing them and is likely to be fired. Managers can and should take any available steps, however. One step is to question unethical activities at every opportunity and to encourage colleagues to speak out. If several managers agree that behavior is unethical, they draw strength from one another. They can implement or can try to implement a policy of competitive bidding for all purchases, including laboratory purchases. They can develop and propose an organization-wide policy on self-dealing and abuse of authority. In short, they must take whatever steps they can to end unethical practices. As moral agents, they cannot close their eyes to such problems.

MISUSE OF INSIDER INFORMATION

Persons in an organization with access to information not available to the public are known as insiders. Ethical problems arise when managers use such information in a manner that is inconsistent with their fiduciary duty, the obligation to be trustworthy. Benefiting oneself or one's associates are examples. Some misuse of confidential information has a salutary effect and must be distinguished. An example is whistleblowing that occurs when internal efforts fail and the manager's moral agency demands external disclosure of information about practices that may affect the safety of patients or the public. Their protection takes precedence over a duty of loyalty to the organization, even if the manager becomes subject to civil or criminal sanctions.

A common misuse of confidential (nonpublic) information occurs when employees (insiders) use it to make advantageous stock market transactions. Historically, health services organizations were largely unaffected because few were traded publicly. Their status has changed dramatically since the late 1960s. Regulation by the Securities and Exchange Commission or its state counterparts does not diminish the seriousness of the unethical conduct inherent in misusing insider information. Again, the law is a minimum that does not necessarily set an appropriate level of ethical behavior. The following case illustrates several ethical problems.

Just Part Owner

Jane Abernathy is the CEO of a large urban not-for-profit nursing facility. She is a voting member of all governing body committees. Following a retreat the governing body's planning committee recommended that rehabilitation become a significant new initiative; for the past several months the capital expenditures committee has considered the purchase of equipment to increase the nursing facility's capacity in rehabilitation. The part-time physician-director of rehabilitation wants to become a full-time employee.

Following an uncle's death 2 years ago, Abernathy inherited 1,000 shares of INCO, Inc., stock. She submits an annual statement of her investments and holdings as part of the governing body's conflict of interest disclosure requirement. The next report is due in 9 months. INCO's last annual report stated that 10 million shares of common stock are publicly held. INCO manufactures rehabilitation equipment similar to that Abernathy's facility is considering.

The capital expenditures committee's draft report includes INCO, Inc., equipment. Abernathy dislikes making private information available to the governing body and is distressed about this apparent need for special disclosure.

In theory Abernathy faces a duality of interests that could lead to a conflict of interest. Also, there is a potential to misuse confidential information to engage in self-dealing if Abernathy recommends purchasing equipment from a manufacturer in which she owns stock. Abernathy's ownership interest is remote, however—a mere .01% of the company's stock. Thus, the personal gain is so small that it is unlikely that Abernathy's decision could be influenced by her stock ownership, or if it were that she would have any measurable benefit. Abernathy's objectivity becomes more suspect as the ownership interest increases. Nevertheless, Abernathy should disclose her holdings in INCO, even though doing so is personally distasteful.

RELATIONSHIPS WITH THE GOVERNING BODY

The CEO is the governing body's agent in achieving the organization's mission. In turn, the CEO selects, hires, evaluates, and retains subordinate managers. The CEO and other managers and staff are moral agents, not only the organization's morally neutral arms and legs.

As previously noted, some sectarian health services organizations require that mid- and senior-level managers be adherents to the religion of the sponsoring organization. This requirement is too restrictive; co-religionists often hold different views about various doctrines or the rigor of their application. An effective corporate culture is built on managers (and other staff) who understand and accept the organization's philosophy. Humanism or nonsectarian philosophies may have values similar to those found in organized religion. Culling for values occurs in recruiting and selecting staff, and it is here that ethical compatibility should be determined. Focusing on congruence of values widens the field from which to recruit competent managers; such diversity inevitably benefits the organization.

The governing body and the CEO and senior management (shown in Figure 7 as "Administration") must define the scope of their respective functions. Figure 7 also suggests the need to distinguish senior and middle management. Governance, administration, and management must understand their respective activities or they will interfere in one another's spheres, with resulting inefficiency and frustration of organizational goals. The diagram is not intended to depict relationships and spheres as isolated. It must contain permeability of ideas and communications, but separateness as well as jointness must be clear.

Early leaders in hospital administration argued that the risk of conflicts of interest that existed when the CEO or members of the medical staff were on the governing body far outweighed any benefit.[1] The current thinking is that the disclosure of potential conflicts of interest prevents or minimizes their actual occurrence. The environment has changed dramatically; by 1996

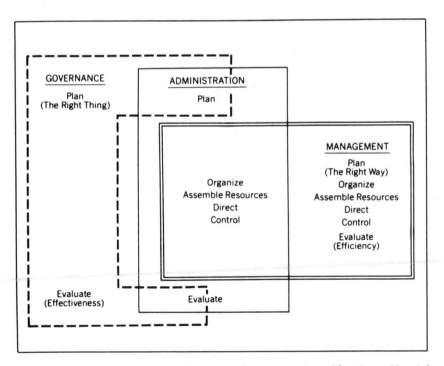

Figure 7. A model of hospital governance, administration, and management. (Reprinted from *Trustee, 34*, p. 6, by permission, June 1981. ©1981, American Hospital Publishing, Inc.)

it was essential that the CEO and medical staff be involved in the governing body. In 1989, 42% of hospital CEOs were full voting members of the governing body, an increase from 38% in 1985.[2] This study found that an average of two physicians with medical privileges at a hospital were members of its governing body.[3]

Anecdotal evidence suggests a trend toward a greater proportion of internal governing body members (senior managers employed by the organization) relative to external members. Internal members are desirable because of their general and organization-specific expertise. The increased potential for conflicts of interest is obvious, however.

Regardless of governing body membership, the CEO and senior managers link governance to the operating components of the organization. As the governing body's agents, they provide it with the information and recommendations upon which macrodecisions are made. This enables senior managers to "sanitize" data and make themselves look good, or to mislead, as occurred in the Cedars of Lebanon case (see Chapter 6). A key issue is how much and what types of information the governing body should receive. The governing body makes this determination. The CEO and senior managers should make recommendations, but governing body members must be sufficiently informed to know which data it needs and how to interpret them. Level of involvement and expertise are special problems in organizations that rely on voluntary governing body members.

It is natural that managers want their performance to be viewed in a good light. Pressures in the external environment may tempt managers to engage in "creative reporting" about their performance. However, managers are obliged to be truthful in governing body interactions, an ethical duty arising from the principle of respect for persons, which applies to all with whom the manager interacts. Deception is disrespectful. This does not mean staff must emphasize unfavorable information; a balanced picture is prudent and desirable. It does mean that the governing body must be informed of problems honestly and in a timely manner. Managers must be alert to understated or misrepresented problems from their subordinates as well. Truthfulness is closely related to whistleblowing, which is discussed in Chapter 8. Standardized and routinized reporting minimizes the potential to manipulate the system or the data.

The following case illustrates the problem of information flow to the governing body.

I Wonder If They Even Care?

Stu White had just returned to his office from a monthly governing body meeting. His assistant, Barbara Jones, noticed that he was agitated and asked, "How was it?" White responded by describing the governing body's chronic problem, something Jones had heard before. "I think I could tell them the moon is made of green cheese and they would believe it! They don't seem to know, or care, what happens in this nursing home!" White described how he did all of the thinking for the governing body. When he came to the facility, he described how there was no reporting system, until he had established one based on his previous experience.

He emphasized that the organization had been lucky to have honest managers because, as he put it, "anybody else could have been hauling it out of here by the carload."

The information flow problem in the case example results from governing body members' lack of awareness or willingness to be fully involved and accountable for the organization, duties that are unquestionably theirs. White is in a powerful position. He works with a governing body that takes little interest in understanding the organization's affairs, and he determines what information it receives. Few managers are involved in such an extreme situation. CEOs and other senior managers possess superior knowledge in at least two respects: They are expert about health services generally and they understand intimately the organization's activities and functioning. Their fiduciary relationship requires that managers be certain that they provide information the governing body needs. They act ethically when they present and interpret information that accurately portrays the organization. White must educate the governing body about its responsibilities. Next, he must help them to identify the data and reports they need to meet those responsibilities.

RELATIONSHIPS WITH THE MEDICAL STAFF

Relations between physicians and the organization and its managers raise several ethical issues that are present whether the organization is designed as a matrix or is organized along the lines of the traditional functional hierarchy. Schulz and Johnson[4] suggest that the CEO's role has evolved from business manager to coordinator to corporate chief to management team leader, the predominant role as of this writing. As a management team leader, the CEO is a partner with physicians. This evolution causes the green-eyeshade mentality of health services managers to become no more than an historical curiosity. In collegial relationships peers identify and solve problems of mutual concern. Regardless of the role and degree of acceptance the CEO has duties and responsibilities that inevitably cause disagreements with physicians.

Managers are ethically (and legally) expected to be aware of clinical practice and to intervene as necessary. This expectation reflects their important ethical responsibilities to protect the interests of patients. This broadened role of managers has positive and negative aspects. Although they are not competent to judge the quality of clinical practice, managers act through experts who are so qualified. This situation is similar to that of a manager responsible for pharmacy or dietetics. Again, the manager relies on technical expertise to assess performance and make decisions. Some physicians react negatively to the slightest hint of such involvement, which they see as interference in clinical decision making. In fact, managerial involvement also serves the physician's best interests because it helps to ensure high-quality medicine. Anecdotal evidence suggests that the more competent physicians are less likely to object to a review of their work. It must be stressed that the manager is not judging quality of care directly but only in cooperation with those clinically competent to do so. Conflicts of duties, perhaps even conflicts of interest, arise because managers must maintain harmonious relationships with physicians while ensuring patients' interests. Physicians are expected to meet the principles of respect for persons, beneficence, and nonmaleficence, but lapses occur.

The manager must be attentive to the needs and activities of physicians because their involvement is essential to patient care. Their clinical service to and relationships with patients are the reason the organization exists. Conflicts with the medical staff result from enforcing medical staff bylaws, resource allocation decisions, and the relationships between physicians and employee staff. Other important responsibilities of senior management are to help the medical staff keep its bylaws current and to assist in enforcing administrative provisions. A typical example of the latter responsibility occurs when a hospital CEO or medical director applies the medical staff bylaws and its rules and regulations to suspend a physician's admitting privileges. This action occurs most often because of tardy completion of medical records. Absent an emergency, such actions use established procedures and are not taken singlehandedly. Because of the independent duty owed to the patient, even exclusively clinical problems cannot be ignored by managers. Clinical and nonclinical managers must act as the need arises. Sometimes mistakes occur, as in the following case example.

Oops!

Dr. M is a graduate of a foreign medical school who has been a successful cardiologist on the staff of a large midwestern hospital for over 20 years. Occasionally, there have been rumors of Dr. M's alcohol abuse and disruptive behavior. Until a month ago, however, the only formal report nursing administration had received was from a registered nurse, who stated that Dr. M had been verbally abusive and had embarrassed her in front of a patient and his family. Recently, nursing administration received two incident reports: one oral, the other written. Both stated that Dr. M had an odor of alcohol about him and seemed mentally and physically impaired. The information was forwarded to the medical director, Dr. G, a hospital employee and a member of the administration.

Dr. G called an emergency meeting of the medical staff executive committee, which the chief operating officer (COO) could not attend because of a professional meeting out of town. After discussing the information but without a formal investigation, the committee agreed to terminate Dr. M's medical staff privileges. A registered letter was sent to Dr. M describing the action and the reasons for it. Another cardiologist was asked to treat Dr. M's hospitalized patients. Upon her return a week later, the COO was aghast to see the letter terminating Dr. M. She realized immediately that Dr. M's privileges should have been suspended, not terminated, pending an investigation.

Dr. M was enraged and immediately retained legal counsel. The hospital withdrew the termination letter 2 weeks after it was sent and reinstated Dr. M's staff privileges pending a full investigation. Dr. M was not placated, however, and filed suit against the members of the executive committee and the hospital, alleging antitrust violations, defamation, and tortious interference with his business relationships.

Dr. G erred in terminating Dr. M's privileges; suspension was the appropriate disciplinary action. Dr. G acted primarily to protect patients; secondarily, he wanted to protect staff. Both actions are ethically correct. However, he mistakenly chose too punitive a disciplinary action. This error was costly for the hospital: public controversy and embarrassment, expensive legal bills, and medical staff disruption and lingering ill will.

The hospital erred in its failure to adequately prepare Dr. G for his duties; furthermore, the hospital failed to require an expedited review process for such actions when patient harm is not imminent. The future holds a greater risk for this hospital, however. Managers and members of the medical staff will be reluctant to act in such cases, perhaps even when the facts are more egregious. Had no action been taken and a patient been harmed because of Dr. M's impairment from alcohol consumption, the public outcry would have been greater, however. The lesson for the hospital is that managers must be prepared for the demands of their jobs.

Dr. M's rights to due process were violated. His anger was justified, but it is not clear that he suffered any significant professional or economic injuries. The termination was rescinded soon after it was imposed. Even if the executive committee had taken the correct disciplinary action, he would have been suspended from admitting patients pending an investigation. Regardless, Dr. M was not treated fairly.

RELATIONS WITH NONPHYSICIAN STAFF

Like staff in nonhealth organizations, health services professionals harbor various goals, objectives, and interests. Their work in the organization is a primary focus of their lives, but the congruence between personal goals and objectives and those of the organization is likely to be less than total. Chapter 3 noted that employees must believe that they and the organization possess the same core principles of working in the patient's best interests. This attitude must be reflected in action, not just in written organizational philosophy and policies. If employees and physicians perceive that the organization places greater value on performance other than that which reflects ethical interaction with patients (e.g., increasing hospital revenues), the principles of respect for persons, beneficence, and nonmaleficence cannot be satisfied. Because the organization can act only through its staff, this lapse is serious. If staff fear that intervening on the patient's behalf jeopardizes their relationship with the organization, they will be discouraged from acting as they should.

The "Uncooperative" RN

Sally Hansen, a registered nurse with 10 years' experience, works nights. At the start of her shift she noted that a urinary catheter had been ordered for a postsurgical male patient with acute urinary retention. Following established procedure, she paged the resident on duty. A first-year resident appeared and told her he would insert the catheter. Hansen accompanied him to the patient's bedside and watched him remove the catheter from its package. He looked at the package, apparently for instructions, but found none. The resident began to insert the catheter into the patient's penis, but faltered. It was clear that he did not know what he was doing and that the patient was in great pain.

The resident turned and asked for assistance, but Hansen refused, saying that inserting a catheter was the job of a properly trained resident. "Really, you shouldn't attempt something you don't know how to do," she said. She also reminded the resident of hospital policy that prohibits a female nurse from performing certain intimate procedures on male patients. The resident yelled at Hansen and stormed off. Hansen paged the chief resident, who catheterized the patient, but offered no explanation when she described the incident with the inexperienced resident.

The next day, Hansen was awakened at home by a call from the vice president for nursing. She told Hansen that the inexperienced resident had filed a formal statement accusing her of insubordination. The resident was adamant about pressing the issue with nursing administration and the chief of his service. The vice president for nursing said she could not be sure as to the outcome.

What was Hansen's proper role in this matter? Where did her duties lie? Clearly, her duties lay with the patient and she acted properly. Even if she had known how to insert the catheter, she was constrained by hospital policy from doing so. Stopping the resident protected the patient from pain and potential injury. A reprimand from nursing administration will greatly diminish Hansen's willingness to intervene on a patient's behalf in the future. The hospital must encourage appropriate action by all staff as it seeks to deliver high-quality care and protect the patient. Teaching is not an issue in this case; the resident was not competent to undertake the procedure—a failure of instruction, not of nursing.

Other issues are present. One is the traditional subservient role of nurses, partly due to sexism. Poor relations between doctors and nurses do not result only from sexism, however. Anecdotal evidence suggests that the problem exists where sexism is not a factor (e.g., male doctors–male nurses, female doctors–female nurses). A second issue is that a resident attempted a procedure that was beyond his competence level. He should have been trained or had the good sense to ask for help from a more senior resident. The third issue is that the limits of residents' clinical activities are unclear. In this regard, the procedures and safeguards in the medical education program may need review. The American Nurses Association's[5] Code for Nurses requires Hansen's action: "[the nurse acts] to safeguard the client and the public when health care and safety are affected by incompetent, unethical, or illegal practice by any person." Implicit in this statement is accountability for one's actions as a nurse—a professional ethic—not merely accountability through the organizational hierarchy.

The organization must support its staff with an unequivocal commitment that encourages them to intervene when a patient is at risk. This policy should be communicated and enforced. Action in such situations may cause some individuals to accuse caregivers of spying on one another. This charge is unfounded. Spying is a negative process, one with no place in health services. The focus here is on an organization-wide effort—an ethic—to protect and cure the patient. If caregivers are able to minimize their ego involvement in the care process and keep their eyes on these goals, this problem will lessen in significance.

Ignoring problems will not solve them. This maxim is especially true if patients are at risk. Such problems can be ignored or covered up for a time, but, as the Watergate political scandal of the 1970s showed, they will come to light eventually. The public reacts to such revelations by assuming that others in the organization knew, yet did nothing. How could such situations occur or be allowed to continue, they wonder. In addition to the moral guidelines of respect for persons and the duty to be honest in all interactions, the likelihood of discovery is a utilitarian reason for recognizing and solving such problems early.

Communicable diseases and other high-risk circumstances raise special issues in the relationship between organization and staff. Both are ethically bound to protect patients and further their interests, but it is ethically unjustifiable for an organization, through its managers, to put clinical staff at risk by failing to train or equip them, for example. High-risk situations should cause managers to consider the need to protect staff from unnecessary risk; failing that, the organization cannot meet its ethical obligations to staff. In turn, staff will be unable to meet their ethical obligations to patients. These issues are discussed in more detail in Chapter 8.

NEW RELATIONSHIPS WITH MEDICAL STAFF

Beginning in the late 1980s significant changes occurred in relationships between physicians and health services organization, a movement led by acute care hospitals. These arrangements are designed to add an economic dimension to relationships that emphasize clinical activities. The *MeSH* (medical staff–hospital) concept began in the 1980s, but gained limited acceptance; then the *joint venture*, which included undertakings such as professional office buildings and lease or purchase and operation of high-technology equipment, became the focus of economic relationships between organizations and practitioners. In the 1990s both concepts were replaced by the *PHO* (physician–hospital organization) and integrated health networks, both of which focus on primary care but seek to deliver a continuum of services to a defined population. The economics of clinical practice must be tied to the organization so that each may assist the other to survive.

Such arrangements are fraught with potential ethical problems. A mildly adversarial relationship between medical staff and managers is useful because it provides checks and balances in maintaining high-quality patient care. This relationship requires that each party remember that its reason for being is to serve and protect the patient. When management and clinical practice are economically bound together, patient interests may suffer. The potential for conflicts of interest is greatly increased if the physicians involved in these arrangements are also part of the governing body. Evidence of actual conflicts of interest and fear of their potential have led to the passage of federal and state laws that regulate certain types of referrals.

APPRAISAL OF MANAGERIAL PERFORMANCE

A principal role of the governing body is appraising the CEO's performance, even as the CEO appraises subordinate managers. W. Edwards Deming rejected management by objectives (MBO) for general use in organizations. He argued that MBO pits managers against one another and leads to internal competition and suboptimization of the affected systems; ultimately, the entire organization is suboptimized. Despite Deming's concerns, MBO continues to be common in organizations.[6] It is argued that in pure form MBO, as first conceptualized by Peter Drucker, is consistent with Deming's theory. Its use, however, has deviated from the original intent.[7]

Despite the controversy, formal appraisal using specific criteria is appropriate for CEOs. They are responsible for the entire organization. Their interests are consistent with its optimization, and appraising them should reflect this consistency. Harvey developed a format in order to use MBO for hospital CEOs.[8] He detailed competencies necessary for managerial effectiveness: planning and organizing, achieving hospital objectives, maintaining the quality of medical services, allocating resources fairly and efficiently, resolving crises, complying with regulations, and promoting the hospital. Harvey's criteria focus on hospital CEOs but could be used in any health services organization in which performance is compared against predetermined measures and standards.

A 1990 report found that 76% of governing bodies in responding hospitals formally evaluate the CEO.[9] Anecdotal evidence suggests that few CEOs are evaluated against specific criteria, however, especially with the specificity described by Harvey.

To avoid conflicts of interest when they are evaluated, CEOs must limit their role to explaining organizational performance. The CEO's performance should be reviewed without the CEO present but with feedback provided later. The CEO is entitled to fairness in the review process, especially if negative outcomes that might result in termination are possible. Problems are minimized if the governing body employs a formal process to evaluate the CEO's performance, one based on predetermined objectives that are to be attained during the period under evaluation.

CEOs evaluate the work of subordinate managers directly or in coordination with other senior managers. This duty includes the evaluation of clinical managers. Some personal and professional relationships interfere with objective appraisal, or, in extreme cases, even day-to-day management.

A Little Too Close

Sue Rosen had been a successful health services executive for more than 20 years. She is currently the CEO of a substance abuse center that provides a full range of in- and outpatient services. Approximately 4 years ago, she experienced significant job-related stress. In addition, she had had emotional problems in her personal life, which became more complex after her divorce, and difficulties with her only child, a daughter.

She recognized her need for professional help and sought the services of Dr. Eisenbard, a clinical psychologist. In addition to his private practice, Eisenbard consulted with several substance abuse centers. Rosen received 32 sessions of intensive therapy over 2 years. Eisenbard was of great assistance and their final session occurred 2 years ago.

Recently, Rosen's clinical director, a clinical psychologist, resigned. Eisenbard responded to a blind advertisement and sent his resume to a post office box. The director of human resources brought the resume to Rosen, who was surprised to receive it. Rosen has high regard for Eisenbard, but is concerned about the implications of his application.

The problem here is obvious: Their previous therapeutic relationship makes it impossible for Rosen to interact effectively with Eisenbard, either as colleagues or as superior–subordinate. Rosen will never feel at ease, and, if needed, disciplinary actions against Eisenbard will be difficult, if not impossible. Eisenbard may not wish to enter into a managerial relationship with Rosen, but at this point he is unaware that she is his potential employer. Regardless of Rosen's high estimate of Eisenbard's professional abilities, this employment relationship should not be undertaken.

Governing bodies should be evaluated, and MBO is also appropriate at this level. Objectivity and comprehensiveness will be enhanced if an external expert assists in the evaluation. An important element of evaluating the performance of governing body members is input from the CEO and other managers who interact with them.

PHYSICIANS AND CREDENTIALING

The process of verifying credentials begins when a physician first applies for medical staff membership and privileges. All aspects of a candidate's education and training, licensure, and clinical preparation are included. Periodic reviews ensure that physicians with independent access to the patient are qualified. Preventing legal actions and bad publicity are important, but the primary reasons to be concerned about competence are the principles of respect for persons, beneficence, and nonmaleficence.

In 1985 the Joint Commission on Accreditation of Healthcare Organizations (Joint Commission) first permitted nonphysician and nondentist independent allied health professionals (IAHPs) to become members of the medical staff. IAHPs are licensed to deliver a limited range of clinical services and include providers such as nurse midwives, clinical psychologists, and podiatrists. Review and delineation of privileges use the same process for all practitioners with independent clinical access to patients. Therefore, IAHPs undergo a similar credentialing process to determine the extent and scope of their clinical privileges. As with physicians and dentists, renewal of privileges depends on demonstrated clinical competence.

Controlling what an independent practitioner does is more difficult when procedures or activities are added to a set of privileges (e.g., when a gastroenterologist wants to use a laser during an endoscopy, or when a general surgeon seeks to perform laparoscopic procedures). Organized efforts to ensure that all such practitioners are qualified and practice at an acceptable level protect patients and further their interests.

FRAUDULENT CREDENTIALS

Occasionally, there are reports about persons claiming to be physicians, but whose credentials are partly or wholly false. The problem of overstated, misrepresented, or false credentials is extensive in the business world, and there is reason to believe health services management is infected with the same

virus. Examples of misrepresented credentials include inflated job titles, responsibilities, and duties; exaggerated or falsified academic preparation and
credentials; and falsified or misleading information about professional
achievement and activities.[10] Such actions are dishonest and unethical.

Even a cursory check by a potential employer will usually uncover nonexistent formal credentials, such as licenses and academic degrees. More subtle and pervasive is the problem of "creative" resume writing. One need only
look at resumes produced by some employment and executive search firms
to realize that it is possible to make trivial management positions appear
significant. Uncovering exaggerated or overstated credentials can be difficult
because specific details of employment must be verified. Even job descriptions
may not adequately reflect what the incumbent actually did in a particular
position. For this reason gray cases may slip through. Egregious examples can
be identified, however.

Managers who encounter an applicant who has presented dishonest credentials have one course of action—exposure and disciplinary action through
the professional society. Appropriate action is less clear when it is discovered
that their current employees have falsified or misrepresented their credentials.
Nevertheless, action is essential. Counseling is a first step, whether or not the
employee is to be retained. Beyond counseling, the action taken should be
proportionate to the seriousness of the problem. Current job performance
and the reasons for the falsified credentials should be considered. Serious
falsifications and misrepresentations must be reported to the professional society and to the authorities if there is criminal behavior.

What action should be taken if one has personally overstated, misrepresented, or falsified qualifications? Managers with such problems should inform their superiors and offer the strongest possible rationale for the action.
This is a sound course of action even when the claimed credential does not
exist but was material to the hiring decision. The employer may not take
drastic action, especially if the reasons for what was done seem compelling.
The employer is likely to consider current job performance. The manager
must be prepared for termination, however. Continued concealment is unacceptable: As one rises to a more senior level, the stakes are higher and the
potential for devastating damage to one's career increases. Misrepresented or
falsified credentials are a burden to the individual because they are likely to
be uncovered eventually and because of the chronic, nagging fear of being
caught. It is better that corrections be made when there is less to lose.

Discovery of significantly misrepresented or falsified credentials should
cause the professional association to take disciplinary action, including expulsion. Representation of a fictitious academic degree or position cannot but
be significant to both employer and professional organization.

Slovenly verification by potential employers breaches their ethical obligations and adds to the ease with which falsified or exaggerated credentials
are used. Inadequate verification is true even when candidates for senior man-

agement positions are considered. The employer is responsible for adequately checking credentials and acting when dishonesty is uncovered.

Employers have an ethical obligation to report the performance of former employees accurately. In the case of serious problems such as drug addiction, specific information should be reported, whether or not it was requested. For less serious problems, a fair and balanced appraisal that reports strengths as well as weaknesses meets ethical obligations.[11]

A Massachusetts case raised questions about ethical behavior when physicians writing references neglected to include information about the character of former residents in anesthesiology.

But Is It Relevant?

The Massachusetts Medical Society plans to investigate three physicians at a leading Boston hospital who wrote highly laudatory letters recommending a colleague only a few days after he had been sentenced to jail for raping a nurse.

The convicted physician was able to use the letters to get a new job as an anesthesiologist at the Children's Hospital in Buffalo, where officials said they were unaware of his legal troubles. [He] was charged last week in another Boston rape case, dating back to 1978, involving patients.

Medical officials say the case, involving physicians at the Brigham and Women's Hospital, is the most striking example they have encountered of how letters of recommendation for hospital jobs have lost their value in recent years, as physicians became cautious about writing anything critical about colleagues for fear of being sued.

Other physicians on the staff of the hospital said they believed the letters were written after consulting with the attorney for the Brigham and Women's Hospital. Because the rape did not occur within the hospital, they suggested that the attorney had advised the physicians that they had no basis for being critical of [the physician's] medical performance.

B.J. Anderson, associate general counsel for the American Medical Association, said that the association advised directors of departments in hospitals to be candid when writing letters of recommendations despite the threat of lawsuits: "Too frequently hospitals that have had a problem with a physician will write a glowing letter because it is easier to export your problems across a state line than to resolve them yourself."[12]

The Massachusetts Medical Society investigated the conduct of the physicians who wrote the letters of recommendation. All three physicians were censured and put on a year's probation. The controversy over the letters prompted appointment of a panel to suggest guidelines for preparing letters of recommendation. Its report advised physicians to follow a Golden Rule of letter writing: "a letter should contain the information known to the writer that he would like to have were he to receive the letter." The report also stated that "information regarding personal character is of great importance in the case of physicians."[13]

Whether or not the physicians who wrote the letters of recommendations violated the letter of the law, they certainly failed to honor its spirit. Any health services organization that might hire the physician would find it relevant that he had been convicted of a crime. This is especially true of a crime such as rape, which involves moral turpitude. As with nonphysician staff and employees, the organization, through its managers, is morally obliged to report relevant information about physicians honestly and objectively.

CONCLUSION

This chapter identified and analyzed ethical problems managers experience in their relationships with the organization and staff. These relationships are analyzed within the context of the manager's ethical obligations to patients. Managers have access to patient and proprietary information, most of which is confidential. This accessibility suggests the potential for inappropriate disclosure, self-dealing, and misuse of insider information.

The unique relationships senior managers, especially CEOs, enjoy with governing bodies and staff are examined within the context of various ethical duties. Managers must act to protect patients when questions of clinical competence arise. Taking this action includes having the policies, procedures, and resources needed to minimize the risk of inadequate practice and to eliminate it should it occur. Managers must establish a culture that emphasizes patient care and safety and must support all staff in their efforts to maintain this focus.

New relationships among organizations and with physicians raise ethical issues, most of which result from the potential for conflicts of interest. Emphasizing the financial aspects makes it easy to forget that the patient is the primary reason for the existence of health services organizations.

The chapter concluded with a examination of falsified or overstated personal qualifications and the obligation of managers to act when these problems come to their attention. Thorough background checks and the provision of honest recommendations assist organizations in their work and maintain the integrity of the profession.

NOTES

1. See, for example, Charles U. Letourneau. (1959). *Hospital trusteeship* (pp. 90–91). Chicago: Starling Publications; Charles U. Letourneau. (1969). *The hospital administrator* (p. 45). Chicago: Starling Publications; and Malcolm T. MacEachern. (1962). *Hospital organization and management* (pp. 87, 97). Berwyn, IL: Physicians' Record Co.
2. Jeffrey Alexander. (1990). *The changing character of hospital governance* (p. 13). Chicago: The Hospital Research and Educational Trust.
3. *Ibid.*, p. 18.
4. Rockwell Schulz, & Alton C. Johnson. (1990). *Management of hospitals and health services.* (3rd ed., pp. 87–95). St. Louis: C.V. Mosby.
5. American Nurses Association. (1985). *Code for nurses.* Kansas City, MO: Author.
6. Edward Marlow, & Richard Schilhavy. (1991, January–February). Expectation issues in management by objectives programs. *IM*, pp. 29–32.
7. Philip E. Quigley. (1993, July). Can management by objectives be compatible with quality? *Industrial Engineering*, pp. 14, 64.
8. James D. Harvey. (1978, Spring). Evaluating the performance of the chief executive officer. *Hospital & Health Services Administration, 23*, 5–21.

9. Daniel R. Longo, Jeffrey Alexander, Paul Earle, & Marni Pahl. (1990, May). Profile of hospital governance: A report from the nation's hospitals. *Trustee, 43*, (no. 5), 7.

10. Physicians are not immune. A study by Gail Sekas and William R. Hutson ([1995]. Misrepresentation of academic accomplishments by applicants for gastroenterology fellowships. *Annals of Internal Medicine, 123*, 38–41) of applicants to a gastroenterology fellowship found that nearly one third of the 53 applicants who said they had published articles in scientific journals misrepresented the articles. Misrepresentations included citations of nonexistent articles in actual journals, articles in nonexistent journals, or articles noted as in press. Review of applicants to an infectious disease fellowship suggested that the problem of misrepresentation is not confined to gastroenterology. The authors of the study posit but do not answer the question of what those discovering the deception should do. They urge that guidelines be developed.

11. Bonnie J. Gray, & Robert K. Landrum. (1983, July–September). Difficulties with being ethical. *Business, 33*, 32.

12. Fox Butterfield. (1981, September 24). Doctors' praise assailed for peer in rape case. *The New York Times*, p. A16.

13. Doctors censured in Massachusetts. (1982, February 4). *The New York Times*, p. D27.

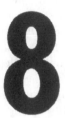

Ethical Issues Regarding
Patients and Community

his chapter identifies the special relationships between managers (and
their organizations) and patients and the community. The personal
duties and obligations of managers and those toward their profession
were noted in Chapter 4 in the context of the moral philosophies and the
ethical principles of respect for persons, beneficence, nonmaleficence, and
justice. The chapter highlighted the need for managers to have a well-defined
personal ethic to guide their decision making on administrative and biomedical ethical problems within the context of the organizational philosophy.

The book's underlying premise that the manager is a moral agent with
independent duties to the patient is reinforced in this chapter. Managers must
juxtapose their relationship with and duty of loyalty to the organization and
patient relationships. The reciprocal duties of colleagues are a part of belonging to a professional group that has expectations and demands certain behavior. In many ways organization and manager are one. Managers must keep
this in mind because their actions and decisions are judged in that
context—they personify the organization. However, there are ethical limits
to what the organization can expect of those working for or affiliated with it.
Managers must know the limits of their personal ethic and must speak out
when the organization infringes upon those limits.

MAINTAINING CONFIDENTIAL INFORMATION

Patient Records
Through their managers, health services organizations are charged with duties
regarding patient information. Medical records are essential for good patient

care and they must be legible, current, complete, and authenticated. The legal duty to maintain their confidentiality and security is met by providing adequate and effective personnel, systems, and procedures in medical records activities and by ensuring that medical staff bylaws and rules and regulations are enforced. Much can be done to prevent or minimize unauthorized access to paper medical records. The control of electronic records raises significant confidentiality issues that must be solved by health services managers.

State legal requirements vary, but individuals working in health services organizations have an ethical duty to ensure the confidentiality and appropriate use of patient information. The most common breach of this ethic occurs when patients are discussed with or in the presence of individuals who have no need to know. A 1995 hospital-based study found significant breaches of patient confidentiality and other types of inappropriate comments such as concerns about a person's ability or desire to provide high-quality patient care, concerns about poor-quality care in the hospital, or derogatory remarks made about patients or their families.[1] Idle talk and gossip about patients are titillating but unacceptable inside and outside the organization.

Conflicts may arise between maintaining confidential information about patients and furthering organizational interests.

Mailing Lists

University Hospital has a very active cardiac medicine section in its department of medicine. Over several decades it has treated thousands of people with heart problems ranging from angina to congestive heart failure. Its patients have been included in several research protocols, many of them funded by the National Institutes of Health or various national heart associations.

Periodic questionnaire surveys are conducted as part of long-term patient follow-up. To complete these surveys, an extensive database and mailing lists are maintained by the cardiac medicine section. On one occasion the development office of University Hospital used the mailing lists to solicit general contributions. On another occasion, it undertook a special fund-raising effort to assist in converting and equipping a cardiac intensive care unit. Contributions by the cardiac program's current and former patients have been excellent, primarily because the program maintains superior rapport with its patients.

The physician-director of the program and her administrative assistant have been approached by a prominent and respected national insurance company that is impressed by the results of the program. It wants to market life insurance to the program's participants. The proposal is attractive because the opportunity to obtain life insurance will benefit present and former patients, many of whom are uninsurable except at very high premiums. The proposal is also attractive because any data obtained by the insurance company will be available to the hospital at cost if the mailing lists are provided to the insurance company.

The physician-director and administrative assistant are enthusiastic about the clinical possibilities in addition to the opportunity to help patients. The director of development views the sale of mailing lists as a way to raise money for the cardiac program's activities. Both he and the physician-director spent an hour trying to convince the CEO that it is appropriate to release the mailing lists for this worthy purpose.

This case suggests the legitimate but opposing and competing considerations that are a part of patient care, research, fund-raising, and a limited duty of general beneficence to help patients solve problems indirectly linked to medical treatment. The case highlights the ethical problems of safeguarding the confidentiality of patient information. Using the information in the way requested violates the confidentiality of patient treatment and diagnosis. Some direct benefits may inure to patients (e.g., opportunity to obtain life insurance) and some indirect benefits may inure to the organization (e.g., improved data for epidemiological studies). Nevertheless, using the mailing lists as suggested serves no valid research purpose, nor does it directly further patients' medical treatment. Data that do not identify patients serve the same epidemiological purposes. The promise of mortality data on insurance purchasers is incidental to the research effort, and the money earned selling the mailing lists is likely to be modest. Regardless, these utilitarian arguments are irrelevant because such uses are incompatible with the principle of respect for persons, which includes confidentiality. The previous use of the lists to solicit contributions was inappropriate and cannot be used to support making the lists available now.

A weightier ethical argument for using mailing lists could be made if all University Hospital patients were included, rather than identifying groups by diagnoses. Mailing to all former patients identifies only that they were patients at University Hospital, but even this activity may raise concerns over confidentiality for some former patients. The problem of mailing lists can be minimized by determining on admission whether patients object to being on mailing lists used for hospital purposes, such as fund-raising.

University Hospital's use of mailing lists must be distinguished from selling or renting them. Patients must be informed if the hospital intends to use a mailing list commercially. Chapter 9 discusses several of the issues incident to obtaining consent in similar situations. Confidentiality concerns change and patients should know that they can ask that their names be removed from a mailing list at any time. Rental or sale of mailing lists in health services settings is fraught with ethical difficulties and is best avoided.

MONITORING CLINICAL ACTIVITIES

Managers are agents of the organization, but as decision makers whose actions have moral implications and as members of a profession, managers are never simply instruments of the organization. Managers have duties to patients independent of those the organization has to the patient or the physician's duties to the patient. Manager's duties are not limited to problems with the business office or the quality of food but extend to clinical activities. In terms of the patient the manager is the organization's conscience.

Nonphysician managers do not judge clinical activities as would a physician. Just as they use technical experts to develop a new computer system or prepare a loss prevention management program, managers rely on experts in nursing and medicine to assist in understanding these activities and their outcomes. Experienced managers have considerable knowledge about clinical medicine, and, in a gross fashion this knowledge enables them to determine when problems are present. Regardless of their clinical sophistication, their purpose is not to be junior physicians but to understand what physicians do and what they need and want. The primary reason to understand clinical activities is to help the organization serve patients.

The health services organization benefits most when involvement is bidirectional—managers should expect and seek physician involvement in administrative decision making. The evidence is clear that hospitals in which physicians participate in management decision making achieve superior results.

An important role of managers in clinical settings is to link the formal and informal organizations. Anecdotal evidence suggests that informal communications are helpful, perhaps critical, in identifying clinical problems, and that they are an important supplement to formal systems. Nursing is especially significant as an informal link. Deficient performance by physicians is often identified initially by nurses. Information provided by them can alert the formal system and be a starting point for further inquiry. Disciplinary actions cannot be based on rumor, however; managers must ensure adequate follow-up and investigation in conjunction with normal quality control and improvement. Should it be necessary, however, the manager must take the action needed to protect the patient. As a moral agent, the prudent, ethical manager cannot ignore situations that jeopardize the patient or the organization. Sometimes, however, the tables are turned, as in the following example.

A Different Kind of Risk

Dr. Sagatius has just returned to his office after seeing the risk manager. He was very upset and slammed the door behind him before slumping into his chair. He wouldn't stand for it, not again, he said to himself. This was the final straw. Hospital administration was not going to push him around!

He thought back to the two previous incidents in the pediatrics unit and considered their similarity. Now there was a third incident; this time a different nurse was involved, however. Another one of his patients had been medicated incorrectly—actually overdosed. Luckily, Dr. Sagatius had been able to intervene once again before serious consequences occurred. The child would have to stay in the hospital several days longer because long-term consequences were possible. He had reported the first two instances to the nurse supervisor. Now he would have to take other action.

The day following the third incident, Dr. Sagatius was asked by the risk manager to stop by her office. While there, he saw the child's medical record lying on her desk. Dr. Sagatius noticed that the risk manager had changed the medication record, which he knew had previously shown the overdose. When he asked the risk manager about it, she said that it did not matter because no apparent harm had come to the child. "Why needlessly upset the parents?" she asked. When Dr. Sagatius protested that this was not honest, the risk manager became hostile and reminded Dr. Sagatius that a malpractice suit would hurt all those affiliated with the hospital, including the doctors, who were almost certain to be sued should this error come to light. She warned him not to discuss what happened with anyone, especially not with the parents.

Dr. Sagatius planned to tell the parents about the overdose, believing that they were owed an explanation for the extra days in the hospital. Also, they had to watch for signs of long-term effects of the overdose and seek medical treatment for the child should they occur.

Dr. Sagatius weighed his options. He knew he had to tell the parents to watch the child closely, even if he did not discuss the overdose. He obtained the parents' phone number.

Dr. Sagatius faces two ethical problems. The first problem concerns the risk manager. Ethically, Dr. Sagatius's primary duty is to protect the interests of his patient, which means that he must provide the parents with the information they need to monitor their child. Providing this information meets the principles of beneficence and nonmaleficence. How can he carry out this duty given the position of the risk manager? The risk manager has violated the principle of respect for persons. In addition, by covering up clinical failures, the risk manager is facilitating a system that violates the principle of nonmaleficence.

The second ethical problem involves the nursing supervisor, who has not acted to prevent a recurrent, serious problem in the pediatrics unit. Such inaction is inconsistent with the principles of beneficence and nonmaleficence. Dr. Sagatius is ethically obligated to report the persistent problem in quality to more senior managers through the medical staff or other appropriate means.

Medical record falsification is rare, even though it is human nature to want to hide failure. Managers' ethical obligations commonly become submerged in the legal dimensions of a problem. As a result, the patient becomes the enemy and those in the organization circle the wagons and move into a defensive posture. Patients and family sense this and are spurred all the more to press for an explanation, a kind word, perhaps even an apology. Lacking these, they become angry, which makes them more likely to sue. This utilitarian argument also supports the unpleasant but preferred course of being forthcoming and honest with injured patients. Anecdotal evidence suggests that patients and families understand that mistakes occur and things go wrong; what they cannot understand is deceit and coldness. Organizations that acknowledge their mistakes and strive to make things right are better served ethically (and legally) than those who fight to the death.

All members of the organization must scrutinize the health services delivered and take action as necessary. If this is seen as "ratting" or being a "stool pigeon," the organization's culture is in need of change. Such a negative interpretation is possible only if one ignores the reason for being of the organization and those who work there. Both exist to further the interests of patients. When problems occur in the delivery of services, the organization and its managers must act to minimize loss and injury and do whatever is possible to make the patient whole. The manager must be involved, as necessary, to eliminate or reduce the recurrence of problems in clinical services.

WHISTLEBLOWING

When an employee reveals information about illegal, inefficient, or wasteful action that endangers the health, safety, or freedom of the public it is called *whistleblowing*.[2] This definition is broad enough to include revelations of mismanagement, including nonfeasance, misfeasance, and malfeasance. As used here, whistleblowing affects the private and public sectors and includes the disclosure of information both within the organization and externally. Reasons for whistleblowing may occur at two levels: activities by individuals and activities by the organization.

An extreme example many health services managers will recognize is that of an organization that harbors a clinical or management staff member whose incompetence or incapacitation is known, except, of course, to those outside of the organization. Despite this knowledge, no action is taken. The organization's culture discourages acting against those "in the club," or the fear of retribution and lack of support in remedying the problem make the price too high. Thus, the problem continues until a catastrophe occurs or the situation becomes intolerable to a critical mass of managers and staff and action is forced. Much of the stimulus is fear of public exposure and the embarrassment or disciplinary action that is likely to result. Such motivation is not the stuff of moral agents, who act because it is right to do so.

Three types of activities are affected by whistleblowing: clear illegality, potential illegality or danger, and the organization's social policy.[3]

Clear illegality occurs when the law is knowingly violated. Examples include falsifying information reported to government, bribing inspectors, making illegal campaign contributions, falsifying audits, deliberately violating labor laws, discriminating in employment because of race or gender, and improperly disposing of hazardous wastes.[4]

The second type of activity affected by whistleblowing involves *potential illegality or danger*. A growing body of regulations and case law protects employee health, patient safety, public health, and the environment. In addition, managers and employees are moral agents, who are morally obligated to take action when there is reason to believe that patients are at risk, regardless of other requirements. In most situations in which whistleblowing occurs or should occur, the whistleblower acts in the belief that a given practice, process, or result is either not in compliance with accepted standards or places the patient unnecessarily at risk. "In any well-run enterprise, management should be seriously concerned about such violations and should welcome warnings by its own employees."[5]

The third type of activity affected by whistleblowing involves the *organization's social policy*. An employee may become concerned about the morality of a management policy and its effect on patients or society. For example, an employee may believe that the net revenue of a not-for-profit health services organization is excessive or spent inappropriately and that too little is used for indigent care. Speaking out or refusing to participate is likely to be protected by conscience clauses in state or federal statutes or by the U.S. Constitution, if state action is involved. Assuming the policy is legal, employee protest raises two issues: the employee's right to free speech and the employee's responsibility as a moral agent. Employees are entitled to the same constitutionally protected right of free speech as are other individuals. Furthermore, as moral agents they have an ethical duty to speak out when policies and actions could or do adversely affect patients or society. The controversy usually arises when an employee exercises the right of free speech or the duty of moral agency by speaking publicly against an organization's lawful policy, thereby harming its reputation and market advantage.[6]

Health services organizations create a paradox when they encourage managers and staff to act responsibly in all situations without causing unnecessary disruption. When the organization or individuals in it act illegally, inefficiently, or wastefully, employees are expected to be loyal and not speak out. This paradox is less easily resolved as organizations become more competitive because employees are asked to deal aggressively with external competitors but to be complacent internally.

In 1986 a significant new dimension was added to whistleblowing when Congress enacted the False Claims Act, which strengthened previous legislation protecting individuals who discover and report fraud in federally funded programs. One provision allows these individuals to sue in the name of the federal government, with the incentive that they will receive 15%–30% of any triple damages and fines that are imposed. Such suits are known as *qui tam* actions (*qui tam*, from the Latin *who as well for the king as for himself sues in the matter*). The vast amounts of money spent by the federal government in programs such as Medicare result in significant potential for fraud. It is likely that many *qui tam* suits will be brought in the health services sector. Such efforts may help managers understand what is acceptable and modify their practices accordingly.

Examples of Whistleblowing

When considering these cases it is important to bear in mind that employees and managers are moral agents with an ethical duty to speak out when policies and actions could or do affect patients or society adversely. This is true regardless of other requirements, such as the law.

How Sweet It Is!

Dr. A. Grace Pierce joined the research staff of Ortho Pharmaceutical Corporation in 1971. In 1975 she was part of a team developing a prescription drug known generically as loperamide. The drug was used to treat acute and chronic diarrhea in infants, children, and older adults. Saccharin was used to make it palatable by masking its bitter taste.

The research team agreed that the formula was unsuitable because it substantially exceeded FDA saccharin limits. Management was informed of this fact, but decided nevertheless to file a new drug application with the FDA. Other members of the research team continued development, but Dr. Pierce refused. Although she was offered work in other projects at no decrease in pay, she resigned her position, apparently believing her refusal had irrevocably damaged her career at Ortho.

Later, she sought relief in the courts, alleging wrongful discharge. The New Jersey Supreme Court ruled that Ortho had not acted illegally and that there were no grounds for a cause of action.[7]

The court placed substantial weight on the fact that there was no imminent harm to the public. The court ruled that the ethic of the Hippocratic oath did not contain a clear mandate of public policy that would have prevented Dr. Pierce from continuing her research.

Similar cases have occurred in organizations that deliver health services, as in the following case.

It's Really Only an X ray

Frances O'Sullivan was an X ray technician employed by several radiologists and a hospital. She brought suit for breach of an employment contract after she was fired. She alleged she was fired for refusal to perform catheterizations, a procedure she had not been trained to perform. O'Sullivan could not legally perform catheterizations in New Jersey, where only licensed nurses and physicians may do so. The issue involved was unique because the plaintiff had been asked to perform an illegal act. The superior court denied the defendant physicians' and hospital's motion to dismiss.[8]

Denying the motion to dismiss meant that O'Sullivan was entitled to a trial on the merits of the case. No report exists that this occurred and it may be assumed that the case was settled out of court. In light of the illegality of what O'Sullivan was asked to do, she acted properly.

Another case is also illustrative.

Don't Speak Now and Forever Hold Your Peace

Linda Rafferty was a psychiatric nurse at a state institution in which the conditions were appalling. The abuses Rafferty claimed to have observed included the staff failing to protect patients from sexual abuse by other patients and from sexual exploitation by outside employees; providing improper nonpsychiatric medical care; allowing patients to keep medications in their rooms; locking up fire extinguishers; leaving blank prescription forms that were signed in advance by physicians in unlocked drawers for nurses to fill out on weekends; and hospital medical staff being chronically absent from work. Rafferty repeatedly complained to her superiors, but resigned when her protests brought no change.

She was hired at another institution, Community Mental Health Center, as supervisor of nurses. Before she was hired, she gave an interview to a Philadelphia newspaper in which she was sharply critical of treatment at the state institution. The morning after the story appeared, she was fired from her new position because "staff members were upset about the article." No other reasons were given until trial, when the Health Center alleged inadequate job performance in addition to the previous reason.

Rafferty brought suit alleging she had been deprived of her constitutional rights. The court ruled that she be reinstated and be awarded over $3,000 in back pay.[9]

These whistleblowing cases resulted in court decisions. The professional literature and popular press frequently report whistleblowing such as that at the University of California Irvine Medical Center. Two senior administrators were fired for allegedly retaliating against three employees who had reported physician misconduct at the center's fertility clinic. Among other allegations, the whistleblowers said that physicians were implanting eggs and embryos into patients without donor consent. An internal investigation corroborated the whistleblowers' allegations and showed that after reporting the wrongdoing they were treated poorly by medical center management and clinic physicians and subsequently fired.[10] Another whistleblower case alleges that 132 research center hospitals conspired to deliberately miscode procedures and manipulate patient records in order to obtain $1 billion in federal reimbursement for the use of investigational devices, which are not covered under Medicare and Medicaid guidelines. The hospitals have argued that diagnosis-related groups (DRGs) pay by diagnosis rather than by products used, and thus payment was due regardless of treatment. The facts of the case suggest that this is a *qui tam* case brought under the federal False Claims Act.[11]

A clear example of a *qui tam* suit can be found in the Pineville (Kentucky) Community Hospital case, in which a new physician found that several of his physician colleagues were not performing some patient histories, physical examinations, and other services listed in patient records. Medical records clerks were writing histories and physicals based on information in the medical records or, occasionally, from interviews with patients. The document created by the clerk became the basis for the physician's bill to Medicare for a comprehensive history and physical. Similarly, on discharge the records clerk used information from the medical record to prepare a discharge summary, which was stamped with the physician's signature. The physician's office used this document to bill Medicare for a discharge examination and treatment plan. After repeated efforts to change the practice, the new physician brought a *qui tam* suit. In settling the case the hospital agreed to pay $2.3 million; each of the two physicians involved in the fraudulent practices paid $100,000. Had the case gone to trial and maximum damages and penalties been awarded, the total recovered from the defendants could have been $31 million. It was alleged that the hospital's administration hindered efforts to end the fraudulent practices. Regrettably, but not unexpectedly, the whistleblower was viewed as the problem by many at the hospital and in the community.[12]

These cases highlight the three significant issues relating to whistleblowing as an ethical problem in health services organizations. The first issue is employee responsibility and accountability, something that applies to all employees, whether or not they are managers. The second issue is fair practices. To encourage responsibility and accountability, due process procedures are necessary to protect employees who consider themselves moral agents and are courageous enough to speak out. Due process regarding employee disciplinary actions (both in terms of procedure and substance) is necessary, whether the organization is one to which federal or state constitutional protections apply. Being bound by such requirements will also encourage others to act when they should. Methods must be developed to balance the individual's duty to the employer against the duty to the public. This can be difficult because "many of the rights and privileges . . . so important to a free society that they are constitutionally protected . . . are vulnerable to abuse through an employer's power."[13] The third issue is how to encourage employees to speak out in appropriate ways in order to meet their independent duty to the patient, without causing unnecessary damage to the indispensable cooperative and trust relationships that exist within the organization as well as between them and their communities.

Negative Aspects of Whistleblowing

Several negative aspects temper what is positive about whistleblowing: Whistleblowers may be incorrect in what they allege to be the facts of management's misconduct. Determining the accuracy of whistleblowing charges is not always easy. The danger exists that incompetent or inadequate employees may become whistleblowers to avoid facing justifiable disciplinary actions. Employees can blow the whistle in unacceptably disruptive ways, regardless of the merits of their protest. Some whistleblowers are not protesting unlawful or unsafe behavior but social policies by management that the employee considers unwise or unethical. The legal definitions of a safe product, danger to health, or improper treatment of employees are often not clear. The efficiency and flexibility of human resources management could be threatened by the creation of legal rights to dissent and legalized review systems. Risks to the desirable autonomy of the private sector are possible because a review of allegations by whistleblowers will expand government's role too deeply into internal business policies.[14]

Courses of Action

Managers with the authority to remedy a problem are morally bound to do so. If persons in authority will not act, there are alternatives consistent with the duty of loyalty managers and staff have to the organization, even if these alternatives ultimately involve public disclosure. It is ethically appropriate to act early, even at the risk of embarrassing an organization, than to await further corruption, with its attendant greater risk of harm to others as well as the organization. The alternatives involve whistleblowing of various types. Regrettably, whistleblowing has a bad connotation for many. It suggests disloyalty to the group, if not to the organization—the person who blows the whistle is considered a "stool pigeon" or informer, a betrayer. Despite its pervasiveness, this reasoning is perverse. How, for example, how could one be considered a traitor by informing senior management of illegal or incompetent actions that risk the health of patients or staff? The perception persists, nonetheless. Changing this perception is a challenge for management.

One type of whistleblowing involves stimulating action by approaching persons in authority directly. Working with persons of like mind—finding allies and strength in numbers—can reinforce and stimulate the need to act. In an environment of fear anonymous communication with persons who are able to remedy the problem may be necessary to produce the desired result.

It is crucial that there be a change in the atmosphere typically found in an organization—the "I win, you lose" (zero-sum) approach to whistleblowing. Responsible reporting will benefit employees and employers, but most important, the patient. As Bowman, Elliston and Lockhart[15] point out, "Directing corrective efforts to (whistleblowers) instead of the policy or practice they protest will not alter the conditions that make whistleblowing necessary." This attitude was pervasive at Pineville when the whistleblower was perceived by many people to be the problem.

Place of Whistleblowing

Leading commercial companies have created ombudsman programs in which one person receives, investigates, and responds to employee complaints. Such programs are important for employees who believe illegal or improper conduct is occurring. The problem is that the ombudsman may lack the authority to solve problems in line departments. The ombudsman may not be empowered to deal with senior managers who actively promote illegal or improper conduct as an organizational imperative.[16]

Even where employees are protected by law, as in federal employment, they fear reprisals. A 1992 survey by the Merit Systems Protection Board found that 50% of employees who said they knew firsthand of illegal acts or waste in federal government failed to report it. Only 13% of whistleblowers were given credit from management for doing the right thing; 71% said their supervisors or upper management became unhappy with them. Of whistle-blowers, 37% said they had experienced or had been threatened with retaliation. The retaliation included poor performance appraisals, being shunned by co-workers and managers, and verbal harassment or intimidation.[17]

The concept of moral agency and the willingness to speak and act as necessary remain central, recurring themes for managers and caregivers alike. Professional dissent is critical to the field of health services administration and the delivery of health services. No morality exists without action; ethics will survive only if people speak their consciences when it matters. Professionals are distinguished by the ability to recognize ethical problems and to act as moral custodians of the organization in which they work.

Organizational Culture

The word whistleblowing is itself unfortunate terminology. Historically, it suggests the work of a police officer who used a whistle to summon assistance in apprehending criminals. It would be far better to make the concept one of highlighting the quality culture, one in which calling attention to a problem is considered positive, not negative.

Managers must work to establish and nurture a culture in which problems of nonfeasance, malfeasance, or misfeasance are easily communicated and action is taken. Such a culture is the ounce of prevention that is worth a pound of cure. The acculturation begins in the recruitment and selection processes and continues with new employee orientation. Later, it must be reinforced by the example of formal and informal leaders.

This culture of responsibility, openness, and commitment on the part of management is essential to developing a meaningful internal policy on whis-tleblowing. Also essential is drafting the principles and policy statements that apply management's intention throughout the organization and communicating the policy to employees. The importance of middle and line managers must be stressed. Not only must they be knowledgeable about the policy but reviews must ensure their adherence to it.

Identifying, communicating, and solving problems are made easier if the elements of fear and fault finding are removed from the equation, an approach that is consistent with the philosophy of W. Edwards Deming. Even Deming recognized that a small percentage of problems is caused by the employee, but that the greatest gain in quality will occur by improving the process. In the case of impairment because of substance abuse or other willful acts with negative effect, however, focusing on the individual is a necessary first step.

Assessing and Improving Quality of Care

Through their organizations, health services managers are charged with the weighty responsibility of assessing and improving the quality of patient care. Managers cannot directly assess clinical quality, but are ethically bound to support and encourage the efforts of experts who can and do. Sometimes, managers must stimulate quality assessment and corrective action. More important, managers are key in leading the organization to adopt the philosophy and concepts of quality improvement and to apply its methods.

Consistent with the manager's duties of beneficence and nonmaleficence is to discourage or actively oppose establishing or continuing a clinical service that exposes patients to unnecessary risk. One source of risk amply demonstrated by research findings is performing a low volume of procedures. Early studies suggested that successful cardiac surgery was correlated positively with the number of procedures and that hospitals performing few procedures had poorer outcomes than hospitals performing many. Patient acuity may have explained some of the difference, but its contribution was not examined specifically. Another explanation may have been that the cardiac surgery programs willing to accept higher-risk patients were those that performed fewer procedures. Absent that explanation, the studies recommended that low-volume/high-risk programs be closed. Data published in 1995 and 1996 support these recommendations and include physician and geographic area volumes, as well as improved outcomes and lower costs.[18]

As one would expect, there have been similar findings in surgery generally. A study of 266,944 patients sponsored by the National Center for Health Services Research (part of the Department of Health and Human Services) and reported in 1984 found that hospitals performing surgical procedures infrequently experienced a substantially higher death rate for patients than hospitals performing high volumes of the same operations. The study found that patients in nine surgical specialties had a 13% greater chance of dying if their operations were performed in hospitals that performed relatively few operations. The study also found that patients in hospitals that performed a low volume of surgeries tended to be hospitalized longer than patients in institutions with a high volume of surgeries. In explaining the findings, one of the authors noted:

> Individual staff members may become more highly qualified because of their increased experience in dealing with patients; organizational routines are more likely to be devised, and their regular use may enhance the performance of all participants; and specialized facilities and equipment may be more likely to be on hand.[19]

Similar results have been obtained in other studies about the value of regionalizing to increase volume by concentrating on certain procedures.[20] A study reported in 1989 confirmed the findings of the earlier studies, although it looked at physician volume rather than hospital volume.[21] Findings such as these have important implications for managers whose organizations either have a low-volume service or are considering undertaking a surgical service that is likely to remain low volume.

Higher-Risk Procedures

Community Hospital was established in 1907 with a grant from a wealthy local industrialist. The star of its long history of educating nurses and physicians is a surgical residency program, a key element of which is cardiac surgery. Two years ago, the cardiac surgery program was set back substantially by the death of the chief of cardiac surgery and the departure of a member of the team. Referrals declined markedly and the volume of open heart procedures dropped to five per month.

The quality assessment department performs special studies for various clinical services. Recently it reviewed mortality data from cardiac surgery and found that mortality rates were more than double the rates found in the literature. The director of quality assessment expressed concern as she discussed the report with the chief executive officer (CEO). She noted that the literature reported an inverse relationship between mortality rates and the number of procedures performed. It seemed that technical competence could be gained only by performing a high volume of procedures.

Soon after, the CEO saw the medical director at lunch. During their conversation, the CEO asked whether he had any reason to believe that the cardiac surgery program was of lower quality than it had been in the past. The medical director replied, "As far as I know, things are fine." When she inquired as to the reason for the concern, the CEO replied that the frequency of performing cardiac procedures had declined and that the literature suggested that this had implications for the quality of care. In fact, the hospital's review had confirmed this information. The medical director said she would look into it. The discussion moved to other matters.

The problem for Community Hospital and its patients is apparent. An ethical problem exists because patients undergoing cardiac surgery there are at higher risk than they would be in a high-volume hospital, and this violates the principle of nonmaleficence. The CEO may not ignore what is happening; to do so is inconsistent with the manager's role as a moral agent as well as that of a professional with an independent duty to protect patients. What is the next step? Discontinuing the program immediately may be politically and economically impossible, but steps must be taken now to gain the support of the medical staff and to apprise the governing body of the problem. Whether or not the medical staff lends its support, the CEO must urge the governing body to suspend the program.

What happens if working within the organization proves fruitless because no one will listen? What if the problem is acknowledged, but the persons in authority will not act? This situation is a significant test of the manager's ethic because it poses a true ethical dilemma: The manager is confronted with conflicting moral duties. On the one hand, information about the cardiac surgery program is confidential and the manager has a duty of loyalty to the organization. On the other hand, organization inaction places patients at special risk. Weighing these conflicting duties should lead the manager to conclude that the higher duty is that of protecting patients. The manager must press and pursue, even to the point of releasing information outside the organization if corrective action is not taken. Going public with such damaging information (whistleblowing) is a last resort and is an act of great moral courage. Whistleblowing will make the manager a pariah in the organization, someone likely to be terminated for what will be seen as an act of betrayal.

The CEO might consider two other options that are more pragmatic but ethically less desirable. One option is to ignore the short-term implications of the decline in quality of care and find ways to build on program strengths to increase volume and quality. Another option is to separate the types of procedures done into those more and less risky and concentrate on performing the former. Both approaches place patients at greater risk. This option seems unconscionable in terms of the principles of beneficence and nonmaleficence, however. Absent an emergency or triage situation, one cannot justify the harm to some (patients) because of benefit to others (surgeons and residents, and hospital income and status). Using patients as a means to an end is morally wrong.

It has been suggested that the prospective payment system (DRGs) will eliminate lower-volume higher-risk programs because these are also likely to incur higher costs. Such reasoning may be faulty. A lower-quality program may be less expensive than one of high quality. These programs might do well financially under DRGs, depending on other variables. If eliminating high-risk programs is justified in terms of quality of care, it must be done directly.

Other issues go beyond reviewing and assuring a clinician's competence: determining the adequacy of support staff and equipment, evaluating the patient's clinical appropriateness for a procedure, and acting when a clinician's abilities decline. Often, the problem is apparent only retrospectively. Some processes allow concurrent quality control.

Operating Beyond His Skill?

Jim Hudson picked up the form that had been delivered by the operating room (OR) scheduling clerk and began to review the procedures scheduled for 2 days hence. Hudson's job is to ensure that surgical packs, equipment, time, and personnel are adequate to meet the demands of surgery. The schedule included a procedure that Hudson had never seen listed before. Looking at the column that showed whether special equipment was needed, Hudson saw a note that the attending surgeon would provide the items. This notation puzzled him because it was the responsibility of the OR supervisor or the purchasing department to provide everything needed for a surgical procedure. Hudson called the chief of surgery, to whom OR staff reported clinically. He was unavailable, but his secretary promised he would return the call.

When the chief of surgery called, he was noncommittal. "If the procedure is scheduled," he said, "it's probably okay for it to be done." The clear implication was that the surgeon would not perform a procedure with inadequate preparation.

Hudson was not sure what to do. Not being a physician, any further action by him would certainly be seen as meddling. Nevertheless, it seemed necessary, perhaps even crucial.

This case focuses on a problem of quality. Similar situations are faced regularly by clinicians. Recent changes will make future monitoring and review even more complex and problematic. Hudson must do more than ponder the problem. Hudson should query the attending surgeon, and if that does not produce satisfactory information, the problem should be taken higher up the administrative hierarchy. Additional information may clear up the questions; it may also cause the procedure to be cancelled.

To obtain routine information on quality of services, health services organizations establish systems to review the content of clinical and administrative activities. Table 2 shows examples of quality measures. The parallels between the two are apparent. It should be stressed, however, that these are primarily objective functions and measures. The judgments and conclusions of individuals reviewing the data are also required. It is these conclusions that trigger action.

MAINTAINING RELATIONS WITH THE COMMUNITY

The health services organization is usually considered quasi-public, regardless of ownership. It has a service orientation and an ethical obligation to meet community health needs. This relationship necessitates building and retaining community confidence and it means taking steps to act in the interests of people in the community who are as yet only potential patients. If potential patients risk acquiring an infection or are in danger because the facility is operating with physical plant or life safety code deficiencies, the organization has special obligations to them.

Table 2. Some measures of hospital quality

Feature	Measures of patient care quality	Measures of administrative quality
Structure	Accreditation Medical staff qualifications Professional staff qualifications Professional staff training Special care unit availability/ utilization	Accreditation Administrative staff qualifications Use of employee development programs Personnel per occupied bed Services provided
Process	Medical staff peer review Average length of stay Autopsy rate Community involvement	Use of management studies Occupancy rate Management planning activities Community involvement
Outcome	Patient outcome Surgical procedures assessment Adjusted death rate Hospital-acquired infections: reported/treated Malpractice suits	Cost per unit of output Staff-hours per patient-day Financial stability
Attitude	Expert evaluation of patient care Patient satisfaction (dissatisfaction)	Expert evaluation of administrative performance Employee satisfaction (dissatisfaction)

Adapted from Grimes, R., & Moseley, S. (1976, Fall). An approach to an index of hospital performance. *Health Services Research, 2,* p. 289.

Protecting the Community

University Hospital plays a unique role in the community. It is a tertiary referral hospital for the region and a major source of health care to the community. In 1977 it experienced an outbreak of legionella (Legionnaires' disease). A number of patients contracted the disease; several died.

Legionella is a bacterial infection of the respiratory tract and lungs that may result in death if not diagnosed and treated early. It is especially dangerous for older adults and people with medical problems that weaken their general resistance. A factor requiring even greater caution on the part of hospital management is that at the time of the outbreaks, the process for identifying the organism in the laboratory took several days. Thus, patients were at greater risk until a confirmatory diagnosis was obtained.

Epidemiological studies showed a relationship between air conditioning cooling towers and the fine aerosol mist they give off and the spread of the disease through the aerosol. Employees exposed directly to the aerosol contracted severe cases of legionella. Chlorinating the water in the cooling towers eliminates the organism. Although a cooling tower was suspected in the 1977 outbreak at University Hospital, the relationship was never confirmed. The hospital's infection control committee did not develop any standing orders or policies after the first outbreak.

In May 1982 there was evidence of another outbreak of legionella. The cooling tower water was immediately chlorinated and the number of new cases dropped dramatically. However, an undetected failure in the chlorination system brought a second outbreak in early June.

When the first cases were detected in May 1982, the hospital administrator was notified. He met with various staff members, including physicians. It was decided that information about the outbreak should be kept from the community, lest a panic and sudden drop in census occur, as well as loss of public confidence. A confidential letter was sent to staff physicians advising them of the problem and asking that they keep in mind the potential for infection when making admissions decisions. Admissions were not limited to emergencies, however, and there was neither a prospective review of elective admissions to determine whether patients at risk for pulmonary infections such as legionella should be sent elsewhere nor a review of indications for and necessity of admission. The medical staff developed a protocol stating that unexplained, acute-onset pneumonias were to be treated immediately with a potent antibiotic known to be effective against legionella. However, no provision was made for effective review to determine that the protocol was actually followed.

The administrator at University Hospital faced several problems, all with ethical dimensions:

1. The medical staff wanted to continue admitting patients.
2. The community could lose confidence in the hospital if it learned that there is an epidemic of a potentially deadly disease.
3. The administrator and management staff could lose face, even their jobs, should the infection become common knowledge.
4. The potential existed for significant legal liability.

Solving this ethical problem is difficult but by no means impossible. Similar situations arise in nursing facilities that are threatened with closure because their physical plants violate fire safety requirements and in hospitals in which outbreaks of meningitis or salmonella occur in the nursery. How does the organization protect current as well as potential patients in such situations? More important, what is the manager's role?

One feature that distinguishes the legionella outbreak from other, similar cases is the difference in duty owed to potential rather than actual patients. The law recognizes a difference. Generally, unless there is a special relationship with potential patients, one has no duty to act on their behalf. In this case, however, there would be a duty to warn elective admissions who are at risk from legionella.

The legal distinction is useful in ethical analysis. The duty to assist actual patients is immediate and more compelling than the duty toward potential patients. Even potential patients should not be put at risk, unless their medical condition puts them at greater risk outside the hospital than inside it. Inpatients who might benefit from a continued stay but who are at greater risk by remaining in the hospital should be discharged. It is incumbent on the managerial and clinical staff to make caregivers understand the obligation to protect the patient.

The argument that the administrator has a duty to protect the reputation of the organization in the community has merit because individuals needing hospitalization should have no fear about receiving it and because of the significant psychological component in health care. Furthermore, individuals may be at greater risk by not obtaining treatment for their medical problems than they are from legionnella. Yet, they may defer care because they are frightened or lack confidence in the facility.

At admission, potential risk becomes actual risk. Emergency admissions pose no ethical problem if an alternative source of care is unavailable and the risk of no care is greater than that of contracting legionnella.

Elective admissions are quite different. At the very least, the organization, led and prompted by its managers, should have developed and applied policies and procedures separating high- from low-risk elective admissions and made special provisions either to send the former group elsewhere or to take special efforts to protect them. Ethically, it could not rely only on the discretion of the admitting physician. As with any quality assessment activity, management has a responsibility to review decision making about care and do so in a fashion consistent with the level of risk. Here, concurrent review is required.

Obvious potential conflicts of interest exist. It is natural for managers to protect their positions and reputations. They do so out of loyalty to the organization, but also out of selfish motives. A typical response is to cover up. Concealment seems an easy way to reduce the risk of personal and professional damage. Experience suggests, however, that from both an ethical and a pragmatic standpoint honesty is the best policy. Rumors will be carried into the community by staff and patients and the potential tarnish to the organization's reputation may last much longer than if the community is informed that there is a problem and that steps are being taken to protect patients from infection. This tactic may raise questions about the cause of and responsibility for the problem, but the community will not distrust the organization. Furthermore, in terms of guiding ethical principles, the organization treats individuals in the community with respect and dignity by being truthful.

CONCLUSION

Managers who are not physicians do not personally judge the quality of clinical activities. They do, however, have responsibility for providing clinical staff with the systems, procedures, and resources required to be effective. The principles of beneficence and nonmaleficence suggest that managers must have enough awareness of what is expected and how that expectation is measured to determine that the goal of delivering quality health services has been met. Managers are remiss in their ethical (and legal) duties if they occupy themselves exclusively with nonclinical activities and claim that clinical matters lie outside their ken and range of responsibilities. Just as they rely on computer programmers or wage and salary experts for reports, advice, and counsel, managers also rely on technical expertise and assistance in judging patient care. The manager is accountable to the governing body for all activities, and this requires active involvement and effective partnerships between managers and clinicians.

This chapter identified and examined several generic ethical problems arising out of the duties owed by managers to patients and community. The duties are not always clear and may be further obscured by accompanying problems, such as bureaucratic inertia and medical staff relations. They become clear if managers focus on the primary reasons for the organization's existence—serving and protecting the patient and community.

NOTES

1. Peter A. Ubel, Margaret M. Zell, David J. Miller, Gary S. Fischer, Darien Peters-Stefani, & Robert M. Arnold. (1995, August). Elevator talk: Observational study of inappropriate comments in a public space. *American Journal of Medicine, 99,* 190–194.

2. James S. Bowman, Frederick A. Elliston, & Paula Lockhart (Eds.). (1984). *Professional dissent: An annotated bibliography and research guide* (Vol. 2, p. 3). New York: Garland Publishing.

3. Alan F. Westin. (1981). *Whistle blowing! Loyalty and dissent in the corporation* (p. 140). New York: McGraw-Hill.

4. *Ibid.,* p. 139.

5. *Ibid.,* p. 140.

6. *Ibid.*

7. Pierce v. Ortho Pharmaceuticals, 84 N.J. 58, 417 A.2d 505 (1980).

8. O'Sullivan v. Mallon et al., 160 N.J. Super. 416, 390 A.2d 149 (1978).

9. Commonwealth of Pennsylvania ex rel. Rafferty et al. v. Philadelphia Psychiatric Center, 356 F. Supp. 500 (E.D. Pa. 1973).

10. Louise Kertesz. (1995, July 3). Execs fired in whistleblower case. *Modern Healthcare,* p. 11.

11. Lisa Scott. (1995, August 21). Whistleblower suit alleges patient records doctored. *Modern Healthcare,* p. 34. Another example of a *qui tam* suit occurred in United States ex rel. Brandimarte v. Wurtzel, Civ. Action No. 94-2398 (E.D. Pa. Nov. 3, 1995), in which defendants settled allegations of making false and fraudulent claims for psychotherapy services under the Medicare and Medicaid programs by paying $500,000 to the United States and $50,000 toward whistleblower's legal fees and costs.

12. Berkeley Rice. (1995, August 7). When a doctor accuses colleagues of health fraud. *Medical Economics*, pp. 172–174, 177–179, 183–184, and 189–190.
13. Lawrence Blades. (1967, December). Employment at will vs. individual freedom: On limiting the abusive exercise of employer power. *Columbia Law Review, 67*, 1407.
14. Westin, pp. 133–136.
15. Bowman et al., p. 4.
16. Westin, p. 144.
17. Stephen Barr. (1993, October 19). Whistleblowers sound alarm on their superiors' reprisals. *The Washington Post*, p. A21.
18. Volume of procedures for physicians, hospitals, and geographic areas linked to outcomes for angioplasty and bypass patients. (1995, July/August). *Research Activities, 186*, 1–3; and Regionalizing cardiac surgery facilities contributes to improved outcomes and lower costs. (1996, January/February). *Research Activities, 190*, 1–2.
19. Spencer Rich. (1984, April 26). Hospitals doing more operations lose fewer patients. *The Washington Post*, p. A2.
20. Harold S. Luft, John P. Bunker, & Alain C. Enthoven. (1979, December). Should operations be regionalized? *New England Journal of Medicine, 301*(25), 1364–1369.
21. Edward L. Hannan, Joseph F. O'Donnell, Harold Kilburn, Jr., Harvey R. Bernard, & Altan Yazici. (1989, July). Investigation of the relationship between volume and mortality for surgical procedures performed in New York State hospitals. *Journal of the American Medical Association, 262*(4), 503–510.

IV

Biomedical Ethical Issues

art IV analyzes consent and issues at the end of life, the biomedical ethical issues most commonly confronted by health services managers and their organizations. Myriad other biomedical ethical issues affect some managers: genetic engineering, screening, and counseling; reproductive technologies; psychosurgery and behavior control; the right to health care; personhood, fetal rights, and abortion; implants and transplants; and mental illness and involuntary commitment. The effect of some of these issues was addressed tangentially in Part III, but space limits prevent considering them further.

The thorny issue of consent is addressed in Chapter 9. Consent affects managers in all types of health services organizations. The law defines acceptable relationships between provider and patient, but for managers this is but a starting point, one that builds upon their moral agency.

Chapter 10 addresses ethical issues arising at the end of life, often called the ethics of death and dying. Changes occurring since the 1970s, many resulting from new technology, raise new issues. The chapter includes defining death, applying life-sustaining treatment (using the example of infants with impairments), withdrawing treatment, and the ethics of intervening in terminal illnesses. All health services organizations are affected by some or all of the ethical issues that arise at the end of life. Like consent, they have major implications for managers.

Consent

onsent is an ethical imperative of great importance to managers and clinicians. In its study of consent the President's Commission for the Study of Ethical Problems in Medicine and Biomedical and Behavioral Research found that patients generally want to be more involved in medical decision making, a finding that suggests both a problem and a goal for health services providers.

The concept of consent evolved to protect individuals from nonconsensual touching. Although the ethical and legal aspects of consent overlap, the legal requirements are only a minimum. In terms of ethics consent is expanded and is based on the principle of respect for persons, specifically, autonomy, which reflects a view of the equality and dignity of human beings. To a lesser extent the concept of consent in ethics reflects the special relationship of trust and confidence between physician and patient and between organization and patient. This fiduciary relationship is supported by the principles of beneficence and nonmaleficence.

According to the law, failure to obtain consent can support a legal action for battery, an intentional tort. Beyond this, an action for negligence can be brought if the physician breaches the duty to communicate information necessary for the patient to give informed consent.

Paternalism stems from beneficence and is the ethical value that competes with patient autonomy in implementing consent. Paternalism arises naturally from the relationship between physician and patient because psychologically, technically, and emotionally, the physician is in a position of superior knowledge and is expected to choose the best course of action for the patient. Historically, the paternalistic nature of physician–patient relations can be traced to the Hippocratic oath. The sense of beneficence and paternalism continues to be the dominant, implicit theme in the practice of medicine. The Principles of Medical Ethics adopted by the American Medical Association (AMA) in 1980 moved organized medicine from paternalism toward autonomy and patient rights, themes amplified by the AMA's Council on Ethical and Judicial Affairs's statement "Fundamental Elements of the Patient-Physician Relationship." Both documents are reproduced in Appendix B.

Specialized codes, such as the Declaration of Helsinki, which guide biomedical research, also recognize the importance of consent. The emphasis on patients' rights or sovereignty in documents such as these are ideals toward which managers and organizations should strive.

LEGAL ASPECTS

Consent must be voluntary, competent, and informed. The law presumes that in an emergency persons want to receive treatment. This presumption is rebutted if treatment is declined by a competent person, or if the person requiring treatment has an advance directive, such as a nonhospital DNR (do-not-resuscitate) order. In addition, if that person's attorney in fact (e.g., someone who holds a durable power of attorney) is present, consent must be obtained. When minors or mentally incompetent persons are patients, and those who speak for them refuse to give consent, the organization is usually successful in persuading the state to allow treatment.

Even in nonemergencies general consent for treatment is implied by the patient's presence and apparent desire to be treated. Noninvasive elective treatment of a routine nature requires only general consent. For invasive, surgical, or special procedures, or when the patient is part of an experiment, special consent is necessary. Oral consent is as legally binding as written consent, but staff changes, faulty memories, and prudence make written consent necessary. General and special consent forms are shown in Figures 8 and 9.

To be *voluntary*, consent must be given without duress that significantly influences the decision. Whether duress is excessive depends on the facts. Threats or force constitute duress. Sometimes, persons have diminished autonomy; military personnel or prisoners are examples. Historically, these settings were important for research involving human subjects. Negative publicity and subsequent public indignation greatly reduced the amount of experimentation performed in such settings, however.

Competent consent means that the person understands the nature and consequences of the course of treatment. The law presumes minor children to be incompetent. In addition, persons whose mental illness or mental disability have resulted in a legal determination of incompetence may not decide about medical treatment or experimentation and others must make such decisions. Judging mental competence is very complex when patients are terminally ill, depressed, or suicidal.

Consent must be *informed*. The law requires full disclosure of the nature of the patient's condition and treatment proposed, alternatives available, and

The George Washington University/Medical Center

Authorization for Medical Care and Treatment
Authorization for Release of Medical Records to Third-Party Payers
Release of Responsibility for Personal Property/Valuables

1. I have come to George Washington University's Hospital for medical treatment. I ask the health care professionals at the Hospital to provide care and treatment for me that they feel is necessary. I consent to undergo routine tests and treatment as part of this care. I understand that I am free to ask a member of my health care team questions about any care, treatment or medicine I am to receive.

2. Because George Washington University's Hospital is a teaching hospital, I understand that my health care team will be made up of hospital personnel and medical students in addition to my attending physician and his/her assistants and designees. Hospital personnel include, but are not limited to, nurses, technicians, interns, residents, and fellows.

3. I understand that as part of my care and treatment, samples of blood, urine, stool and tissues may be removed from me from time to time. I permit the University to so use leftover blood, urine, stool and tissues for research. (If I do not want the University to so use leftover portions, I may stop the University from doing so by writing "no" in the following block and writing my initials after it [   ].) If additional samples are needed for the research, I will be asked at that time.

4. I am aware that the practice of medicine is not an exact science and admit that no one has given me any promises or guarantees about the result of any care or treatment I am to receive or examinations I am to undergo.

5. I agree to the University's and/or my physician sending copies of my medical records (or information from my medical records) to my insurance provider(s) or other sources of payment, which may include my employers. I understand that this information will be sent when it is needed for payment of my medical bills. I release and forever discharge The George Washington University, its employees and agents and my attending physician from any liability resulting from the release of my medical records or information from them for payment purposes.

6. **Release of Responsibility for Personal Property/Valuables:** I understand the George Washington University is not responsible for any personal property or valuables that I keep with me while I am at the hospital, even if placed in a hospital provided locker. Personal property includes, but is not limited to, clothing, shoes and baggage. Valuables include, but are not limited to, money, credit cards, dentures, eyeglasses, hearing aids and jewelry. I understand, therefore, that I should send my valuables and as much of my property as possible home with my family/friends. I realize that I can request the University's Cashier's Office to store valuables I cannot send home.

7. I agree that photographs of me may be taken during treatment and utilized for research, teaching or other scientific purposes as long as my identity is not disclosed: ☐ YES   ☐ NO

8. I am currently a Tissue/Organ donor: ☐ YES   ☐ NO

EMERGENCY UNIT PATIENTS ONLY

9. I understand that it may be helpful for my personal physician to be involved in the care I receive while I am in The George Washington University Emergency Unit. I therefore allow an Emergency Unit physician to contact my personal physician, Dr. _____ . (If I do not wish my physician to be contacted, I may stop the University from doing so by writing "no" in the following block and writing my initials after it. [   ].)

10. I agree to the University's sending copies of my Emergency Unit record to my personal physician named above. (If I do not wish the University to send a copy to my physician, I may stop the University from doing so by writing "no" in the following block and writing my initials after it. [   ].)

DISCHARGE TIME 10:30 A.M.

AFFIRMATION

I have read this form and understand it. All of my questions about what it says have been answered. A am signing it of my own free will. I understand that by signing it, I am agreeing to it.

_____
Signature of patient (or parent, legal guardian or next-of-kin. Please indicate which)

_____
Date/Time

_____
Witness to affirmation and signature

_____
Date/Time

Figure 8.   A general consent form. (From The George Washington University Medical Center, Washington, DC. © 1996. Reprinted with permission.)

I, Haskell Karp, request and authorize Dr. Denton A. Cooley and such other surgeons as he may designate to perform upon me, in St. Luke's Episcopal Hospital of Houston, Texas, cardiac surgery for advanced cardiac decompensation and myocardial insufficiency as a result of numerous coronary occlusions. The risk of this surgery has been explained to me. In the event cardiac function cannot be restored by excision of destroyed heart muscle and plastic reconstruction of the ventricle and death seems imminent, I authorize Dr. Cooley and his staff to remove my diseased heart and insert a mechanical cardiac substitute. I understand that this mechanical device will not be permanent and ultimately will require a replacement by a heart transplant. I realize that this device has been tested in the laboratory but has not been used to sustain a human being and that no assurance of success can be made. I expect the surgeons to exercise every effort to preserve my life through any of these means. No assurance has been made by anyone as to the results that may be obtained.

I understand that the operating surgeon will be occupied solely with the surgery and that the administration of the anesthetic(s) is an independent function. I hereby request and authorize Dr. Arthur S. Keats, or others he may designate, to administer such anesthetics as he or they may deem advisable.

I hereby consent to the photographing of the operation to be performed, including appropriate portions of my body, for medical, scientific, and educational purposes.

_____   _____
Signature   Date

Figure 9.   A special consent form. (From *Karp v. Cooley*, 349 F. Supp. 827 [S.D. Texas 1972]; aff'd, 493 F2d 408 [5th Cir. 1974], cert. denied, 419 U.S. 845 [1974].)

likely consequences and difficulties that may result from treatment or non-treatment. The courts are about evenly split between those that hold that patients should receive as much information as the reasonable physician would provide under the same or similar circumstances and those that use a standard based on what the reasonable patient would want to know. A legal criterion used by a few courts—and one oriented to patient sovereignty—is what that particular patient would have wanted to know.

Historically, cases involving Jehovah's Witnesses, a religion that prohibits homologous transfusions of whole blood or components, have been problematic for hospitals. Potential legal liability for transfusing or not transfusing the patient has resulted in a number of court cases. In older cases courts often overrode the patient's wishes and ordered transfusions when patients, especially mothers, were charged with significant family responsibilities. Such cases show that judges considered more than liberty rights (autonomy) when important societal interests were present. Developments in bloodless medicine and surgery in the 1960s and 1970s were spurred in the mid-1980s by problems with the blood supply, such as transmission of the human immunodeficiency virus (HIV). The result of these developments has been a complete rethinking of the use of blood and blood products—transfusions are avoided, if possible. In addition, landmark decisions such as *Cruzan v. Missouri Department of Health*, which is discussed in Chapter 10, have recognized a constitutional right to refuse treatment.[1]

Thus, on the basis of either the common law right of bodily self-determination or the Fourteenth Amendment's guarantee of individual liberty, competent adults, incompetent adults who had clearly expressed their wishes, and even older minors with adult-like decision-making capacity have had their right to refuse unwanted blood transfusions recognized.

As for minor children generally, although parents may not deprive their children of necessary care, if the parents have a choice between two or more effective treatment options, the state has no *parens patriae* interest in mandating treatment entailing the use of blood simply because it is the popular or standard approach. If the child's health problem can be effectively managed without the use of homologous blood, the parents should be free to choose that treatment option without governmental interference.[2]

An ethic that emphasizes autonomy and respect for persons can significantly affect the patient–caregiver relationship. Fully expressed, patients alone choose the level of involvement they want. The President's Commission stated that patient sovereignty with complete participation in the process is a desirable, if not a readily achievable, goal.[3] The principle of respect for persons cannot be realized, nor participation achieved, absent truthfulness and the organization's consistent efforts. Autonomy means patients may not agree with caregivers' recommendations and assessments. Sometimes, clinicians and organizations find this concept threatening.

Some patients do not wish to participate in decision making. Whether explicitly or implicitly, they want to remain ignorant of their medical problems and be excluded from decision-making processes. They prefer a paternalistic relationship and they choose to delegate decision-making and allow persons caring for them to do what they think best. This relationship is not the one between patient and caregivers envisioned by the President's Commission, but patients' autonomy is also violated if they are forced to participate. Caregivers and managers should consider a decision not to participate to be an acceptable choice and work to make it a reality.

The law contains a concept called *therapeutic privilege*, which permits physicians to withhold information from patients when the physician believes it serves patients' best interests. States recognize therapeutic privilege in several ways, and a general rule is difficult to state. Some criteria reference the danger full disclosure may cause to a patient's physical or mental health; other criteria focus on the patient's best interests.[4] Such paternalism is supported by the principles of beneficence and nonmaleficence. The therapeutic privilege exception is pragmatic and avails physicians of a range of actions. It is desirable that physicians possess the latitude to make such judgments, especially if the alternative is probable harm to the patient. In these cases, beneficence takes precedence.

Ethical Aspects

The premise for a discussion of the ethics of consent is that the ethical standard is significantly higher than the legal standard. This expectation arises from exercising the principles of respect for persons (autonomy) and nonmaleficence, which are based on Kantian deontology (see Chapter 1), natural law, and rule utilitarianism, and is supported by virtue ethics.

The nuances inherent in duress and inducement are important in determining whether consent is *voluntary*. In these cases ethical considerations and duties extend well beyond the standard in the law. Can patients suffering from a fatal disease make medical decisions voluntarily? Are patients' decisions free of duress if they fear losing their physicians' friendship and loyalty because they prefer an option the physician opposes? Clinical staff talk about "bad" patients, patients who are uncooperative. Such patients are not intentionally harmed or mistreated, but they may not receive the same attention as "good" or pliable patients. Patients sense this attitude and it affects their volition. Patients are also heavily influenced by family and friends and may make decisions because of them. Similarly, family members may ask clinicians to behave in ways that are unwanted by an incompetent patient or that, under the principle of beneficence, do not serve the patient's interests.

Given such considerations, consent may never be voluntary. It has been argued that patients' personal freedom to accept or reject medical treatment has been so reduced that it is only a right to veto unwanted procedures.[5] The complex relationships in medical care preclude simple answers and easy determinations as to the voluntariness of consent. It is critical that managerial and clinical staff understand this and make every effort to further patient autonomy.

In determining the voluntariness of consent, some groups present special problems. For example, healthy persons with diminished autonomy—soldiers, prisoners, even students—may be asked to participate in a nontherapeutic experiment, one with no benefit to them. Because their status limits autonomy, is their consent voluntary? Voluntariness may also be reduced through inducements that cause prudence to be cast aside. Money or other incentives may be offered to participate in a potentially dangerous experiment; for example, indigent persons may be persuaded by money. Students are unique in this regard and may fit into several categories. Often, they are economically disadvantaged. In addition, some instructors encourage students to participate in experiments by exempting them from other, seemingly more onerous requirements such as examinations. Occasionally, there is implicit, or even explicit, coercion by faculty who control the students' academic (and sometimes economic) destiny and who unethically use this position to coerce consent.

Ethical considerations regarding whether one is *competent* to consent are usually easier than those regarding voluntariness. Competence is assumed in adults. Medical personnel can usually determine when a patient's mental capacity is questionable and obtain an expert opinion. Absent such evidence, there should be an explicit assumption in the organization's policies that patients are autonomous in making decisions. It is incumbent on managers to assist in this process through education and the support provided by appropriate systems and procedures.

The third element of consent is that it be *informed*. (Some commentators inaccurately refer to the concept of "informed consent" as though it is the only criterion to consent.) Because of the complexity of informed consent, whether the patient was *adequately informed* receives the most attention. Several states have enacted statutes to ensure that patients obtain adequate information for medical decisions. A Virginia law concerning informed consent was prompted by reports that physicians performed radical mastectomies when removal of malignancy would suffice, and it was claimed that women were not provided with enough information to make an intelligent choice. When introduced, the proposal raised questions among a number of groups, including the American Cancer Society, which stressed that the emphasis should be placed on improved education about the disease and alternative methods of treatment, rather than on a legislative enactment.[6]

Wait a Little Longer, We'll Do it Then

The emergency department at County Hospital has a typical caseload: some true emergencies and urgent medical conditions, but lots of sniffles and other nonemergencies. It contracts with an emergency medicine group, but administrative activities, including systems, procedures, and personnel, are managed by the hospital. The process for obtaining consent is typical: Unconscious patients are treated as indicated. Competent patients who are able to communicate sign a consent form authorizing treatment. Parents and next of kin are involved as needed and as available.

Early one afternoon, a conscious, middle-aged man who had been in a car accident was brought in. He was diagnosed with internal injuries that required immediate exploratory surgery. He was asked to sign the consent form but refused on the grounds that as a Christian Scientist to receive medical treatment violated his religious beliefs. He asked for a Christian Science practitioner.

The physician-director of the emergency department was paged, and, after reviewing the chart, she felt certain she could obtain his consent for surgery. She discussed the situation with the patient, who clearly understood that without surgery death was likely. He continued to refuse and repeatedly asked for a Christian Science practitioner. The director left the treatment area very agitated; her mouth and chin shook in anger. She said, "This man is throwing his life away, all in the name of some religion that denies scientific medicine to its followers. I can't believe he's doing it!" She turned to the nurse and whispered, "Let me know when he's unconscious and we'll save his life, despite his silly ideas."

Such deception rides roughshod over the patient's clearly expressed wishes. The patient is competent, he has been informed, and his refusal is voluntary. In addition to violating the principle of respect for persons (autonomy), the physician is ignoring the AMA's Principles of Medical Ethics and the AMA's Council on Ethical and Judicial Affairs's Fundamental Elements of the Patient–Physician Relationship. Such methods are unconscionable.

The organizational philosophy should consider the issues presented here prospectively. The results could reflect the approach used for Baby Boy Doe, whose case was discussed in Chapter 1. In that chapter it was suggested that the organization might have intervened by petitioning a court to order lifesaving surgery. Such intervention gives less weight to the principle of respect for persons (autonomy) and more to beneficence (and its corollary, utility) and paternalism. Increasing focus on liberty rights such as autonomy by the courts make it unlikely that the Christian Scientist will be forced to undergo surgery, which is true even if he has a family that is dependent on him. The principle of nonmaleficence also supports action by the hospital. However, forcing treatment is paternalistic and significantly limits individual autonomy. The competing ethical principles of such cases pose ethical dilemmas to organizations and managers.

Role of the Organization

What is the organization's role? Patients should give informed, voluntary, and competent consent before treatment—a simple ethical concept. As is often true, difficulties arise in operationalizing the concept; it is in instances such as these that the criteria may be more often violated than met. Since the 1970s organizations have focused greater attention on consent. This emphasis reflects more a fear of legal problems than a desire to do what is ethically correct. Before the 1970s organizations were less concerned about consent because they adopted and amplified the historical paternalistic view of the patient.

Policies and procedures consistent with the organizational philosophy must at minimum be established for obtaining consent, and their application must be systematically monitored. If the philosophy emphasizes patients' rights, actions and efforts to guarantee those rights will be encouraged and actions and efforts to contravene them will be restricted. Specific means exist for allowing patients to assert their rights, but these means are costly and can result in adversarial relationships. One method is to provide an advocate for each patient. Another is to establish an ombudsman office to review problems.

Often, the circumstances of consent are complicated because of the many parties involved (e.g., providers, patient, family), as in the following example.

When Is Consent Consent?

Henry Franklin was an emergency admission to University Hospital. He was diagnosed with mild cardiac failure by an attending physician. Because he was 78 years old and had complicating medical problems, a dispute arose as to the proper course of treatment. The consulting cardiologist recommended that Franklin be treated medically and given the best quality of life possible. The cardiologist estimated that Franklin had 6 months to live.

The cardiac surgeons had a different view. They recommended replacing the aortic and mitral valves and estimated that this procedure would provide at least 2 years of useful life. When the options were described to Franklin, he was told the probability of surviving the surgery was 50%. He decided he would work with the cardiologist.

After hearing his decision, the surgeons intervened directly with Franklin's family. The family agreed with the surgeons and placed great pressure on Franklin. He finally agreed to the procedure. Franklin's body did not withstand the rigors of surgery and he died in the operating room.

Even if informed and competent, Franklin's final decision was made under duress; the circumstances were coercive. In such situations family and physicians press for what they assert are the patient's best interests. However, sometimes both groups are driven by motives that conflict with the patient's self-expressed decision. Family may have various psychological and financial motives; physicians may act out of technological daring or hubris.

The challenge managers face is ensuring patient autonomy. Patients may choose a course of action that is not their first choice or even in their best interests as they view them because they defer to the wishes of others. They may fear abandonment or caregivers' anger if they choose a course of action other than what caregivers want, or what they think caregivers want. An added complexity is that patients are often uncertain about what to do; they vacillate between wanting and not wanting aggressive treatment. Preserving patient autonomy in these circumstances is difficult, perhaps impossible, but must be attempted nonetheless.

The surgeons played an important role in the Franklin case. They may have allowed bravado to cloud good judgment, especially given the probability of success. Franklin's family were also important, and health services organizations interfere at their peril in situations that reflect family dynamics, even though their duty lies with the patient.

What is the role of the organization in determining that patients have consented in a way that meets ethical criteria? Obvious coercion is likely to be noticed by staff. A patient advocate program may minimize duress. Complicating efforts to ensure that consent meets the criteria is that the private attending physician has an independent ethical duty to inform patients about the procedure's nature, consequences, risks, and alternatives. The attending physician also primarily determines that the patient is competent to give consent and does so voluntarily. Some health services organizations see their ethical duty as independently determining or verifying that the criteria of consent have been met. Others ask only that patients sign an authorization that verifies that they have been informed about the procedure by the physician and that permits the hospital to participate in rendering the care to which patients have consented.

Unless it is certain that patients have been informed about the treatment in a way that meets organizational criteria, the ethically preferred course is that staff be involved, at least to the extent of verifying that the patient is informed and competent. The manager must fulfill the organization's positive ethical duty to monitor consent, which includes a process that entails forms and procedures to assist and guide staff as necessary. Physician and nonphysician staff will also benefit from education about the ethical (and legal) dimensions of consent.

The case of Henry Franklin is distinguishable from that of the Christian Scientist. Franklin had had more time to consider his decision, which was likely influenced by his age. The other patient was middle aged, with decades of productive and enjoyable years remaining. Beyond these apparent differences, both cases raise questions about patient autonomy and its relationship to the principles of beneficence and nonmaleficence. The weight given these principles in the organizational philosophy determines the outcome.

Managers of nursing facilities face ethical issues regarding consent similar to those of their counterparts in acute care hospitals. Decision making in nursing facilities is more likely to be complicated by factors such as competence or abandonment of patients. Thus, the process requires special attention.

I Intend to Be Independent

Oliver Harris is 82 years old and has been a resident at Five Oaks Nursing Home for 7 years. When he first sought admission, Harris had been evaluated and found to be only marginally in need of the care provided at Five Oaks. Because he was a private pay patient, management decided to admit him. For 5 years his health was such that he needed minimal nursing care. In Year 6 he showed evidence of dementia. Medical evaluation found that he had experienced several minor strokes. Harris was physically active and had always done a great deal of walking in the facility. He liked to visit other patients as he went around the facility. His declining medical condition resulted in several falls, which caused cuts and bruises, but as yet no broken bones.

Harris's case was discussed at a staff conference. It was the consensus that he be physically restrained so that he could not ambulate independently, but this was possible under federal guidelines only with an order from Harris's physician. Staff doubted the physician would agree, but they believed that if he continued to walk unassisted it was only a matter of time before he fell and broke a bone. The issue was discussed with Harris, but he was adamant that he not be restrained. His daughter agreed that physical restraint was wise. Staff also believe that even if his physician ordered restraints, Harris would fight them.

Staff and management face a dilemma: How can they meet their duty of nonmaleficence to Harris while maximizing his autonomy under the principle of respect for persons? Harris is competent to decide about restraints. It is also clear that he is risking his well-being. A major fracture is likely to result in rapid deterioration of Harris's general health. The staff do not seem very creative in finding a way to allow him to ambulate safely. Such options should be explored first. Alternatively, various possibilities should be tested for short periods. If all efforts fail, and Harris cannot be persuaded to accept restraints, he should be allowed to ambulate freely in the facility.

MEDICAL EDUCATION

The case of Richard Weidner in Chapter 7 involved problems of consent in the context of medical education. Weidner was admitted to the hospital for a cardiac catheterization following recurrent chest pain. His cardiologist told him she would perform the procedure, but it was actually carried out by a cardiology resident. The misrepresentation violated Weidner's right to autonomy and informed decision making and angered him greatly.

Medical education is a primary source of problems in consent, especially as to patient knowledge about who will perform a procedure. In January 1978 a medical practice task force established by the New York State Assembly issued a report. The conclusions of the task force were not based on statistical evidence of harm to patients caused by residents performing surgery but on interviews with chiefs of surgery, attending surgeons, residents, and anesthesiologists at 34 hospitals in New York State. It reported the following:

- Private surgical patients in teaching hospitals are usually not operated on by the attending surgeon they retained, but by residents. Between 50% and 85% of the surgery in teaching hospitals is done by residents.
- Although most residents operated only under the close supervision of attending surgeons, some residents performed surgery without supervision, and some attending surgeons left the room while the operation was still in progress or before the incision was closed.
- Most patients are unaware of the degree to which residents participate in their surgery, and consent forms that name the attending surgeon and "such assistants as he shall select" do not give patients meaningful notice that a resident may do the actual cutting or suturing.[7]

The authors stressed there was no evidence that allowing residents to be active participants in surgery caused harm to patients. However, other researchers are less certain. They suggest that harm to patients from care rendered by physicians in training may be much more common than is generally known.[8] Whether harm occurs is a utilitarian consideration. Kantians do not consider outcomes but only determine whether actions meet the criterion of respect for persons. Misleading patients or lying to them violates this principle.

Recommendations to the New York State Assembly resulting from the report focused on providing the disclosure necessary for informed consent and having sufficient supervision to ensure patient safety. The task force recommended that physicians be required to obtain the patient's consent for each person who participates in the surgery. It also recommended that vague phrases such as "such assistants as the surgeon may select" be deleted from consent forms. The recommendations encouraged adequate supervision by limiting the number of patients a surgeon could treat and the number of operating rooms that surgeons could reserve at one time.[9]

The AMA and the American College of Surgeons (ACS) have addressed the question of medical education and consent. They agree that if a resident rather than the surgeon retained by the patient actually performs the surgery, the patient must be made aware of that fact and consent to the substitution. *Report of the Council on Ethical and Judicial Affairs of the* AMA states the following:

A surgeon who allows a substitute to operate on his or her patient without the patient's knowledge and consent is deceitful. The patient is entitled to choose his or her own physician and should be permitted to acquiesce in or refuse to accept the substitution.

Under the normal and customary arrangement with patients, and with reference to the usual form of consent to operation, the operating surgeon is obligated to perform the operation but may be assisted by residents or other surgeons. With the consent of the patient, it is not unethical for the operating surgeon to delegate the performance of certain aspects of the operation to the assistant provided this is done under the surgeon's participatory supervision, i.e., the surgeon must scrub. If a resident or other physician is to perform the operation under nonparticipatory supervision, it is necessary to make a full disclosure of this fact to the patient, and this should be evidenced by an appropriate statement contained in the consent. Under these circumstances, it is the resident or other physician who becomes the operating surgeon.[10]

In its Statements on Principles, the ACS delineates the following:

A surgeon may delegate part of the care of patients to associates or residents under his or her direction, because modern surgery is often a team effort. However, the surgeon's personal responsibility must not be delegated or evaded. It is proper for the responsible surgeon to delegate the performance of part of a given operation to assistants, provided the surgeon is an active participant throughout the essential part of the operation. If a resident is to operate upon and take care of the patient, under the general supervision of an attending surgeon who will not participate actively, the patient should be so informed and consent thereto.

It is unethical to mislead a patient as to the identity of the doctor who performs the surgery.[11]

These statements are unequivocal. The patient must be informed about a resident's participation. Regrettably, the evidence suggests that these principles are regularly violated. Learning by doing is most apparent in training surgeons and in educating residents in medicine. Ethically, there is no difference between a surgical resident wielding a scalpel and a medical resident ordering a medication for unsuspecting patients.

Consent in settings in which medical education occurs is paid inadequate attention. It is an area in which patient autonomy is often breached and in which organizations, through their managers, must substantially improve performance. Medical education and patient consent are compatible. Most patients will cooperate when they know that physicians in training will play a role in their care.[12] If patients are so unwilling to permit residents to treat them that they seek care elsewhere, this is their right. If this right is ignored, ethical commitment to patient rights and autonomy is lacking.

CONCLUSION

This chapter addressed ethical issues raised by consent. Health services organizations and their managers should consider legal requirements as a minimum. It is on the basis of ethical principles that the organization should build a strong relationship with the patient. This independent relationship is the basis for the autonomy and respect owed to the patient.

Operationalizing the President's Commission's finding that patients' desire to be further involved in the consent process will require managerial attention to consent processes—not an easy task. Doing so means overcoming a long history of medical paternalism and educating patients as well as encouraging and assisting them to become involved.

A significant ethical problem is providing information about treatment to patients in health services organizations in which teaching occurs. Managers face many barriers in convincing attending staff that fully informing patients will not lead to diminished "clinical material" for teaching. No evidence suggests that many patients will refuse to participate after they have been informed, and there is every reason to believe that patients will overwhelmingly agree to the involvement of medical and surgical residents in their treatment.

NOTES

1. Donald T. Ridley. (1995, February). Working with Jehovah's Witnesses on treatment issues. *Hospital Law Newsletter, 12*(4), 6.
2. *Ibid.*
3. President's Commission for the Study of Ethical Problems in Medicine and Biomedical and Behavioral Research. (1982). *Making health care decisions* (Vol. 1). Washington, DC: U.S. Government Printing Office.
4. *Ibid.*, Vol. 3, p. 201.
5. Jay Katz. (1977, Winter). Informed consent—A fairy tale. *University of Pittsburgh Law Review, 39*, 137–174.
6. Breast cancer law opposed in Richmond. (1983, August 12). *The Washington Post*, p. 84.
7. Margaret Keller Holmes. (1980, May). Ghost surgery. *Bulletin of the New York Academy of Medicine, 56*(no. 4), 414.
8. Toby Cohen. (1983, September 20). The high cost of bad medicine. *The Washington Post*, p. A15.
9. Holmes, p. 415.
10. American Medical Association Council on Ethical and Judicial Affairs. (1994). *Code of medical ethics: Current opinions with annotations* (pp. 121–122). Chicago: Author.
11. American College of Surgeons. (1994, February). *Statements on principles* (Rev. ed.). Chicago: Author.
12. Martin L. Kempner. (1979). Some moral issues concerning current ways of dealing with surgical patients. *Bulletin of the New York Academy of Medicine, 55* (no. 1), 62–68.

10

Decisions at the End of Life

D ying and death are fundamental to human existence. As in abortion, the ethical questions involved prompt emotional responses from the public and many health professionals. Ethical issues in death and dying arise in various ways (e.g., treating neonates with severe disabilities who are unlikely to survive; caring for children or adults who are terminally ill, who are often unable to express personal autonomy).

Technology is at the heart of the matter. Since the 1970s developments such as renal dialysis, mechanical ventilation, and intensive care units have made it possible to postpone the end of life. Similar developments allow neonates who would have died in the 1980s to survive. Sometimes an ethical dilemma occurs when a person asks the organization to assist in achieving pain-free death. A great deal has been written about the questions raised by such technology, but few widely accepted courses of action have been identified.

Adding complexity to these ethical issues is that they are poorly developed in the law. Deliberately shortening a patient's life raises obvious ethical and legal questions. Judges and juries are reluctant to convict, even when violent means have been used to end the painful life of someone with terminal illness.

Chapter 9 noted that the President's Commission for the study of Ethical Problems in Medicine and Biomedical and Behavioral Research recommended a physician–patient relationship that maximizes patient sovereignty, with the patient fully participating in the decision process. Often, by the time crucial medical decisions must be made, the patient can no longer participate effectively and may not be competent. A medical ethic dedicated to preserving life and staving off death controls, and it is typical that the technological imperative results in expending all efforts, many times with only marginal results. The economic and psychological costs are obvious.

Many managers feel ill at ease even discussing death and dying. They are likely to consider decision making at the end of life to be clinical, a situation in which they play no role. Certainly, physicians are the lead actors in these dramas, but the effect of such issues on the organization requires that managers be knowledgeable about them and participate in developing and implementing policies and procedures. Managers also must be involved in committee activities.

Life-prolonging and life-sustaining treatments were distinguished in the mid-1980s; since then, the two concepts have merged and are simply called life-sustaining treatments. *Life sustaining* means "any treatment that serves to prolong life without reversing the underlying medical condition. Life-sustaining treatment may include, but is not limited to, mechanical ventilation, renal dialysis, chemotherapy, antibiotics, and artificial nutrition and hydration."[1] Care must be exercised in reading material about end-of-life issues to ensure that the writer's intent is understood.

DEATH DEFINED

Historically, death has been defined as the stoppage of blood circulation and the cessation of circulation-dependent animal and vital functions, such as respiration and pulsation. New technology proved this definition to be inadequate. Table 3 summarizes definitions of death. Definitions that are based in law and theology provide limited help to contemporary clinicians.

In 1968 a Harvard Medical School committee defined irreversible coma. This important step solved some problems but created others. The original Harvard criteria were accompanied by a report stating that the patient's condition can be determined only by a physician and that when the condition is found to be hopeless certain steps are recommended, as follows:

> Death is declared and *then* the respirator is turned off. The decision to do this and the responsibility for it are to be taken by the physician-in-charge, in consultation with one or more physicians who have been directly involved in the case. It is unsound and undesirable to force the family to make the decision.[2]

This quotation is noteworthy because of the changes in society's attitudes and perceptions that have occurred since 1968, including emphasis on patient autonomy and natural death act determinations, family involvement in decision making, and establishment of institutional ethics committees (IECs). These changes diminish the centrality and primacy of the physician's role.

About the time the Harvard criteria were issued, one of the first court cases dealing with brain death was decided in Virginia.[3] This case raised issues of consent, appropriate criteria and process for determining death, conflicts of interest, beneficence, nonmaleficence, and organizational philosophy and managerial ethics. The physicians involved sought to use a brain death standard, but failed to meet the Harvard criteria in two ways: They did not use

Table 3. Definition of death

Concept of death	Locus of death	Criteria of death
(Philosophical or theological judgment of the essentially significant change at death)	(Place to look to determine whether a person has died)	(Measurements physicians or other officials use to determine whether a person is dead—to be determined by scientific empirical study)
1. Irreversible loss of flow of vital fluids (i.e., the blood and breath)	Heart and lungs	Visual observation of respiration, perhaps with the use of a mirror Feeling of the pulse, possibly supported by electrocardiogram
2. Irreversible loss of the soul from the body	Pineal body (?) (according to Descartes) Respiratory tract (?)	Observation of breath (?)
3. Irreversible loss of the capacity for bodily integration	Brain	Unreceptivity and unresponsivity No movements or breathing No reflexes (except spinal reflexes) Flat electroencephalogram (to be used as confirmatory evidence) All tests to be repeated 24 hours later (excluded conditions: hypothermia and central nervous system depression by drug)
4. Irreversible loss of consciousness or the capacity for social interaction	Probably the neocortex	Electroencephalogram

Note: Death is defined as a complete change in the status of a living entity characterized by the irreversible loss of those characteristics that are essentially significant to it. The possible concepts, loci, and criteria of death are much more complex than the ones provided here. These concepts are meant to be simplified models of types of positions being taken in the current debate. It is obvious that those who believe that death means the irreversible loss of the capacity for bodily integration (3) or the irreversible loss of consciousness (4) have no reservations about pronouncing death when the heart and lungs have ceased to function. This is because they are willing to use loss of heart and lung activity as shortcut criteria for death, believing that once the heart and lungs have stopped, the brain or neocortex will necessarily stop as well.

Adapted from Veatch, R.M. (1976). *Death, dying, and the biological revolution: Our last quest for responsibility* (p. 53). New Haven: Yale University Press. © Yale University Press. Used with permission. This table has been modified using material from the 1989 second edition.

an electroencephalogram to verify brain activity and the respirator was turned off *before* the patient was pronounced dead. Despite these lapses, the court accepted a determination of brain death, thus making legal history.

The Harvard criteria have proved reliable, but not without difficulty. The President's Commission[4] summarized the criticisms in the following way:

- The phrase "irreversible coma" is misleading as applied to the cases at hand. "Coma" is a condition of a living person, and a body without any brain functions is dead and thus *beyond* coma.
- The writers of these (Harvard) criteria did not realize that the spinal cord reflexes actually persist or return quite commonly after the brain has completely and permanently ceased functioning.
- "Unreceptivity" is not amenable to testing in an unresponsive body without consciousness.
- The need to adequately test brainstem reflexes, especially apnea, and to exclude drug and metabolic intoxication as possible causes of coma, are not sufficiently explicit and precise.
- Although all individuals who meet "Harvard criteria" are dead (irreversible cessation of all functions of the entire brain), there are many individuals who are dead but do not maintain circulation long enough to have a 24-hour observation period.

The term "brain death" is now in common use and "(T)he three cardinal findings . . . are coma or unresponsiveness, absence of brainstem reflexes, and apnea." [5] By 1995 the Uniform Determination of Death Act developed by the National Conference of Commissioners on Uniform State Laws had been enacted in 31 states, the District of Columbia, and the Virgin Islands. The act reads as follows:

> An individual who has sustained either (1) irreversible cessation of circulatory and respiratory functions, or (2) irreversible cessation of all functions of the entire brain, including the brain stem, is dead. A determination of death must be made in accordance with accepted medical standards.[6]

The definition of brain death is endorsed by the American Academy of Neurology.[7]

As scientific developments permit increasingly sophisticated assessments of a patient's condition, especially prognosis, brain death criteria may be superseded by those that incorporate psychosocial factors. Prominent among the criteria proposed is the capacity or potential capacity for social interaction. This definition raises ethical issues and puts in jeopardy persons with no capacity for normal social interaction (e.g., persons with significant mental retardation). A definition that includes a lack of the potential for normal social interaction was applied when infants with mental retardation, such as Baby Boy Doe, were allowed to die. Although federal regulations since the 1980s specifically prohibit applying quality-of-life criteria to infants with disabilities who have life-threatening medical conditions, the evidence that quality-of-life criteria are commonly used in decision making for other types of patients is ample.

ADVANCE DIRECTIVES

When the federal Patient Self Determination Act (PSDA) of 1989 took effect December 1, 1991, efforts to achieve patient participation in and control of their health care decisions gained a significant impetus. PSDA requires that hospitals, nursing facilities, hospices, home health agencies, and health maintenance organizations that participate in Medicare and Medicaid give all patients written information about their rights under state law to accept or refuse medical or surgical treatment and to formulate advance directives. Adult patients must also be given the provider's written policies about implementing these rights. Medical records must document whether a patient has executed an advance directive. Providers must also educate their staffs and the community about advance directives. Despite PSDA and widespread state legislation, problems continue in operationalizing patient involvement in decision making about advance directives and relatively few patients execute them.

Living Wills

The living will was developed so that persons unable to participate in decision making could guide caregivers. The concept of living wills is several decades old and has been publicized extensively by an organization called Choice in Dying. The words *living* and *will* seem contradictory. Traditionally, a will is the legal mechanism by which a deceased person's wishes are carried out. Living wills allow persons unable to communicate with caregivers to express their wishes about treatment. In theory living wills allow persons to limit what is done for and to them and to control the technological imperative regardless of its potential benefit. Absent legislation or case law living wills have no legal status; patients must rely on the willingness of caregivers to follow the directives in them. The sample living will form shown in Figure 10 is useful only in states without specific requirements.

Natural Death Act Statutes

Interest in living wills and public reaction to cases in which seemingly excessive treatment was provided led to rapid enactment of state laws recognizing the patient's right to control treatment processes. These laws are variously called living wills laws, natural death acts, or death with dignity laws. In early 1983 there were 14 states with such laws; by 1985 there were 35 states and the District of Columbia; and by 1996 the total number was 47.[8] The Virginia form is shown in Figure 11.

Generally, the laws recognize a patient's right to direct physicians to withhold or withdraw life-sustaining treatment. When the patient meets stat-

To My Family, My Physician, My Lawyer, And All Others Whom It May Concern

Death is as much a reality as birth, growth, and aging—it is the one certainty of life. In anticipation of decisions that may have to be made about my own dying and as an expression of my right to refuse treatment, I, _____, being of sound mind, make
(print name)
this statement of my wishes and instructions concerning treatment.

By means of this document, which I intend to be legally binding, I direct my physician and other care providers, my family, and any surrogate designated by me or appointed by a court, to carry out my wishes. If I become unable, by reason of physical or mental incapacity, to make decisions about my medical care, let this document provide the guidance and authority needed to make any and all such decisions.

If I am permanently unconscious or there is no reasonable expectation of my recovery from a seriously incapacitating or lethal illness or condition, I do not wish to be kept alive by artificial means. I request that I be given all care necessary to keep me comfortable and free of pain, even if pain-relieving medications may hasten my death, and I direct that no life-sustaining treatment be provided except as I or my surrogate specifically authorize.

This request may appear to place a heavy responsibility upon you, but by making this decision according to my strong convictions, I intend to ease that burden. I am acting after careful consideration and with understanding of the consequences of your carrying out my wishes. *List optional specific provisions in the space below.*

How to Use Your Living Will

The Living Will should clearly state your preferences about life-sustaining treatment. You may wish to add specific statements to the Living Will in the space provided for that purpose. Such statements might concern:

- Cardiopulmonary resuscitation
- Artificial or invasive measures for providing nutrition and hydration
- Kidney dialysis

- Mechanical or artificial respiration
- Blood transfusion
- Surgery (such as amputation)
- Antibiotics

You may also wish to indicate any preferences you may have about such matters as dying at home.

Important Points to Remember

- Sign and date your Living Will.
- Your two witnesses should not be blood relatives, your spouse, potential beneficiaries of your estate or your health care proxy.
- Discuss your Living Will with your doctors; and give them copies of your Living Will for inclusion in your medical file, so they will know whom to contact in the event something happens to you.
- Make photocopies of your Living Will and give them to anyone who may be making decisions for you if you are unable to make them yourself.

- Place the original in a safe, accessible place, so that it can be located if needed—not in a safe deposit box.
- Look over your Living Will periodically (at least every five years), initial and redate it so that it will be clear that your wishes have not changed.

Figure 10. A sample living will. (From Choice in Dying, Inc., 250 W. 57th Street, New York, New York. Reprinted with permission.)

Written Natural Death Act Declaration

A declaration executed pursuant to this article may, but need not, be in one of the following forms, and may include other specific directions including, but not limited to, a designation of another person to make the treatment decision for the declarant should he be (i) diagnosed as suffering from a terminal condition and (ii) comatose, incompetent or otherwise mentally or physically incapable of communication. Should any other specific directions be held to be invalid, such invalidity shall not affect the declaration.

Declaration made this _____ day of _____ (month, year).

I, _____, willfully and voluntarily make known my desire and do hereby declare:

CHOOSE ONLY ONE OF THE NEXT TWO
PARAGRAPHS AND CROSS THROUGH THE OTHER

If at any time I should have a terminal condition and my attending physician has determined that there can be no recovery from such condition, my death is imminent, and I am comatose, incompetent, or otherwise mentally or physically incapable of communication, I designate .... to make a decision on my behalf as to whether life-prolonging procedures shall be withheld or withdrawn. In the event that my designee decides that such procedures should be withheld or withdrawn, I wish to be permitted to die naturally with only the administration of medication or the performance of any medical procedure deemed necessary to provide me with comfort care or to alleviate pain.

If at any time I should have a terminal condition and my attending physician has determined that there can be no recovery from such condition and my death is imminent, where the application of life-prolonging procedures would serve only to artificially prolong the dying process, I direct that such procedures be withheld or withdrawn, and that I be permitted to die naturally with only the administration of medication or the performance of any medical procedure deemed necessary to provide me with comfort care or to alleviate pain.

In the absence of my ability to give directions regarding the use of such life-prolonging procedures, it is my intention that this declaration shall be honored by my family and physician as the final expression of my legal right to refuse medical or surgical treatment and accept the consequences of such refusal.

I understand the full import of this declaration and I am emotionally and mentally competent to make this declaration.

_____

(Signed)
The declarant is known to me and I believe him or her to be of sound mind.

_____

Witness

_____

Witness

Figure 11.   Suggested form of Written Natural Death Act Declaration adopted by the State of Virginia. (From *Code of Virginia* 1950, 1990 Cumulative Supplement vol. 7A. Title 54.1, Article 9, section 2984, 197–198.)

utory requirements, the directives are legally binding on caregivers. The laws tend to be drafted narrowly and apply when a physician has determined that the patient who signed the declaration is terminally ill and has no prospect of recovery. In some states the directives must be reaffirmed when patients know they are terminally ill. Some laws include penalties against caregivers and the organization if directives are ignored. In addition to statutes, appeals court and state supreme court decisions affect how the laws are interpreted and how life-sustaining treatment is withheld or withdrawn.

These laws solve some of the issues of control (autonomy), patient role, and, to an extent, organizational and provider efforts to comply with the patient's wishes. Even when there is an advance directive, caregivers may be unlikely to follow it. Fragmentation of care among several health services providers and organizations further complicates patients' use of advance directives and poses a special challenge to managers in the organization to which the patient has been transferred. For example, an advance directive in effect in a nursing facility medical record may not be transferred to the hospital with the patient. A study of older patients hospitalized for acute illnesses found that in 75% of cases the medical record did not indicate that physicians had consulted the patient's living will or designated proxy before making treatment decisions, including whether to resuscitate. This failure was attributable to several factors, such as nursing facilities failed to transfer the information, patients were not asked or did not volunteer the information, and the hospital staff failed to ask or to ensure that such documents were part of the record. Once documented in the hospital record, advance directives influenced treatment decisions in 86% of cases involving patients who were judged incompetent.[9]

Other problems regarding advance directives also occur, for example, determining mental status and whether the patient comprehends the effect of what is being done, and establishing the presence of a terminal illness. Of course, the ethical dilemma remains for organizations in which the patient has not met statutory requirements or no statute and no advance directive exist.

The challenge for the organization is to provide processes that promote the completion of advance directives. A study conducted in the mid-1990s suggested that completion rates for advance directives can be markedly improved by altering the time when information is distributed to patients entering hospitals for planned admissions. Patients were far more likely to complete an advance directive at a hospital that distributed information several days before admission rather than only on the day of admission. Patients were much more likely to read the information provided when it was available before hospitalization. The most common reason given for not completing an advance directive was that it was not seen or was not read, a more common problem in hospitals that did not provide information in advance.[10] Another study suggested that providing reminders, education, and feedback to attending physicians and a new documentation form used by physicians for advance directives can greatly increase the percentage of patients who have advance directives. The study also found that 87% of physician-attested directives agreed with the treatment preferences of patients interviewed. Other results showed that physicians' attitudes and interest in advance directives improved.[11] Other research suggests that changes in the care of dying patients may not have kept pace with national recommendations, in part because many physicians and nurses disagreed with and may have been unaware of some key guidelines, such as the permissibility of withdrawing treatments.[12]

Substituted Judgment

Various types of health care surrogates are available whose judgments substitute for those of someone who is incompetent to make a decision because they are too young or have a physical or mental infirmity. Historically, surrogates were appointed by courts upon a petition that a person had no advance directive and was incompetent to make health care decisions. To avoid the cost and delays of court proceedings states began enacting laws that established a priority list of relatives who could make decisions for a person without an advance directive. By March 1996 the District of Columbia and 24 states had authorized surrogate decision making in such circumstances.[13]

Powers of attorney are another type of decision making by a surrogate. They occur before the fact and are delegations of authority made by an individual. Powers of attorney may be general or limited. They are *durable* when the grant of authority extends beyond the point the person granting it becomes incapacitated. Different names are used, but, in effect, health care agents and surrogate decision makers have been granted durable powers of attorney for health care. These are limited powers of attorney that enable a surrogate to make legally binding decisions on behalf of the person who has granted the power of attorney. By 1996, 48 states and the District of Columbia had enacted statutes specifically recognizing the appointment of health care agents.[14] Figure 12 is a sample form appointing a health care agent. Care must be taken to meet state requirements.

Do-Not-Resuscitate Orders

The do-not-resuscitate (DNR) order is another type of advance directive, albeit typically much closer to the point of service delivery. Most patients have neither living wills nor advance directives that comply with the state's requirements. This fact emphasizes the organization's need for policies and processes about resuscitating patients who are terminally ill and patients for whom life continuation decisions must be made (e.g., patients in persistent vegetative states [PVS]).* Typically, organizations have DNR policies affirming the legal right of a patient (or a surrogate, as appropriate) to direct care-

---

*The word *permanent* is used instead of *persistent* after a vegetative state has continued for longer than 1 year.

Durable Power of Attorney
for Health Care Decisions

To effect my wishes, I designate _____,
residing at _____(Phone #) _____,
(or if he or she shall for any reason fail to act, _____
(Phone #) _____, residing at _____)
as my health care surrogate—that is, my attorney-in-fact regarding any and all health care decisions to be made for me, including the decision to refuse life-sustaining treatment—if I am unable to make such decisions myself. This power shall remain effective during and not be affected by my subsequent illness, disability or incapacity. My surrogate shall have authority to interpret my Living Will, and shall make decisions about my health care as specified in my instructions or, when my wishes are not clear, as the surrogate believes to be in my best interests. I release and agree to hold harmless my health care surrogate from any and all claims whatsoever arising from decisions made in good faith in the exercise of this power.

I sign this document knowingly, voluntarily, and   Witness _____
after careful deliberation, this _____ day of _____,   Printed Name _____
19____.   Address _____

_____   Witness _____
           (signature)   Printed Name _____
Address _____   Address _____

_____
I do hereby certify that the within document was
executed and acknowledged before me by the principal   Copies of this document have been given to:
this _____ day of _____, 19____.

_____
Notary Public

The Durable Power of Attorney for Health Care

This optional feature permits you to name a surrogate decision maker (also known as a proxy, health agent or attorney-in-fact), someone to make health care decisions on your behalf if you lose that ability. As this person should act according to your preferences and in your best interests, you should select this person with care and make certain that he or she knows what your wishes are and about your Living Will.

You should not name someone who is a witness to your Living Will. You may want to name an alternate agent in case the first person you select is unable or unwilling to serve. If you do name a surrogate decision maker, the form must be notarized. (It is a good idea to notarize the document in any case.)

Figure 12.   A sample durable power of attorney for health care decisions. (From Choice in Dying, Inc., 250 W. 57th Street, New York, New York. Reprinted with permission.)

givers. The DNR policy should identify the chemical and mechanical technologies included and the specific instances in which they will be applied. Patients with DNR orders may require surgery and anesthesia management for palliative care, for relief of pain or distress, or to improve the patient's quality of life. This order presents unique ethical problems that should be addressed prospectively by the organization.[15]

Developments in the 1990s are nonhospital DNR orders, which allow people to refuse resuscitation in medical emergencies. In early 1996 statutes in 27 states recognized nonhospital DNR orders.[16] Often, these are known as emergency medical services do-not-resuscitate orders, or EMS DNR. These orders make the patient's wishes legally binding in the home or a similar setting and override state laws that require EMS technicians to undertake cardiopulmonary resuscitation (CPR).

A study of three Houston teaching hospitals without DNR policies reported inconsistent application of DNR orders.[17] The study found that some patients with DNR orders underwent chemotherapy and surgery and were admitted to the intensive care unit. Some patients with DNR orders received inadequate hydration and nutrition. Staff are often confused about what type of care patients with DNR orders should receive, perhaps because they disagree with decisions made about patients. The study found that in 10% of cases no decision had been reached about keeping the patient alive. This finding indicates that efforts to decide about resuscitation before a crisis commonly fail. In most no-decision cases the subject of DNR had not been broached with the patient or family. Other studies of DNR orders report similar findings.[18] A key aspect of DNR is whether patient wishes about CPR are clear to physicians. One study found that in nearly one of three cases the patient's preference not to be given CPR was at odds with the doctor's perception of what the patient wanted.[19]

Another dimension of DNR orders is whether they are written equitably for patients with different diseases but similar prognoses. A study reported in 1995 found that DNR orders are written more often for older patients, women, and patients with dementia or incontinence and less often for patients who are African American, had Medicaid insurance, or were in rural hospitals.[20] Similar disparities were found in an earlier study in which DNR orders were much more likely to be written for patients with AIDS or inoperable lung cancer than for patients with other diseases with equally poor prognoses, such as cirrhosis or heart failure.[21] Neither study assigned causes for the differences.

Veatch[22] considers the more important problem to be that of forgoing treatment because the physician assumes it is not in a patient's interest or because the physician believes the patient would not want it. Such actions do not consider the autonomy of the patient, either as an independent decision maker or as an involved participant. Veatch's concerns and research findings suggest that significant ethical problems exist involving DNR orders for patients with terminal illnesses in hospitals.

Summary

It has been suggested that the widespread use of advance directives, such as natural death act declarations, may encourage systematic rationing of health care to older adults. If a right to die becomes a duty to die, the living will and its progeny, the natural death act declaration, will become a Franken-stein's monster. Indeed, the suggestion by former Governor Richard Lamm of Colorado, as well as by officials at the U.S. Department of Health and Human Services (DHHS), that older people should be required to have living wills raised a storm of protest. Regardless of true motives, such suggestions are often seen as motivated by economics.

The organization must be alert to the ethical issues of advance directives, which are present regardless of a natural death act statute or a living will. Health services organizations and their managers must consider these issues prospectively and develop policies that respect patients' wishes, consistent with the organizational philosophy.

Euthanasia

The terms *natural death* or *death with dignity* should not be confused with *euthanasia*. The first two terms mean that a patient or surrogate has directed that life not be extended artificially and that life-sustaining treatment be withheld or withdrawn. *Euthanasia* comes from the Greek *eu* and *thanatos*, or good death. Used in the context of the Hippocratic tradition, which pro-hibits physicians from administering a deadly drug, euthanasia describes care that makes an inevitable death pain-free. Artificial means need not be used to extend life.

Euthanasia is, however, often used to describe situations in which active steps cause death (e.g., mercy killing). Such use blurs important distinctions. Providing comfort care and pain control without purposefully hastening death allows persons to experience a pain-free death and helps them die naturally, with dignity. To minimize confusion, however, this discussion uses the com-mon, bastardized definition.

Morphia Somnolence

Henrietta Morrow was diagnosed with inoperable cancer 18 months ago. Chemotherapy was ineffective. The lymph system had spread the cancer throughout her body, and Morrow was in severe pain. Initially, she had received home hospice care. As the disease worsened she became an inpatient at the hospice. She was expected to live less than 3 months.

Morrow received nutrition, hydration, and comfort care. The morphine used for pain control was increased as the disease progressed and her pain worsened. A staff member asked the medical director about the depressant effect that morphine would have on Morrow's respiration. She worried about depressing respiration so much that death would result. Her concern was expressed in both legal and ethical contexts. The medical director assured her that there were no legal problems and described the ethical considerations, including ordinary versus extraordinary care, active and passive euthanasia, voluntary versus involuntary euthanasia, and the principle of double effect.

Ordinary Versus Extraordinary Care

Hastening or bringing about death by increasing the morphine beyond that needed to control pain would be euthanasia, an unethical and illegal act. For Morrow, comfort care and pain relief are ordinary care. Further chemotherapy, however, would be extraordinary. Historically, hydration and nutrition were considered ordinary, a hotly contested distinction. The principle of non-maleficence provides a distinction:

> Ordinary means are all medicines, treatments, and operations which offer reasonable hope of benefit and which can be obtained and used without excessive expense, pain, or other inconvenience. Extraordinary means are all medicines, treatments, and operations which cannot be obtained or used without excessive expense, pain, or inconvenience, or which, if used, would not offer a reasonable hope of benefit.[23]

Ordinary and *extraordinary* should not be interpreted to mean usual and unusual, respectively. This interpretation could be confusing, primarily because there is variation even among similar hospitals as to which treatments are usual or unusual. The usual emergency treatment in a shock trauma unit is different from that provided in a community hospital. Instead, the measure is hope of benefit as compared with excessiveness of expense, pain, or other inconvenience. Absent hope of benefit, any medicine, treatment, or operation is extraordinary. If there is hope of benefit, using the same medicines, treatments, and operations is not excessive.

In the 1980s the ethics literature began to suggest that the correct focus was benefits to and burdens on the patient, the proportionality of treatment. Some writers suggest that *proportionate* and *disproportionate* are clearer and more descriptive than *ordinary* and *extraordinary*. The criteria used to measure proportionate and disproportionate care are similar to those for ordinary and extraordinary, but are stated somewhat differently. The type of treatment, its complexity or risk, cost, and appropriateness are studied and compared with results to be expected, taking into account the state of sick persons and their physical and moral resources.[24] Using this calculus it is ethical to provide the treatment if the potential benefit justifies the burden. Like ordinary and extraordinary, proportionate and disproportionate are primarily qualitative measures of the treatment. Summarized, ordinary/extraordinary and proportionate/disproportionate mean "Does the benefit justify the burden?"

Types of Euthanasia

Euthanasia has four permutations: voluntary active, voluntary passive, involuntary active, and involuntary passive. *Voluntary* means that the person has freely consented. *Involuntary* means that the person either has not freely consented or cannot freely consent, but is presumed to want to die. *Active* means that positive steps are taken to bring about death, an action that should be called killing. *Passive* means that nothing is done to hasten death; the natural course of the disease causes death. All types of euthanasia include comfort care and pain control.

Active or Passive Euthanasia The case of Henrietta Morrow raises questions about the concept of euthanasia: Does increased morphine for pain control constitute euthanasia that is active or passive or voluntary or involuntary? *Active euthanasia* occurs when the patient's death is purposely hastened. Giving Morrow an overdose—more morphine than was needed to control pain—would be active euthanasia, both unethical and illegal. *Passive euthanasia* occurs when the patient is allowed to die and no extraordinary means are used to prolong life, or when extraordinary means for prolonging life are withdrawn and the patient is allowed to die. Withholding or withdrawing life-sustaining treatment does not preclude comfort care and pain control. Artificially provided nutrition and hydration can be extraordinary (disproportionate) care, however, if they offer no hope of benefit.

Voluntary or Involuntary Euthanasia　*Voluntary* and *involuntary* euthanasia refer to patient decisions about treatment. It is unknown whether Morrow is aware that increasing the morphine might shorten her life and, if knowing, that she agrees. It is reasonable to assume that she prefers to live pain-free despite the other effects of morphine. However, the organization that emphasizes patient autonomy will involve, to the greatest extent possible, the competent patient in decisions concerning all treatment, including pain control.

Rule of Double Effect

The Morrow case raises the issue of the moral rule of double effect (RDE). Like ordinary and extraordinary care, double effect is a subset of nonmaleficence.

> According to classical formulations of the RDE, four conditions or elements must be satisfied for an act with a double effect to be justified. Each is a necessary condition, and together they form sufficient conditions of morally permissible action.
>
> 1. *The nature of the act*—The act must be good, or at least morally neutral (independent of its consequences).
> 2. *The agent's intention*—The agent intends only the good effect. The bad effect can be foreseen, tolerated, and permitted, but it must not be intended.
> 3. *The distinction between means and effects*—The bad effect must not be a means to the good effect. If the good effect were the direct causal result of the bad effect, the agent would intend the bad effect in pursuit of the good effect.
> 4. *Proportionality between the good effect and the bad effect*—The good effect must outweigh the bad effect. The bad effect is permissible only if a proportionate reason is present that compensates for permitting the foreseen bad effect.[25]

The principle of double effect allows ethical use of morphine, even in increasing quantities, to ease Morrow's pain.

PATIENT DECISION-MAKING PROCESS

Competent Patients

Persons who are competent have an ethical and a legal right to decide what treatments they will accept. This precept applies equally to withholding and withdrawing treatment. Consent is discussed in Chapter 9. Anecdotal evidence suggests that staff find it easier to withhold than to withdraw treatment. The reluctance to discontinue treatment seems based more on fear of legal liability than a search for the ethically best choice.

The Henninger Case   Decided by the New York Supreme Court, the appellate division in New York State, this case involved G. Ross Henninger, an 85-year-old man who was confused, depressed, and irritable, and was hospitalized for treatment of fever and infection. These problems were compounded by a stroke, arthritis, heart disease, and hardening of the arteries. The court stated it would not "go against (Henninger's) wishes and order this 85-year-old person to be operated on, or be force fed, or to be restrained for the rest of his natural life." [26] The decision followed a hearing in which attorneys for Henninger and the nursing facility where he lived petitioned the court to determine the legality of the facility allowing him to starve to death, which was his wish. Henninger died the day following the decision.

The case of Henrietta Morrow suggests that decisions about death and dying are similar in all types of health services organizations. An aging population and the prospect of the human immunodeficiency virus as a chronic rather than an acute medical problem are two important reasons that nursing facilities, hospices, and home health agencies should prospectively address the issues of end-of-life decisions. This focus entails a review from organizational philosophy down to operational policies. The philosophy and policies regarding matters such as life-continuation decisions and artificial hydration and nutrition should be communicated to patients and potential patients and their families.

Somebody Changed the Rules!

In 1986 Ruth Mittlemann was admitted to the Hebrew Home, a nursing facility. Mittlemann had amyotrophic lateral sclerosis (ALS), or Lou Gehrig's disease. Her condition deteriorated gradually. By late 1989 it was clear that she would soon be unable to swallow and thus could not take food and water by mouth. Before entering the facility, Mittlemann had executed a living will expressly stating that she did not want to receive artificial hydration or nutrition; she wished to be kept comfortable and treated for pain when she could no longer swallow. At the time Mittlemann entered the Hebrew Home, her living will posed no problem because the facility had no organizational policy on this issue.

In early 1988 the Hebrew Home's board of trustees began work on a policy regarding artificial nutrition and hydration. It was the most rancorous issue the board ever considered. Several members resigned because of the intense debate, which sometimes degenerated into personal attacks. The result was a policy adopted in late 1988, which stated that the sanctity of life had to be respected and that only if death were imminent could patients or their surrogates direct that such basic human care as food and water be stopped.

Mittlemann learned of this new policy only when she was informed that it would be necessary to place a nasogastric tube so that she could be hydrated and fed. She protested vehemently and reaffirmed her living will. She did not want to move to another nursing facility in the area; she liked where she was living. She objected only to being forced to receive treatment that she did not want.

On its face, this change is fundamentally unfair to Mittlemann. She is caught up in a situation not of her making and beyond her control. The organization is also caught up in an awkward situation: Acceding to her wishes causes it to violate its newly developed philosophy about the sanctity of life.

The principle of respect for persons—specifically, fidelity—governs the Mittleman case. The organization is obliged to apprise patients of policies that affect them. Because the Hebrew Home had no written policy on artificial hydration and nutrition when Mittlemann was admitted, the trust she placed in the organization when she chose it would be violated. Moving her elsewhere does not eliminate the home's duty. As distasteful as it may be to the organization and its board, Mittlemann's situation must be an exception to the policy.

Formerly Competent Patients

In theory patients retain the right to determine what care they receive and when it will be discontinued. However, treatment processes, even for competent inpatients, often become psychologically and physically overwhelming. The processes and the persons who apply them dominate; the patient quickly loses control. Patients (or their advocates) may be forced to bring legal action to reassert their autonomy.

Instructions from a Formerly Competent Patient

Constance Emerson lived a full life. She had been active in the community. She worked as a volunteer at Homer House, a noted settlement house, where she developed educational programs for children of working mothers. Emerson is age 92 and lives in a nursing facility. In 1988 she fell and sustained a cerebral hemorrhage. Her mental faculties remain impaired even after extensive therapy.

After her injury, Emerson's husband cared for her until his own health deteriorated and it became impossible for him to continue caring for her. Emerson has long had diabetes. She requires a special diet and insulin. She eats only soft foods or liquids and is bedridden, blind, and deaf. Emerson experiences occasional respiratory infections that respond well to treatment. Her heart is strong. Except for mild arthritis, she feels no pain. She sometimes recognizes her husband when he visits, but her speech is often unintelligible.

Three years before her injury, Emerson gave a talk on the miseries of prolonging life for older adults who are dying. Having experienced the agony of deterioration in her relatives, she made an eloquent plea for a "dignified and simple way to choose death." She showed the manuscript to her husband and mentioned publishing it, but had not done so. Her husband now fears speaking to her about what she had written or how she feels about her life because she might infer that he wants her to die. The Emersons' son visits her weekly and feels they should not disturb the care she is receiving.[27]

This case illustrates the ethical problems associated with caring for infirm older people who are no longer competent. The care provided to Emerson maintains her, but nothing can be done to reverse the injury to her brain. She is not terminally ill. The care she requires and receives is usual for her condition and would fit the definition of ordinary care. The evidence as to Emerson's views about people in her situation is several years old. Her incompetence precludes knowing her current wishes. Even if Emerson could direct her care or had an advance directive, she could not order the organization to assist her in ending her life. She is not terminally ill; discontinuing treatment is unethical.

Applying these criteria to the case of Constance Emerson, who needs a special diet, insulin, and occasional antibiotics, leads to the conclusion that nothing being done is extraordinary. All care offers reasonable hope of benefit without excessive expense, pain, or inconvenience. Reasonable hope of benefit is not based on an expectation that she will regain her former mental and physical condition, but that she will live the life of a 92-year-old woman who has sustained head injury.

It is instructive to apply the final definition of death in Table 3 (see p. 173) to Emerson. Is she "alive" if a social interaction criterion is applied? The case notes that she sometimes recognizes her husband when he visits. Whether she has the capacity for social interaction could be determined. If she is not capable of social interaction, this definition of death would allow her to die by withholding antibiotics or insulin. Whether it is ethical to do so absent an advance directive is another question. Given the facts in this case, the only ethical action is to continue hydration, nutrition, and medication.

Noncompetent Adult Patients

In re Quinlan Karen Ann Quinlan was 21 years old in mid-1975 when she became comatose after ingesting an overdose of alcohol and tranquilizers. The New Jersey Supreme Court overturned a trial court ruling and permitted Karen's father to be appointed her guardian.[28] The court authorized Quinlan to discontinue all extraordinary measures to sustain life if the family and physicians agreed that there was no reasonable possibility that Karen would emerge from her vegetative state and if there was consultation with the hospital ethics committee. This ruling was among the earliest enunciations of an ethics committee's role, and it stimulated New Jersey hospitals to establish these committees. The context of the opinion makes it clear that the court intended that the committee would be a prognosis committee, a rather different role from that which ethics committees have assumed.

After her father ordered the respirator disconnected, Karen was weaned successfully by physicians and she breathed unaided. She was discharged to a nursing facility, where she remained until her death in mid-1985. When she died, she weighed 66 pounds and her body was locked in a fetal position.

In addition to the New Jersey courts, courts in Massachusetts and New York have been especially active in cases similar to the Quinlan case. The cases have been brought by families seeking to regain control from the organization or by managers wanting protection from legal claims. Not all such cases follow the Quinlan case. Some patients have received continued treatment absent hope of benefit. In other situations painful treatment of little benefit was withheld. With court guidance health services organizations are attempting to solve the problem of when to discontinue life support. The courts are a necessary final arbiter in settling legal questions that arise, especially when there is dissonance in the ethics of those involved, including the organization. By defining limits of the law, court decisions aid persons and organizations in developing and refining their ethic.

In re Cruzan   One of the most important cases of the 1990s is that involving Nancy Cruzan, a young adult who sustained severe injuries (including cerebral contusions compounded by significant anoxia) in a 1983 automobile accident. Initially, Cruzan was in a coma, but she progressed to an unconscious state and was subsequently diagnosed as being in PVS. To ease feeding and further her recovery, a permanent gastrostomy tube provided hydration and nutrition. When it became apparent that Cruzan had virtually no chance of regaining her mental faculties, her parents asked the Missouri state hospital caring for her to end artificial hydration and nutrition. The staff refused to do so without court approval. The parents successfully sought authorization from a state trial court, which found that someone in Cruzan's condition had a fundamental right under state and federal constitutions to refuse treatment or direct the withdrawal of "death-prolonging procedures." On appeal, the Missouri Supreme Court reversed the trial court's decision.

The Missouri Supreme Court recognized a right to refuse treatment in the common law doctrine of informed consent, but did not consider it applicable. It also declined to read into the state constitution a broad right to privacy that would support an unrestricted right to refuse treatment and expressed doubt that the U.S. Constitution embodied such a right. The court then decided that the state living will statute embodied a policy strongly favoring preservation of life and that Cruzan's statements to her housemate that she would not want to continue her life unless she could live "halfway normally" were unreliable in determining her intent.[29] The Court rejected the argument that her parents were entitled to order termination of medical treatment, concluding that no person can make that choice on behalf of an incompetent person absent the formalities required by the state's living will statute or clear and convincing evidence of the patient's wishes.

The U.S. Supreme Court agreed to review the case to determine whether Cruzan had a right under the U.S. Constitution that would require the hospital to withdraw life-sustaining treatment. On June 25, 1990 the U.S. Supreme Court affirmed the Missouri decision.[30] It held that the U.S. Constitution does not forbid Missouri to require that evidence of an incompetent person's wishes as to withdrawal of life-sustaining treatment be proved by clear and convincing evidence. The Court distinguished the rights of competent persons, who it assumed have a constitutionally protected right to refuse life-sustaining hydration and nutrition, from the rights of incompetent persons. It noted that although the Missouri Supreme Court had in effect recognized that under certain circumstances a surrogate may act for the patient in electing to withdraw hydration and nutrition and thus cause death, the state had established a procedural safeguard to ensure that the surrogate's action conforms as closely as possible to the wishes expressed by the patient while competent. The Court granted broad latitude to the states to protect and preserve human life and recognized their right to require a standard of "clear and convincing evidence" as to the person's intentions regarding life-continuation decisions. It noted that the state is entitled to guard against potential abuses by surrogates who may not act to protect the patient's interests. In addition, states may decline to judge the quality of a person's life and simply assert an unqualified interest in the preservation of human life to be weighed against the constitutionally protected interests of the individual. The Cruzan case makes it clear that the Court is unwilling to extend to incompetent persons (through surrogates) the same constitutional right of self-determination available to competent persons. The Court found it appropriate that the state establish procedures and safeguards for such decisions. Considerable weight was placed on the fact that the state had a law regarding how such matters should be solved. The Court did not outline the range of actions a legislature could take.

In November 1990 Cruzan's parents were granted a second hearing in state court, which Missouri did not oppose. New evidence convinced the judge that Nancy Cruzan would not have wanted to live in PVS. On December 14, 1990 he ordered the feeding tube removed. Anti-euthanasia groups unsuccessfully sought to intervene and Cruzan died of dehydration December 26, 1990, 8 years after her accident.[31]

The Cruzan case makes it clear that states have the authority and the responsibility to legislate processes for such situations and that the Court granted them broad latitude. Health services organizations are guided by state law. In addition, they shoulder a special burden: advising patients about their legal rights regarding advance directives. The organization must go beyond informing and assisting patients to actually ensuring that that guidance is part of the medical record and is applied in the process of care. The research finding that most hospitals place the burden of preparing advance directives on patients and that few advise patients about their use indicates that much work remains to be done. Health services organizations meet that challenge as part of their commitment to the principles of respect for persons, beneficence, and nonmaleficence.

Cases such as Henninger and Cruzan have fueled the debate about whether health services organizations and their clinical staff are ethically and legally obliged to administer food and water artificially to patients who are terminally ill or in PVS. When patients must be sedated or restrained to endure tube feedings or intravenous lines the burdens are significant and it must be asked whether care in this context is required.[32] Another way to state the issue is that providing life-sustaining food and water for this type of patient is extraordinary (disproportionate) care, although under usual circumstances nutrition and hydration are ordinary (proportionate) care.

Some individuals will ask whether feeding and hydrating patients who are terminally ill or in PVS is or should ever be considered extraordinary (disproportionate) care. The AMA addressed this issue in the mid-1980s when it stated that it was not unethical for physicians to discontinue "life-prolonging" medical treatment from patients with terminal illness or irreversible coma when the physician determined that the burdens of treatment outweighed its benefits. Treatment was defined to include medication and artificially or technologically supplied respiration, nutrition, or hydration.[33] Protests were made by people who feared that the new policy might cause physicians to discontinue nutrition and hydration when *they* considered it in the patient's best interests, even though patients believed their interests were furthered by continuing these treatments but could not communicate this decision. The AMA has maintained this position but with much greater emphasis on patient autonomy and surrogate decision making, where necessary, rather than on physician determinations of benefits and burdens.[34]

A common question for patients denied hydration and nutrition has been whether it is inhumane treatment because of the pain they were believed to experience. The issue may not be settled for all. The weight of evidence seems to be that prolonged dehydration and starvation produce no pain and that ice chips or swabs will relieve the limited discomfort from a dry mouth. Problems with excessive secretions, edema, or incontinence can be alleviated.[35] As Sullivan[36] stated,

> In the setting of hydration and starvation, death can occur from a multitude of causes. Arrhythmia, infection, and circulatory system collapse due to volume depletion are common terminal events. The clinical course of each should be rapid and, ideally, not associated with perceived discomfort by the patient.

Some organizations insist on continuing hydration even though nutrition is stopped. This action seems pointless.

Objections to this ethic are heard less often in the mid-1990s, although most people are likely to find themselves discomforted by failing to provide food and water because these are the staples of human existence. Regardless of the direction the debate takes at the theoretical level, an ethic must be applied at the bedside. What is the ethically correct action for a particular patient? Thus, the debate may begin anew.

Infants

The Baby Doe cases added an important dimension to what began with the Quinlan case. The name Baby Doe derives from court proceedings in several states in the early 1980s. All cases were similar to the case of Baby Boy Doe described in Chapter 1 and involved parents who decided to forgo life-sustaining treatment of their newborn infants with treatable genetic anomalies. Publicity surrounding the subsequent deaths of two such infants prompted DHHS to issue regulations in April 1982 prohibiting hospitals that receive federal funds from withholding life-sustaining treatment from infants with disabilities. Authority for this action was claimed in Section 504 of the Rehabilitation Act of 1973 (PL 93-112), which prohibits discrimination on the basis of handicap. The regulations were challenged by health services organizations on procedural grounds, and an injunction suspending implementation was issued. Another attempt to promulgate a modified version of the regulations followed in 1983. Like the first regulations, they mandated telephone hotlines to report alleged cases of withholding life-sustaining treatment from newborns with serious illnesses. Signs containing information about the need to treat such newborns had to be posted. For providers, the hotlines were the most hated and controversial requirement. Opponents claimed the regulations turned providers into spies and stool pigeons. An important modification in the 1983 revision was that impossible or futile acts or therapies that merely prolonged the dying of an infant born terminally ill were not required. Opponents successfully obtained judicial relief preventing implementation.

In June 1985 the U.S. Supreme Court agreed to hear a Justice Department appeal of a lower court decision that invalidated the Baby Doe regulations. This was surprising because the actions of Congress and DHHS had eliminated the need for the first regulations. In June 1986 the high court agreed with the lower court in an opinion that struck down the Baby Doe rules. It agreed that Section 504 of the Rehabilitation Act of 1973 did not empower the DHHS to force hospitals to treat infants with severe disabilities over parental objections. The Court's decision displeased some disability advocacy groups, who claimed that there are major enforcement problems with the Child Abuse Amendments of 1984 (PL 98-457), both procedurally and because of a basic antidisability bias held by some physicians and child protective services agencies. They contended that these biases will result in a do-not-treat decision in large numbers of cases.

Child Abuse Amendments

The original controversy surrounding the Baby Doe cases prompted Congress to address directly the question of newborns with serious disabilities. The Child Abuse Amendments of 1984 became law on October 9. The regulations established treatment and reporting guidelines for care of newborns with significant disabilities. Withholding *medically indicated treatment* from infants with disabilities is illegal except when

> in the treating physician's(s') reasonable medical judgment (i) the infant is chronically and irreversibly comatose; (ii) the provision of such treatment would merely prolong dying, not be effective in ameliorating or correcting all of the infant's life-threatening con-

ditions, or otherwise be futile in terms of survival of the infant; or (iii) the provision of such treatment would be virtually futile in terms of the survival of the infant and the treatment itself under such circumstances would be inhumane.[37]

The definition of medically indicated treatment includes appropriate care, such as nutrition and hydration, as well as medication.[38]

Under the law appropriate health services organizations must designate persons who will report suspected problems to state child protective services agencies. The agencies coordinate and consult with those persons and, after notification of cases of suspected medical neglect, may initiate legal action.

PHYSICIAN-ASSISTED SUICIDE

Definition and Legal Background

What is being called physician-assisted suicide became a prominent ethical and legal issue in 1990. Physician-assisted suicide fits none of the types of euthanasia described earlier in this chapter. It has characteristics of voluntary, active euthanasia, but differs in a critical aspect. Physician-assisted suicide occurs when the physician provides the means, medical advice, and assurance that the suicide will be successful. The patient performs the act that leads to death. Broadly defined it is a good death because it is likely to be pain free; it is not, however, euthanasia, as defined earlier. Physical disability prevents some individuals from committing suicide; they are candidates for voluntary, active euthanasia, should it become legal. The mental competence of individuals who are to be assisted in suicide must be ensured.

Legalizing physician-assisted suicide was considered in initiatives on ballots in Washington State (1991) and California (1992). Both initiatives were rejected, a result resoundingly inconsistent with polls showing that, by a large majority, Americans favor physician help in ending the lives of people who are terminally ill. In 1994 Oregon voters narrowly (52% to 48%) enacted a physician-assisted suicide law, which remains unimplemented because of a court challenge. The law permits physicians to prescribe but not administer medications for competent patients. Among the requirements are only 6 months of life remaining; a second opinion about the patient's medical condition; multiple oral and written requests; and two waiting periods. Physicians must report participation to the state health division, but those who act in good faith within the law are protected from both professional discipline and legal liability.[39] It is too early to know if these West Coast developments suggest a nationwide trend; several other states are considering similar legislation.

Statutes in 33 states criminalize assisted suicide; in 10 states and the District of Columbia the common law is used for the same purpose.[40] Some of these laws have been challenged in federal court. In March 1996 the California-based 9th Circuit Court of Appeals ruled that the Washington state law that made physician-assisted suicide a felony was a denial of due process of law under the 14th Amendment to the U.S. Constitution. The court of appeals' reasoning relied heavily on the Supreme Court's abortion cases, which were found to have compelling similarities.[41] A month later, the New York-based 2nd Circuit Court of Appeals ruled that terminally ill people have the same right to hasten death by taking drugs as they do by refusing artificial life support, thus striking down a New York state law. The ruling was based on the equal protection clause of the 14th Amendment.[42] The issue of physician-assisted suicide is likely to be heard by the Supreme Court in the near future.

The Case of "Dr. Death"

Although seldom discussed, it has been understood that the preeminent role of the physician is to "comfort always," especially when little else can be done. This ethic has never included assisting in suicide, however. Sometimes, for example, efforts to eliminate pain caused too much morphine to be administered, but this unintended effect of comfort care was never an ethical issue. The Hippocratic tradition considers it to be unethical for physicians to deliberately cause death, whether requested by the patient or for a noble purpose such as pain relief. This prohibition gave no weight to the patient's wishes and is reflected in laws against homicide as well as laws in many states that make it illegal to assist in a suicide. Surveys of physicians reported in 1996 found that a majority of physicians in Michigan (Dr. Jack Kevorkian's home state) and Oregon favor the legalization of assisted suicide, although a sizable minority in Oregon objects to legalization and participation on moral grounds.[43] Similarly, in 1995, 12% of responding physicians in Washington State reported receiving one or more explicit requests from patients for physician-assisted suicide; 4% had received one or more requests for euthanasia.[44]

In 1990, 54-year-old Janet Adkins, a woman with early-stage Alzheimer's disease, feared losing her memory and the ability to engage in normal activities. She sought the help of Dr. Jack Kevorkian, a retired pathologist, to assist her in committing suicide before her mental abilities were so impaired that she could no longer make a rational decision.[45] Kevorkian had gained national prominence earlier that year at a press conference in which he showed a device he had designed to enable persons who wanted to die to self-administer toxic chemicals, after initial assistance from a physician. Commentators have criticized the action and the help given to Adkins by Kevorkian as procedurally flawed, and have questioned Adkins's competence because of her diagnosis.[46] This case brought to the public's attention the issue of active, voluntary euthanasia and the right to an assisted suicide.

In the first several assisted suicides Kevorkian played a much more active role by starting a saline iv. The patient then initiated the flow of potassium chloride and barbiturates that caused death. Changes occurred as Kevorkian, or "Dr. Death" as his critics call him, continued to assist in suicides. Kevorkian lost his medical license. Because he could no longer legally obtain the needed chemicals, he changed to carbon monoxide, which is breathed through a mask placed on the face of the patient, who then initiates the flow of gas. Kevorkian began to videotape conversations held prior to assisting the suicide in which the "patients" answered questions that documented their state of mind as well as their desire to die. By the end of 1996 Kevorkian had assisted over 40 persons to commit suicide. Several of these cases are pending in the criminal justice system. All of Kevorkian's assisted suicides have occurred in Michigan, a state that initially had no law against the practice. Hastily passed legislation outlawing assisted suicide did not stop him and he continued to help people to die.

Kevorkian was criticized on professional and ethical grounds, including accusations that he did not know his "patients"; he was unqualified to diagnose or understand illnesses because he is a pathologist; he had a conflict of interest because of his desire to publicize himself and (initially) his suicide machine; he assisted persons who did not have terminal illness; and he made no effort, nor was he qualified to judge, the competence of the persons he assisted. Kevorkian has stated that he hopes to establish a clinic, called an *obitorium*, for persons with terminal illness in order to assist those who want to commit suicide.

One of Kevorkian's stated goals is to test the limits of patient autonomy. His primary defense seems to be that the law criminalizing assisted suicide is an unconstitutional interference in the right to privacy. This defense uses reasoning similar to that used in *Roe v. Wade*, the Supreme Court decision that found a constitutional right to privacy protected a woman's decision to abort her pregnancy in the first trimester from state interference. Assisted suicide seems to present an even stronger case for individual autonomy as expressed in the right to privacy because no other life (i.e., a fetus) is involved. In the case of assisted suicide, however, experts disagree.[47,48] In mid-1995 the U.S. Supreme Court declined to review various appeals regarding Kevorkian's activities.[49]

Dutch Practice

International comparisons are instructive. The Netherlands is the vanguard of aid in dying. Euthanasia and assisted suicide continue to be illegal there, but a February 1993 law permits physicians to euthanize *and* assist in suicides if certain rules are adhered to, as follows:

- *Voluntary*—request must be of the patient's free will with no pressure from others; requests cannot come from others
- *Alternatives*—patient must be well-informed and able to consider alternatives
- *Certain decision*—patient must have a "lasting longing for death," impulsive requests or those made while depressed cannot be considered
- *Suffering*—suffering must be perpetual, unbearable, and hopeless (terminal illness)

- *Consultation*—physician must consult at least one other physician with experience in euthanasia
- *Reporting*—a well-documented written report must be filed with the coroner[50]

Only a small minority of Dutch physicians (11%) said they would not participate in euthanasia or physician-assisted suicide.[51] The survey of physicians in Oregon mentioned earlier found a much greater reluctance to participate in physician-assisted suicide, with 31% stating they would be unwilling to do so on moral grounds.[52]

Evidence exists that euthanasia and physician-assisted suicides occurred before the law changed. A 1990 government study found that 2% of all deaths were the result of these means. The same study found that in 1,000 other cases a patient's life was ended without an explicit recent request to die.[53] The study also showed that in 1990 death was hastened for 16,850 patients, of whom 8,750 died by withholding or withdrawing treatment and 8,100 died by administering pain-killing drugs. Consent was obtained from only 3,100 of the patients in the second group. No consent had been obtained from the others. Thus, a majority were killed without their consent.[54]

Soon after the February 1993 law was passed the Dutch government reported that it would consider broadening euthanasia guidelines to allow the killing of patients unable to request it such as newborns with profound disabilities and persons who are mentally incompetent.[55] This action would sanction *involuntary* active euthanasia—a significant change.

It is arguable that the Dutch law only recognizes existing practice—*de facto* became *de jure*. However, that a western European democratic government is willing to publicly acknowledge this development will raise ethical concerns for many people. Seemingly begun as an effort to enhance individual self-determination, the Dutch experience suggests that euthanasia is by no means limited to persons who request it. This troubling precedent highlights the slippery slope, which philosophers define as one exception leading to other, more easily accepted exceptions.

Issues for Physicians

The primary issue for physicians is that their profession is being turned on its head. Those who play the traditional role of the guardians of life may now be asked to induce death. Proposals that physicians aid in dying have been roundly condemned by organized medicine. However, given that only a small percentage of Dutch physicians state that they are morally opposed to euthanasia and assisted suicide, this reaction may be overstated. Nevertheless, the question of aid in dying raises significant moral questions and necessitates a thorough reexamination of the physician–patient relationship. At the very least, it would be unacceptable to require physicians to provide aid in dying if they are morally opposed to this activity. The American tradition of the overriding importance of personal conscience in such matters must govern. Perhaps a new medical specialty, thanatology, will be recognized.

Demedicalizing aid in dying reduces the number of ethical issues for the medical profession but simultaneously raises others. German law, for example, effectively makes it illegal for physicians to assist in suicides. However, because neither suicide nor assisting the suicide of persons who are capable of exercising control over their actions *and* who have made a freely responsible choice to commit suicide are illegal, unique societal views about suicide and aid in dying have developed in Germany.[56]

Issues for the Organization

It is noteworthy that none of Kevorkian's assisted suicides occurred in a health services organization. Most of his "patients" were ambulatory, and several different settings were used. Usually, the "patients" he assisted would not be the type who would be hospitalized when a question of aid in dying arose. A hospital that provided home health or home hospice services would encounter the issue as defined by Kevorkian, however.

Common situations for hospitals and nursing facilities are patients in PVS, patients who are bedridden with a terminal illness, or patients who in other ways are too ill to be transferred. What are their rights as compared with the organization's? The importance of an organizational philosophy with specific attention to aid in dying is clear, again, because legally and ethically the organization cannot be forced to participate in activities that compromise its ethic.

Economics of Euthanasia and Physician-Assisted Suicide

Economic incentives in fee-for-service medicine err on the side of too much care, and the physician's and organization's interests in voluntary or involuntary passive euthanasia is limited to questions of the futility, or hope of benefit, from continued treatment. New forms of payment and new organizational arrangements will change the incentives for health services organizations, even as they become less able to meet the costs of services. Hospitals have already experienced a form of capitation in diagnosis-related groups, which have the incentive to limit services. Cost shifting is increasingly difficult for hospitals. Thus, they are forced to reduce costs, which can be accomplished through greater productivity—achieving the same results with fewer resources—or by changing the content of care, easily done by providing aid in dying.

When physicians were less affected by cost-reduction pressures, they counterbalanced an organization's efforts to limit services. Traditional relationships are changing rapidly, however. This change will attach prominence to questions of aid in dying as arrangements that economically bind physicians and organizations, especially hospitals, become increasingly common. Networks and alliances are the logical extension and the private sector is working hard to establish them. The economic oneness of physician and organization raises numerous ethical issues.

Any fixed sum payment scheme (e.g., capitation) provides an incentive to minimize the number and range of services, especially those that are costly. The implications of such incentives are the same for private insurers and government. The words used are different—government is likely to use euphemisms such as "quality of life," whereas insurers are likely to more overtly focus on costs. The issue is the same for both, however—how can costs be controlled? Such incentives cause an inherent conflict of interest between providing services that might be in the best interests of the patient and holding to a fixed monetary limit. The result is that certain services (especially those that are high cost) are likely to be withheld and that services will be withdrawn from persons who are deemed to have a poor quality of life or prognosis. Systems in the United States in which capitation or global budgets are used may not take positive steps to end life, but may simply deny care of certain types because it is uneconomic or because it has little effect on quality of life. In such cases Oregon's priority list for Medicaid beneficiaries is instructive.

As framed, the debate on decisions at the end of life focuses on negative rights. Freedom from unwanted health services is a negative ethical and legal right grounded in the right to be free from unwanted interference. Simply stated, this right is called autonomy. No positive right to die exists—persons cannot compel others to aid them in dying, nor can anyone be required to aid another in dying. As yet, aid in dying is not reimbursable.

ASSISTED SUICIDE AND THE ORGANIZATION

In late 1983 a dramatic case highlighting several of the concepts described earlier began in California. Elizabeth Bouvia, who has cerebral palsy, entered county-owned Riverside General Hospital and asked that the staff aid her in fasting until she died. She was unable to move and required assistance in all physical activities. Bouvia entered the hospital to receive the hygienic care and drugs necessary to facilitate a painless death by starvation. A court injunction prevented the hospital from discharging her. To ensure adequate nutrition, hospital staff inserted a nasogastric feeding tube, allegedly against her wishes. She asserted that she had reached a competent and rational decision, one her lawyer argued was protected by the constitutional right to privacy and self-determination. Her mental competence was confirmed by several psychiatrists.

After a hearing on whether the hospital would be forced to assist Bouvia in her suicide, the court ruled that "despite her right to commit suicide, which is not illegal in California, she could not ask society in the person of the hospital staff to help her because she was not a terminal patient." [57] Notably, California has criminal penalties against aiding and abetting a suicide. The court distinguished Bouvia from people with terminal illnesses. In January 1984 the California Supreme Court refused to hear her appeal. [58]

The decision permitted the hospital to force-feed Bouvia. She was discharged from Riverside General on April 7, 1984, and was hospitalized in Tijuana, México.[59] It was reported that she had reconsidered her decision to die and would return to the United States for medical treatment. Her lawyer maintained that she still wished to die, despite the fact that she had been accepted for care somewhere in California on the condition that she not stop eating.[60]

After a year in the new institution and a subsequent stay of several months at an acute care hospital, where a morphine pump was installed for pain control, Bouvia was admitted to Los Angeles County-High Desert Hospital in late 1985. As at Riverside General Hospital, and against her wishes, the staff inserted a permanent feeding tube. Court action by Bouvia initially resulted in the court's refusal to order discontinuation of the forced feeding. On appeal, however, the case was remanded, with instructions to consider her request further. As a result, tube feeding was discontinued and Bouvia was discharged. Her attorney stated, "She's promised to continue to eat her liquid diet. I know she would welcome death . . . but she has renounced [suicide]."[61] In May 1986 she was hospitalized at Los Angeles County-University of Southern California Medical Center, where she was treated for chronic pain.[62] In June 1986 the California Supreme Court affirmed a lower court decision allowing her to die by refusing force-feeding (at the time she was accepting a liquid diet). The hospital had argued that removing the tube would officially endorse suicide.[63] Since that time, Bouvia has shunned publicity.

In addition to highlighting the problems of the nonterminally ill, the case of Elizabeth Bouvia delineates the clash between organizational philosophy (here with both ethical and legal justification) and patient autonomy. Bouvia's problem was not that the facilities where she was treated refused to discharge her; instead, her difficulty was finding a facility that would admit her. Institutions that agreed to admit her insisted on doing everything they could to maintain or improve her physical condition—thus the force-feeding. Several state courts have specifically addressed this issue. By late 1989, 16 states permitted withholding or withdrawing tube feeding; 3 states prohibit such actions under certain circumstances.[64]

The Bouvia case suggests the limit of what patients can ask of health services organizations. At least in California, the law determines what the organization and its managers can do and the obligation to obey the law guarantees a minimum performance. The ethics reflected in the organization's philosophy determine the extent to which it relies on a higher standard. The law is different in other states such as New York and New Jersey, and this difference reinforces the organization's need to be aware of state law and, more important, to address such issues prospectively.

Conclusion

Ethical issues arising from end-of-life decisions are among the most common health services organizations and their clinical and managerial staffs encounter. Technology is central to the ethical and legal problems concerning death and dying. New technology may solve some problems, but if history is a guide, technology is as likely to create ethical dilemmas as it is to solve them. For treatments such as tube feedings, which extend life using low technology, the issue is more basic. Food and water are fundamental to human existence. However, it is likely that both will be seen as extraordinary treatment when continuing to provide them artificially offers no hope of benefit.

Continued attention to the implications of technology for patient autonomy and the principle of nonmaleficence are necessary if the organization is to fulfill its mission in the context of its philosophy. This role is a primary one for managers, who are moral agents at the same time that they function as employees of the organization.

The law regarding the criminality of aiding and abetting suicide will need to change before a case such as that of Janet Adkins has implications for health services managers. It is possible, however, that like abortion, suicide will be defined by courts or legislatures as a privacy issue. If so, health services organizations and their managers will be forced to grapple with the ethical implications of assisted suicide.

The incentives resulting from cost constraints and the increasingly interlocking economic interests of physicians and organizations, whether or not under health care reform, will cause a major reassessment of aid in dying. Numerous questions must be answered: Must physicians meet their patients' demands for aid in dying through active means? Is it reasonable (or wise) to ask those committed to preserving and extending life to become thanatologists? Have patients who cannot assist in suicide a right to voluntary active euthanasia? And, for health services managers, is there a role for the organization to aid in dying, regardless of how the current controversy is resolved? At minimum, health services managers must assure that a right to die does not become a duty to die.

NOTES

1. American Medical Association, Council on Ethical and Judicial Affairs. (1994). *Code of medical ethics: Current opinions with annotations* (pp. 36–38). Chicago: Author.

2. A definition of irreversible coma. Report of the Harvard Medical School Ad Hoc Committee to Examine the Definition of Brain Death. (1968, August). *Journal of the American Medical Association, 205*(6), 337–338.

3. Robert M. Veatch. (1972, November). Brain death: Welcome definition or dangerous judgment? *Hastings Center Report, 2*(6), 10.

4. President's Commission for the Study of Ethical Problems in Medicine and Biomedical and Behavioral Research. (1981). *Defining death: Medical, legal and ethical issues in the determination of death* (p. 25). Washington, DC: U.S. Government Printing Office.

5. Eelco F.M. Wijdicks. (1995, May). Determining brain death in adults. *Neurology, 45*, 1003–1011.

6. *Uniform laws annotated*, Vol. 12, *Civil procedural and remedial laws*. (1995, pp. 441–445). St. Paul, MN: West Publishing.

7. The American Academy of Neurology adopted the National Conference of Commissioners on Uniform State Laws' definition on August 3, 1978. The definition states that "for legal and medical purposes an individual with irreversible cessation of all function of the brain, including the brain stem, is dead. Determination of death under this act shall be made in accordance with reasonable medical standards." Personal communication from the American Academy of Neurology, May 17, 1996.

8. Choice in Dying, Inc. (1996, March). *State statutes governing living wills and appointment of health care agents.* New York: Author.

9. R. Sean Morrison, Ellen Olson, Kristan R. Mertz, & Diane E. Meier. (1995, August 9). The inaccessibility of advance directives on transfer from ambulatory to acute care settings. *Journal of the American Medical Association, 274*(6), 478–482.

10. Anna Maria Cugliari, Tracy Miller, & Jeffery Sobal. (1995, September 25). Factors promoting completion of advance directives in the hospital. *Archives of Internal Medicine, 155,* 1893–1898.

11. Brendan M. Reilly, Michael Wagner, C. Richard Magnussen, James Ross, Louis Papa, & Jeffrey Ash. (1995, November 27). Promoting inpatient directives about life-sustaining treatments in a community hospital. *Archives of Internal Medicine, 155,* 2317–2323.

12. Mildred Z. Solomon, Lydia O'Donnell, Bruce Jennings, Vivian Guilfoy, Susan M. Wolf, Kathleen Nolan, Rebecca Jackson, Dieter Koch-Weser, & Strachan Donnelley. (1993, January). Decisions near the end of life: Professional views on life-sustaining treatments. *American Journal of Public Health, 83*(1), 14–21.

13. Choice in Dying, Inc. (1996, March). *State statutes governing surrogate decision-making.* New York: Author.

14. Choice in Dying, Inc. (1996, March). *State statutes governing living wills and appointment of health care agents.* New York: Author.

15. Bonnie S. Jacobson. (1994, September). Ethical dilemmas of do-not-resuscitate orders in surgery. *AORN Journal, 60*(3) 449–452; Proposed AORN position statement on perioperative care of patients with do-not-resuscitate (DNR) orders. (1994, October). *AORN Journal, 60*(4), 648, 650; and Statement of the American College of Surgeons on advance directives by patients: "Do not resuscitate" in the operating room. (1994, September). *ACS Bulletin,* p. 29. Judith O. Margolis, Brian J. McGrath, Peter S. Kussin, & Debra A. Schwinn. (1995). Do not resuscitate (DNR) orders during surgery: Ethical foundations for institutional policies in the United States. *Anesthesia and Analgesia, 80,* 806–809.

16. Personal communication. (1996, February). New York: Choice in Dying, Inc.

17. Andrew L. Evans, & Baruch A. Brody. (1985, April). The do-not-resuscitate order in teaching hospitals. *Journal of the American Medical Association, 253*(15), 2236–2239.

18. Susanna E. Bedell, & Thomas L. Delbanco. (1984, April). Choices about cardiopulmonary resuscitation in the hospital: When do physicians talk with patients? *New England Journal of Medicine, 320*(17), 1089–1093.

19. Joan M. Teno, Rosemarie B. Hakim, William A. Knaus, Neil S. Wenger, Russell S. Phillips, Albert W. Wu, Peter Layde, Alfred F. Connors, Neal V. Dawson, & Joanne Lynn, for the SUPPORT Investigators. (1995, April). Preferences for

cardiopulmonary resuscitation: Physician–patient agreement and hospital resource use. *Journal of General Internal Medicine, 10*, 179–186.

20. Neil S. Wenger, Marjorie L. Pearson, Katherine A. Desmond, Ellen R. Harrison, Lisa V. Rubenstein, William H. Rogers, & Katherine L. Kahn. (1995, October 23). Epidemiology of do-not-resuscitate orders: Disparity by age, diagnosis, gender, race, and functional impairment. *Archives of Internal Medicine, 155*, 2056–2062.

21. Robert M. Wachter, John M. Luce, Norman Hearst, & Bernard Lo. (1989, September). Decisions about resuscitation: Inequities among patients with different diseases but similar prognoses. *Annals of Internal Medicine, 111*(no. 6), 525–532.

22. Susan Morse. (1985, July 15). Final requests: Preparing for death. *The Washington Post*, p. B5.

23. Gerald Kelly. (1951, December). The duty to preserve life. *Theological Studies, 12*, 550.

24. Vatican Congregation for the Doctrine of the Faith. (1980, June 26). *Declaration on euthanasia*. Vatican City, Italy: Author.

25. Tom L. Beauchamp, & James F. Childress. (1994). *Principles of biomedical ethics* (4th ed., p. 207). New York: Oxford University Press.

26. Patient's right to starve upheld. (1984, February 3). *The Washington Post*, p. A20.

27. Robert M. Veatch. (1977). *Case studies in medical ethics* (pp. 340–341). Cambridge, MA: Harvard University Press.

28. In re Quinlan, 70 N.J. 10, 355 A.2d 647 (1976).

29. Susan M. Wolf. (1990, January–February). Nancy Beth Cruzan: In no voice at all. *Hastings Center Report, 20*(1), 39.

30. Cruzan v. Director, Missouri Department of Health et al. 110 S. Ct. 2841 (1990).

31. Malcolm Gladwell. (1990, December 27). Woman in right to die case succumbs. *The Washington Post*, p. A3.

32. Joanne Lynn, & James F. Childress. (1983, October). Must patients always be given food and water? *Hastings Center Report, 13*(5), 17–21; John J. Paris, & Anne B. Fletcher. (1983, October). Infant Doe regulations and the absolute requirements to use nourishment and fluids for the dying infant. *Law, Medicine & Health Care, 11*, 210–213.

33. American Hospital Association. (1986, March 15). *Withholding and withdrawing life-prolonging medical treatment*. Chicago: Author.

34. American Medical Association, Council on Ethical and Judicial Affairs. (1994). *Code of medical ethics: Current opinions with annotations* (pp. 36–38). Chicago: Author.

35. Robert J. Sullivan, Jr. (1993, April). Accepting death without artificial nutrition or hydration. *Journal of General Internal Medicine, 8*, 222.

36. *Ibid.*

37. Department of Health and Human Services, Office of Human Development Services. Final Rule, Child Abuse and Neglect Prevention and Treatment Program, 45 C.F.R. § 1340 (April 15, 1985).

38. *Ibid.*

39. Melinda A. Lee, & Susan W. Tolle. (1996, January 15). Oregon's assisted suicide vote: The silver lining. *Annals of Internal Medicine, 124*(2), 267–269.

40. Choice in Dying, Inc. (1996, March). *Assisted suicide laws in the United States.* New York: Author.
41. Henry Weinstein. (1996, March 7). Appeals court in West strikes down prohibition against doctor-aided suicides. *The Washington Post,* p. A5.
42. Joan Biskupic. (1996, April 3). U.S. appeals court overturns New York assisted-suicide ban. *The Washington Post,* p. A1.
43. Jerald G. Bachman, Kirsten H. Alcser, David J. Doukas, Richard L. Lichtenstein, Amy D. Corning, & Howard Brody. (1996, February 1). Attitudes of Michigan physicians and the public toward legalizing physician-assisted suicide and voluntary euthanasia. *New England Journal of Medicine, 334*(5), 303–309; Melinda A. Lee, Heidi D. Nelson, Virginia P. Tilden, Linda Ganzini, Terri A. Schmidt, & Susan W. Tolle. (1996, February 1). Legalizing assisted suicide—views of physicians in Oregon. *New England Journal of Medicine, 334*(5), 310–315.
44. Anthony L. Back, Jeffrey I. Wallace, Helene E. Starks, & Robert A. Pearlman. (1996, March 27). Physician-assisted suicide and euthanasia in Washington State: Patient requests and physician responses. *Journal of the American Medical Association, 275*(12), 919–925.
45. Victor Cohn. (1990, June 12). An assisted suicide: Is it the first step toward euthanasia? *The Washington Post,* Health Section.
46. Nancy Gibbs. (1990, June 18). Dr. Death's suicide machine. *Time,* pp. 69–70.
47. Arguing that assisted suicide is unconstitutional is Yale Kamisar. (1993, May–June). Are laws against assisted suicide unconstitutional? *Hastings Center Report, 23*(3), 32–41.
48. Arguing that assisted suicide is constitutional is Robert A. Sedler. (1993, September–October). The Constitution and hastening inevitable death. *Hastings Center Report, 23*(5), 20–25.
49. Frank J. Murray. (1995, April 25). High court won't touch Michigan suicide-aid ban. *The Washington Times,* p. A1.
50. Marlise Simons. (1993, February 10). Dutch Parliament approves law permitting euthanasia. *The New York Times,* p. A10.
51. *Ibid.*
52. Melinda A. Lee, Heidi D. Nelson, Virginia P. Tilden, Linda Ganzini, Terri A. Schmidt, & Susan W. Tolle. (1996, February 1). Legalizing assisted suicide—views of physicians in Oregon. *New England Journal of Medicine, 334*(5), 310–315.
53. Marlise Simons. (1993, February 10). Dutch Parliament approves law permitting euthanasia. *The New York Times,* p. A10.
54. John Keown. (1991, November 5). Dutch slide down euthanasia's slippery slope. *The Wall Street Journal,* p. A18.
55. Dutch may broaden euthanasia guidelines. (1993, February 17). *The New York Times,* p. A3.
56. Margaret P. Battin. (1992, March–April). Assisted suicide: Can we learn from Germany? *Hastings Center Report, 22*(2), 44–51.
57. Jay Matthews. (1983, December 17). Judge rejects palsy victim's bid to starve. *The Washington Post,* p. A3.
58. California Supreme Court rejects appeal by Bouvia to starve. (1984, January 20). *The Washington Post,* p. A15.

59. Patient repeatedly calls off her effort to starve to death. (1985, April 24). *The New York Times*, p. B15.
60. The latest word. (1985, August). *Hastings Center Report, 15*(no. 4), 36.
61. Doctors stop force-feeding of quadraplegic who sued. (1986, April 18). *The Washington Post*, p. A12.
62. Bouvia moves to another CA hospital. (1986, May 30). *Hospital Week*, pp. 21–23.
63. Right to refuse forced feeding upheld in court. (1986, June 6). *The Washington Post*, p. A8.
64. Tinker Ready. (1989, December 18). Medical groups back plaintiffs in right-to-die case. *Healthweek*, pp. 6–8.

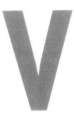

Emerging Ethical Issues

Ore changes in the management of health services organizations have occurred since the 1970s than occurred from 1900 to 1970. Change is the
future, and may occur at an accelerating pace. New managerial challenges
mean greater demands on organizational philosophies and cultures and the manager's
personal ethic. Managers with an ill-defined personal ethic will feel adrift in a world
that seems to have few solid foundations.

Chapter 11 examines marketing and managed care in a competitive environment,
Chapter 12 analyzes the impact of human immunodeficiency virus (HIV) and acquired
immunodeficiency syndrome (AIDS) on health services organizations, and Chapter 13
focuses on resource allocation and social responsibility. These areas have grown in
importance since the 1980s, and their ethical implications require special attention.

The competitive environment has convinced the managers of most health services
organizations that marketing is essential if the organizations are to survive. The marketing function is not new to these leaders. Applying it in a more commercial and
entrepreneurial manner is new, however, and many managers are uncertain of the
ethical implications, especially if they manage not-for-profit organizations. Managed
care has emerged as the primary means by which health services delivery will be organized and financed well into the next millennium. Like marketing, managed care is
not new to health services, but its increasing prevalence, coupled with quality and cost
pressures, raise complex ethical issues that will challenge management.

HIV and AIDS and the ethical issues they raise affect and will continue to affect
all types of health services organizations. They became major ethical issues in the
1980s. Gratefully, the shrillness that marked discussion of them is largely gone. The
managerial and ethical implications continue and both raise some of the most complex
problems health services managers will address.

Health services managers cannot but be aware of the increasingly ominous struggle for resources that is occurring at all levels of society. The organization is a micro-
cosm of this struggle. Given the importance of health services in providing critical
services to society, persons who manage the organization play a central role as arbiters
of resource allocation. The ethical implications are enormous.

11

Ethics in Marketing and Managed Care

MARKETING

Although the elements of marketing—product, place, promotion, and pricing—have been applied to health services with apparent ease, the purposes and the context of health services differ from the typical business enterprise.

In the 1920s President Calvin Coolidge noted that the business of America is business. This premise remains accurate: The United States continues to be a bastion of capitalism. Unique among its businesses is the health services industry. Health services differ from other enterprises in purpose, type of service provided, orientation, and motives. Unlike most other enterprises, health services providers may be affiliated with a specific religion and may have not-for-profit tax status. Health services organizations are also unique in that they are intimately involved with several professions and provide services that comprise significant emotional and psychological dimensions. Health services organizations are social enterprises with an economic dimension rather than economic enterprises with a social dimension.

Cunningham[1] noted that marketing in traditional business enterprise differs from marketing of health services because the former markets to create demand for its products and to promote and sell goods and services aggressively. This distinction is sometimes blurred. All health services organizations market, and have always done so. This is especially true for acute care hospitals and is increasingly true in managed care and nursing facilities. Historically, marketing occurred in several ways, including community "health days" and press releases, but the milieu of the competitive marketplace requires that marketing become systematic, focused, and much more aggressive.

NEED VERSUS DEMAND

Opinions vary when the role of marketing is assessed: Is demand being created or is it being met? Important to answering this question is disagreement about which types of health services demand are meritorious, a value-laden concept in itself. Few persons would disagree that it is important to create consumer demand for hypertension or colorectal cancer screening. The desirability of such efforts is tempered by calculating costs and benefits. Depending on the population and the disease, screening may be unacceptably expensive when measured by the number of true positives found and the morbidity and mortality prevented.

Both price and nonprice competition may increase demand, but it is generally agreed that competition in and of itself is desirable. Despite acceptance of competition, disagreement as to whether the demand created is appropriate continues to be an issue. In addition, some conditions that require medical intervention may be treated with more than one type of therapy. Coronary artery bypass surgery for patients with mild or moderate symptoms of heart disease is an example of an expensive therapy that some patients might avoid. Cardiac surgeons stress the procedure's usefulness for occluded coronary arteries and relief of angina. The cardiologists and internists who are inclined to treat such patients medically rely on data that show similar long-term results for patients in some categories when managed with a medical regimen instead of surgery. Cost differences are enormous. A National Heart Institute study reported in the early 1980s estimated that of the 200,000 bypass procedures performed each year, about 25,000 could be forgone, with a savings of $15,000–$40,000 per procedure.[2]

Other diagnoses have been involved in similar controversies about treatment. Prostate cancer is an example. Following early detection using the prostate-specific antigen test the standard therapy is to treat all malignant prostate tumors aggressively with surgery or with a 7-week course of radiation therapy. The result is that men who would neither die from nor likely even notice small prostate tumors endure treatment that often invites complications, such as incontinence, impotence, injury, and sometimes death. The watchful waiting, or expectant management, approach has been proposed as a less detrimental alternative. Both entail closely monitoring the progression of a small, slow-growing tumor and initiating treatment only when necessary. Such an approach is appropriate for men who may not live another 10 years, such as those over age 75 or those with severe heart disease or diabetes. The cost and quality of life differences are obvious.[3]

Contrasted with the objective need to intervene in the case of coronary artery disease are situations that are more subjective. Cosmetic surgery is often cited as an example of an "unnecessary" medical service. It is claimed that face lifts, tummy tucks, and silicone implants waste medical resources—regardless of payment source—and that these resources should be available for other health uses. This is a subjective definition of need. Reasonable persons could reach different conclusions as to what patients "need" and how or whether the demand that arises from that need should be met by the health care system. Perhaps activities such as cosmetic surgery should not be defined as health services at all but as consumer services similar to haircutting and bodybuilding that happen to use elements of the health care system.

Epidemiologic studies should be used to develop data about populations. These data reveal the incidence and prevalence of diseases as well as psychological and physical concerns of the population that may fall outside the more traditional definitions of disease. The real problem in terms of assessing need and demand arises when persons judging such data apply their value systems to determine the problem's importance. These judgments cause the process to be less than objective whether it affects decisions in determining what to study or what is to be done with the results. In turn, these decisions affect the choice of regimens and decisions whether to treat.

The debate about need is most heated when issues of marketing ethics are included, especially if marketing is to be used to affect demand or to encourage persons to seek elective procedures. Physical or psychological conditions about which an individual is either unaware or unwilling to seek treatment represent potential demand for medical services. Conditions for which no help is sought because of financial barriers also represent potential demand; examples include dental care, hammer toes, hemorrhoids, cataracts, and psychiatric services.

Troubling in this debate is the suggestion that meeting potential demand is unethical. If one applies the admittedly broad World Health Organization definition of health,* then all efforts to improve health are beneficial. It is instructive to consider wellness (prevention) activities. The possibilities for organizational involvement are almost limitless because every facet of life could be affected to improve general health and prevent medical problems. In addition to wellness activities there are questions of how to treat demand for services that may seem foolish to some observers. Should people be denied cosmetic surgery simply because other people judge such procedures to be trivial or because what they seek to correct is not life threatening? Such infringements on individual autonomy are greater than the public will accept.

It is not clear how and by whom need and demand are to be judged. Despite the presence of the occasional hypochondriac or Munchausen's syndrome patient, demand for services should be accepted as rational. In looking at demand for medical services, it is most useful to focus attention on "typical" patients. When "typical" patients hear about new medical problems or treatment and diagnostic possibilities, they respond rationally. The "worried well" are persons who are not clinically ill but properly concerned about their health and the quality of their lives. Their decisions about elective proced-

---

*"Health is a state of complete physical, mental, and social well-being and not merely the absence of disease or infirmity."[17]

ures are cost–benefit analyses. It is when publicly funded programs use cost–benefit analyses to make macroallocation decisions that services formerly provided may become unavailable. The Oregon example of prioritizing health services in its Medicaid program is thus instructive and rational when resources are inadequate.

Responsible Marketing

How does the health services organization market to patients and potential patients consistent with its ethical obligation to avoid creating "unnecessary" demand, while simultaneously meeting its obligation to seek out and serve those who might be in need? The American Hospital Association (AHA) has developed a statement on proper health care facilities' advertising, a major element of marketing. The statement should be used to educate the public about services and health care, provide public accountability, gain public and medical staff support, maintain or increase market share, and recruit employees. Advertising must be truthful, fair, accurate, complete, and sensitive to the public's health care needs and not raise unrealistic expectations. Comparisons between facilities must be objective and fully substantiated.[4]

Few individuals would dispute that the above description is one of responsible marketing. If profits and return on investment are the primary reasons for their existence, organizations will take a very different view of what is responsible marketing as well as what is appropriate competition. This is the difference between giving people whatever they want and tempering desires and potential demand with efforts to judge value and usefulness. This view of the patient involves elements of paternalism, but it should be consistent with the statement of purpose in the organization's mission statement.

Demarketing to Avoid Bankruptcy

CEO Chris Hines had finally gotten down far enough in the stack of papers on her desk to get to last month's emergency department (ED) activity report. She had already digested the grim news about the continued financial hemorrhage affecting Community Hospital. The current deficit was $500,000—and it was only the fourth month of the fiscal year. Because Community Hospital served largely inner city patients, many of whom were uninsured or whose care was paid by a chronically underfunded Medicaid program, there seemed to be little hope that the financial situation would improve.

Hines knew that over 40% of Community Hospital's admissions came through the ED, and that about half of those admissions arrived by taxi, private automobile, or on foot. The other half came in via the ambulance service owned by the city. Hines had tried to implement a plan to increase elective admissions, thus improving the payer mix, by encouraging her attending physicians to bring their patients to Community. Her effort failed. Next, Hines tried to work with city officials to implement a new ambulance routing system that would give Community a chance to improve its financial condition. Unsympathetic city officials refused to assist this effort.

Hines knew that Community Hospital's endowment would carry the hospital for approximately 3 more years, but that it would have to close if it was not breaking even by then. Because the city was uncooperative, Hines concluded that the key to survival lay with reducing the number of uninsured and Medicaid patients admitted through the ED.

Hines spoke with several marketing consultants, one of whom offered to do *pro bono* work for Community Hospital. He seized upon the idea of "demarketing" the ED. He reasoned that it was the fine reputation enjoyed by Community Hospital's ED that was largely responsible for the 50% of ED patients who arrived other than by city ambulance. He listed the following ways the ED could be made less attractive to potential patients: reducing ED staffing to a minimum; closing the parking lot near the ED; reducing housekeeping services so that the physical plant would be dirty and unkempt; deferring nonsafety-related maintenance; changing triage policies, procedures, and staffing to increase waiting time for nonemergency patients; using staff who were most likely to be rude and inconsiderate; and encouraging rumors that closure of the ED was imminent.

The consultant knew that there might be repercussions beyond the ED, but Community was desperate, and he believed extreme action was necessary.

In analyzing this case, one must first ask whether there were other steps Hines and her managers could have taken to improve the financial condition of Community Hospital. Examples include closing the ED rather than demarketing it (a more honest solution); undertaking other, more remunerative medical care activities to offset the ED losses; or opening less costly primary care clinics to care for the worried well and other nonemergency medical problems coming into the ED.

Assuming, however, that such options were unavailable, the demarketing strategy raises two ethical issues. First, the steps contemplated are likely to negatively affect the quality of care in the ED. Beyond staffing and the physical aspects directly affected, the psychological effects on ED staff, with a probable ripple effect on inpatient care, will negatively affect morale and ultimately the quality of care. Such actions violate the principles of beneficence and nonmaleficence.

A second ethical issue raised is that of justice. People in the community are caught between the city bureaucracy and the efforts of Community Hospital to remain financially viable. They may have little choice but to endure the indignities and reduction in quality of care that would result from the demarketing strategy. Deliberately adding insult to injury should give all concerned a great deal of discomfort. Another dimension of justice is the unfairness associated with forcing the remaining ED staff to work under such conditions. They will bear the brunt of angry patients and the dilapidated, depressing environment of the ED.

The fact that the declining financial condition of Community Hospital might have resulted in many of the same changes in the ED eventually does not justify deliberately undertaking them in the manner contemplated. Desperate managers may commit desperate acts, but this does not justify them morally.

FUTURE OF COMPETITION

A political science theory suggests that over time enemies begin to take on one another's attributes. This concern deeply troubles the not-for-profit sector of the health services system, which views itself as holding and furthering values different from those in the for-profit sector. They fear that competition for market share and the focus on financial considerations and economic survival will cause them to lose sight of their humanitarian and charitable motives.

In this regard payment systems are especially significant. The advent of reimbursement using diagnosis-related groups (DRGs) for hospitalized Medicare beneficiaries was the opening round of what is proving to be a complete reassessment of payment schemes. Competitive and cost-cutting pressures are causing a rapid shift away from fee-for-service to various forms of fixed payment for services. Physician and organizational providers are becoming aligned in relationships that add a significant amount of complexity to traditional ethical problems and raise several new ones.

Some writers suggest that the pressures of fixed-fee reimbursement will lead to an adversarial relationship between patients and organizations (and perhaps the physician), and that patients' interests will be overrun by the demands of efficiency and economic survival. Such results are possible under any payment system or ownership and will occur whenever caregivers and managers lose sight of their reason for being. Doing more with less need not be at variance with efforts to operationalize the principles of respect for persons, beneficence, nonmaleficence, and justice. It remains for all who are involved in organizing, planning, and delivering health services to keep these principles firmly in mind.

COMPETITION AND HUMAN RESOURCES POLICY

Competition has implications for hiring practices.

Hiring the Competition

The two nursing facilities in town are highly competitive. This competition has caused them to oppose one another's certificates of need applications to the point of suing one another. The chief operating officers (COOs) of the nursing facilities have been friends since before they joined their respective nursing facilities. They play golf monthly. The COO of one nursing facility is fired because of political intrigue on the board of directors. The other COO offers to hire him as a consultant.

Codes of ethics do not cover this set of circumstances. The fired COO is privy to proprietary information that could give the other nursing facility an unfair competitive advantage. In theory, it is possible that the fired COO could consult on matters that would not require him to reveal or use proprietary information. Given the history of the two organizations this is unlikely. The ethically superior answer would be to not hire the former competing manager. Short of that, it may be possible to avoid using the competitor's proprietary information, something that could be determined only by looking at the specifics of the case.

Does a fired manager have any duty to a former employer? Managers have an ethical duty to keep proprietary information confidential after they sever relations with an employer. This duty of confidentiality continues until events have overtaken the confidential information. If there were no duty of confidentiality, organizations could be held hostage by former employees.

Managers would be among the first to agree that this is an undesirable situation from both managerial and professional perspectives.

MANAGED CARE

The primary ethical issue that arises in managed care is conflict of interest. The potential for conflicts of interest is inherent in managed care because the goals, purposes, and objectives of management and personnel may be at variance with the interests of enrollees. The tension between the managed care organization (MCO) and its enrollees and potential enrollees occurs as early as initial marketing, when benefits packages and market segments are identified. The potential for conflicts of interest is unavoidable, but their presence and consequent negative effects can be minimized if they are recognized by clinicians and managers. Enrollees also must be alert to the potential for conflicts of interest.

How do conflicts of interest affect the marketing of an MCO? The potential conflicts of interest that are present when no relationship exists between the provider and those at whom marketing is directed can lead to actual conflicts. This potential for conflicts is exacerbated because some MCOs, especially not-for-profit health maintenance organizations (HMOs), maintain a self-image that they are more public service oriented and are on a higher moral plane than the "typical" health services organization. Historically, the perception of prepaid health plans and HMOs has been that they are a "purer" delivery system, a system untainted by the profit motive and one through which members gain access to high-quality medical services at modest cost. The field is changing as the number of for-profit MCOs and HMOs increases. The historical perception remains, however. To the extent that marketing ignores or purposely excludes high-risk groups ("cream skimming"), there may be variance between historic and current mission and purpose.

Adverse Selection and Marketing Managed Care

The marketing strategy must consider whether to minimize significant clinical strengths that provider components may possess. If the MCO is or is perceived to be a leader in treating a complex or high-cost medical condition and this fact becomes known, adverse selection is likely, and the MCO will be inundated with persons requiring that treatment. If higher quality results in higher costs, the MCO falls into a vicious cycle. An MCO's reputation for high-quality results encourages more high-risk persons who need expensive care to join. Straining against this adverse selection may cause quality to decline for other enrollees, or the MCO may be forced to restrict benefits or increase premiums. Thus, if the MCO is to survive, marketers may be required to minimize references to superb care of specific types and to focus instead on developing a reputation that the MCO delivers general medical services of high quality but that there are no "centers of excellence."

The following case suggests the potential for problems if an MCO is perceived to be especially effective in treating certain types of patients.

I Want to See Dr. Nightengale

Dr. Nightengale is a pediatrician with HMO, Inc., located in a medium-size city. She has had no specialty training beyond her residency, but she has developed into an adept diagnostician, often diagnosing cases that baffle her colleagues.

At the last open enrollment, management noted that an unexpectedly large number of families with young children enrolled. As is typical, HMO, Inc., limits in-area, out-of-plan services, and restricts referrals to subspecialists. Dr. Nightengale uses subspecialists more often than her colleagues, but she achieves excellent results. The new member survey showed that for many families, the presence of excellent pediatric care was an important factor in making their decision to join HMO, Inc. A few named Dr. Nightengale specifically.

Management expressed fears that such perceptions might cause an adverse selection problem. Management even suggested that to protect the organization's financial position a special review of Dr. Nightengale's use of subspecialists should be undertaken. Some thought this was an overreaction. They agreed to take a "wait and see" approach. If there were problems, they would talk to her.

Another example of adverse selection occurred in treating persons who are HIV positive. An HMO in the Washington, D.C., area has achieved a deserved reputation for providing high-quality care to this group. This knowledge has been disseminated throughout the community and high-risk individuals are enrolling disproportionately. No data have been compiled by the HMO showing higher costs for enrollees with HIV. However, it is generally agreed that hospitalization and high-cost drug therapies as HIV progresses to frank AIDS will make care expensive, although less expensive sources of care are increasingly available. Sicker enrollees require more care, which places an MCO with disproportionate numbers of such persons at financial risk and, in terms of its survival, at a competitive disadvantage.

Service Utilization in Managed Care Organizations

Managers, staff, and clinicians in the MCO bureaucracy seek to maximize position, power, income, and rewards with the least disruption of the organization's homeostasis. Achieving these goals, especially that of maximizing income, may minimize service, whether or not that is consistent with the contract between the MCO and the payer. The bureaucratic response may even be at variance with the MCO's long-term survival needs. To regain or retain their health, enrollees want to pay as little as necessary but obtain all needed services—at the least they want value for their premium. When enrollees use services efficiently and stay well at minimum cost, MCO and enrollee goals are congruent. The situation is rarely that simple, however.

The primary source of potential conflicts of interests is in utilization of services. Enrollees may be divided into two groups: light and moderate users of services and heavy users. The MCO's interests and the interests of light and moderate users are generally congruent; to be competitive, the MCO must control heavy users. Even moderate users are potential financial threats to MCOs in a competitive environment, and to cut costs the MCO may seek to transform them into light users. The potential for conflicts of interest is clear.

How do potential conflicts of interests, as shown by incongruent goals of MCO and enrollee, become true conflicts? The MCO's marketing will stress access to primary and specialty services and minimize limits on services. Enrollees may be constrained by limited hours, services, and having too few clinical staff to meet demand, thus purposely creating queues. Waits for appointments will reduce operating costs, especially for the 85% of medical complaints that are self-limiting. The public is unlikely to endorse a deliberate strategy of deferring treatment, regardless of the clinical and economic soundness of such a policy. MCOs have an escape valve for these pressures by providing advice nurse consultation and treating walk-ins during office hours. In the late 1980s a furor resulted when the CEO of a large East Coast HMO stated publicly that the HMO used a deliberate policy of allowing queues, noting their value in reducing demand for certain services, especially self-limiting conditions. Such policies may cause disenrollment in the long term, but are effective in the short term.

Physician Incentives and Disincentives

For the enrollee, the more subtle and potentially more serious constraints imposed by MCOs are directed at affiliated physicians. Conflicts of interest are possible both between MCO and enrollee and between physician and enrollee. The Hippocratic oath requires physicians to act in the patient's best interests. The AMA's Principles of Medical Ethics state: "A physician shall be dedicated to providing competent medical services with compassion and respect for human dignity," and "A physician shall deal honestly with patients and colleagues." [5] These ethical guidelines suggest that patients' interests be at the forefront as physicians choose the level and content of care.

MCOs, however, determine the context that facilitates or inhibits physician responses. Initially, there is a self-selection bias when physicians choose where to practice or with whom they will contract. Physicians who cannot accept the rules imposed by an MCO will look elsewhere. Once a physician joins an MCO, management can use a range of actions to modify behavior, including financial disincentives and incentives, peer pressure, nonrenewal, and dismissal. MCOs can limit referrals, especially outside the MCO; strictly control hospitalizations; establish quotas on the number of enrollees who must be seen, as in a staff model HMO; and use a system of peer review. Peer pressure plays an important role in most constraints. Constraints are positive when they encourage judicious, but appropriate use of resources. This may account in part for the use of fewer ancillary services and hospital days by MCOs than by fee-for-service providers.

Financial incentives and disincentives are high-risk propositions in terms of conflicts of interest, and among these, physician-at-risk or capitated payments are among the most problematic. Bonuses may be based on use of ancillary services, referrals, and hospitalizations. Thus, they may be either incentives or disincentives. The effect of a potential bonus can be insidious in that the physician's decision-making process may be affected subconsciously or in ways not fully appreciated by the physician or others, but especially not by the patient. Another problem with bonuses is that staff begin to view them as a usual and expected part of their compensation, and failing to pay them is likely to result in lower morale or other, more negative consequences.

When do constraints become excessive and deny members needed services? When do constraints violate the principles of nonmaleficence and beneficence? Such questions are not easily answered because they are a function of the MCO's willingness, prompted by its managers acting as moral agents, to institute the safeguards that balance competitiveness and financial factors with protecting enrollees.

Other Constraints in Managed Care Organizations

Besides physician-oriented constraints, other types of constraints are found in the organizational and managerial functioning of MCOs. By employing a complicated process (e.g., significant committee involvement and several levels of review), the MCO may be slow to approve use of new procedures, techniques, or equipment that raise costs. Such complexities may be prevalent more often in not-for-profit than in investor-owned MCOs. The complex processes operating in not-for-profit MCOs may be a function of a greater degree of democracy and not a deliberate effort to diminish access. The effect may be the same, however. For-profit MCOs tend to use a narrower management pyramid that gives the CEO more authority. A complex management structure in the investor-owned MCO is less likely to diminish its ability to conserve resources to the potential detriment of enrollees.

MCOs may forgo purchasing high-technology equipment, or they may contract with physicians and hospitals without such equipment. For example, the higher operating costs of teaching hospitals place them at a competitive disadvantage, which means they are less likely to have contracts with MCOs. Such strategies lower costs. If lower costs enhance financial integrity and guarantee the continued availability of services to enrollees, all parties' interests are congruent. A conflict arises, however, between enrollees who might have benefited from access to the technology and the MCO.

Controls on access such as using primary care physicians as gatekeepers or case managers, limiting out-of-plan services, and specifying dollar limits on referrals and consultations help MCOs curtail costs. Those in competitive environments, however, must show that enrollees who need services get them (or at least create such a perception) lest they lose market share. In addition, indirect and retrospective controls on access occur through use of utilization review, which is conducted on resource consumption patterns of various types of services by physicians, but focus on those that are high cost. Controls risk malpractice suits and negative publicity should limiting access and utilization be perceived as resulting in poor outcomes.

Dissatisfaction regarding access to treatment was reflected in a study of nonelderly sick enrollees. Those in managed care were almost twice as likely (22% vs. 13%) to state that they experienced major or minor problems obtaining treatment they or their physicians thought was necessary. The managed care group experienced greater difficulty (21% vs. 15%) than the fee-for-service group in seeing a specialist in the past year when one was needed.[6] Data such as these support widespread anecdotal impressions that there is a cost–quality trade off in managed care. In addition, the media regularly reports horror stories that describe alleged denials of (usually specialty) care to enrollees who suffer significant morbidity or death as a result.[7]

Utilization review and financial incentives and disincentives for physicians are likely to be interim steps in the evolution of managed care, which itself is likely to be only a way station in the evolution to direct contracting between employers or other groups and health services providers. Financial incentives and disincentives to enrollees are common and likely to become more important. Ultimately, however, *managed care* will become *managed lives*. Health care costs can best be controlled by reducing health risks, which inevitably means affecting lifestyles. Lifestyle initiatives may be economic, such as charging higher premiums for people with unhealthy habits; medical, such as early detection of disease or disenrolling noncompliant enrollees; or legal, such as providers or MCOs lobbying for passage of laws that promote healthful activities or limit those that are unhealthy.[8] In its latter stages this evolution will bring us to an Orwellian relationship with MCOs.

Minimizing Conflicts of Interest and Other Conflicts

How do MCOs and their managers prevent or minimize conflicts of interest? An indispensable first step is a willingness to acknowledge that potential conflicts of interest are inherent in the relationship between MCOs and enrollees as well as that between physicians and the MCO and physicians and enrollees. Awareness permits avoidance or minimization. It is also obvious that third parties have legitimate interests in physician–patient encounters, but as third-party demands for information and control increase "physicians must reassert their own moral authority and that of their patients."[9] Without the active cooperation of health services managers, such a task is likely to be impossible.

A system of checks and balances is also needed. One solution appoints an ombudsman or customer relations specialist to assist enrollees. In addition, there should be due process procedures for persons who wish to have a decision reviewed. Federally qualified HMOs must have an effective grievance procedure for enrollees. This requirement provides some protection. To be effective, however, enrollees must know that a problem has occurred; lack of knowledge is especially problematic when subtle quality of care issues arise. Enrollees are protected if they are able to participate effectively and if management is enlightened and the education and personal characteristics of staff involved are adequate.

MCOs may use the managing physician or gatekeeper concept to limit services provided to enrollees. Such roles are certain to cause conflicts between physicians' ethical obligations to foster the best interests of their patients and the economic expectations and constraints imposed on them by the MCO.[10] Internal audits of MCO utilization data or external data from similar MCOs enable management to determine whether utilization is within acceptable limits. Comparisons such as these alert managers to problems in the delivery of services that may result from conflicts of interest. Awareness of the way in which conflicts of interest arise will help prevent them or minimize their effect. Such activities are essential if managers are to meet their ethical obligations to enrollees.

Mixing managed care employed medical staff with voluntary fee-for-service physicians raises a number of difficult questions, as in the following case.

Practice Pattern Problems Persist

Cedars-Sinai is a 400-bed community hospital located in a large East Coast metropolitan area. It has a reputation as a high-quality, low-cost provider. The medical staff at Cedars-Sinai comprise board-certified physicians who are overwhelmingly solo practitioners or part of two- or three-physician practices. No single- or multispecialty group practices are affiliated with Cedars-Sinai. Medical staff matters are handled cautiously and conservatively by hospital administration.

In 1987 a large West Coast HMO established a presence and grew rapidly. Because of its fine reputation, Cedars-Sinai has become a leading provider of services for the HMO and many of the HMO's physician-employees have admitting privileges. Almost 20% of Cedars-Sinai's patient days come from the HMO.

Following a review of the HMO's utilization patterns a West Coast consultant noted the large difference in hospital days per 1,000 enrollees between East and West Coast branches of the HMO. The HMO's clinical director was asked to assess how many days of care and, consequently, how many premium dollars could be saved with various levels of progress toward the West Coast utilization.

Word of this study came to the attention of Cedars-Sinai's CEO, who was immediately alarmed by the implications. She knew that reducing lengths of stay in any significant way by moving utilization patterns toward the West Coast experience would send shock waves through the majority of the members of her medical staff—the voluntary, fee-for-service physicians. The consequences of such a disparity in patient–day utilization patterns could be a decision by her medical staff leadership not to reappoint the HMO's physician-employees to the medical staff because her voluntary medical staff would judge that the lengths of stay were inappropriately short and risked patient morbidity and mortality.

The CEO faces a true ethical dilemma: She has a duty of loyalty (fiduciary obligation) to the organization, but she also has a duty of beneficence to patients who are treated in the hospital and potential patients in the community. Major disruptions caused by medical staff conflict will surely have a negative effect on the financial situation of the hospital. Yet, decreasing lengths of stay consistent with quality of care and patient safety is desirable from the standpoint of patients and payers and meets the hospital's social responsibility as well. An evolutionary push toward shorter lengths of stay may meet the needs of both groups although neither will consider it very desirable.

Long-Term Cost Savings of Managed Care

As this book publishes, it is generally agreed that managed care has shown that it can reduce health services costs, at least as measured by payments to providers. It is more accurate to say that managed care *may* save costs, depending on the specifics of the situation and the assumptions. To state that managed care *always* saves money perpetuates a myth. The best explanation of why this is a myth is that there is significant evidence that the current cost savings in managed care occur because other payers subsidize the deep discounts demanded and received by MCOs. Absent cross-subsidies, managed care could not show the savings claimed. One large HMO operator, U.S. Healthcare, doubled its profit margin in 2 years, not as the result of productivity or quality enhancement, but by cutting fees paid to doctors and hospitals by 12%–20%. Increasingly, U.S. Healthcare is asking them to share financial risk through capitation.[11]

Managed competition was the cornerstone of the Clinton health plan. "Managed" in that context was a euphemism for government regulation and control. Given that basic benefits packages were mandated and that providers were highly regulated, savings might have occurred, at least in the short term, but with significant economic costs to providers of services and great noneconomic costs to users, especially in the long term.

By every measure the evidence that managed competition will reduce costs is far from clear, and the federal watchdog General Accounting Office has found little empirical evidence as to the cost savings of managed care.[12] In addition, a report on an aggressive attempt to direct most military retirees and dependents into managed care found that there were "(H)igher costs from enhanced benefits, induced demand, and the significant expense for administration and profit."[13] An earlier study found that a demonstration program in California and Hawaii would save the government $300 million over a projected 5-year period.[14]

Other evidence exists that HMOs do not save money. Researchers have found that the effect of HMOs on premiums in employment-based health plans was to increase them. The study compared the weighted average HMO and fee-for-service premium in firms that offer HMOs to the premium of fee-for-service–only firms and found that offering an HMO raises the average premium for family coverage health insurance by $25.14 per month and for single coverage by $3.68 per month.[15] HMOs may have other advantages, but these findings suggest that decreased cost is not among them.

A Congressional Budget Office (CBO) report stated that "the most efficient health maintenance organizations cut patients' use of health services by 19.6% while maintaining levels of care roughly comparable to other types of health plans."[16] Although seemingly contradictory, the language appears to hinge on how services and care were defined. However, there were two important caveats: The first caveat is that the finding applies only to staff and group model HMOs—those that employ physicians; this level of savings is not found in independent practice association-model HMOs, a type proving to be very popular among enrollees. The second caveat is that the CBO concluded that even if all insured people switched to such HMOs health care costs would not decrease 19.6% because administrative costs, pricing decisions, and doctor and hospital fees would also be factors. The study also questioned whether the successes of prepaid care among relatively younger, healthier individuals, who have tended to choose HMOs, can be replicated among sicker patients, who have tended to choose fee-for-service insurance. One significant unknown is the amount spent out-of-pocket by HMO enrollees for health services because of aspects of their plan such as coverage shortcomings and access to specialty referrals.

CONCLUSION

The competitive environment in the field of health services brought with it the perception that marketing was essential. Almost universally during the 1980s health services organizations engaged in marketing, at least at the level of building name recognition. For the not-for-profit organization especially, the question of whether to market raised a host of ethical issues that began with the basic question of the propriety of marketing itself and extended to issues such as creating demand and distinguishing among various types of demand.

Hospitals with large amounts of uncompensated care may see offering better reimbursed services, such as rehabilitation and cosmetic surgery, as ways to offset these losses. "No margin, no mission" is an oft-repeated justification for such actions, if one is needed. More fiscally sound hospitals must ask themselves whether they are meeting a general duty under the principle of justice to offer unprofitable but necessary services that benefit the wider community.

As with all activities undertaken by the health services organization, philosophy and mission statement provide an ethical context for marketing. Managers have a duty under the principle of respect for persons to be honest and keep the promises their marketing makes. The principle of justice suggests that careful attention must be paid to the groups and medical conditions at which marketing is focused. Non–MCO health services organizations potentially experience the same ethical problems.

It behooves health services managers to read beyond the headlines and to be especially skeptical of claims that certain remedies are universal cures. Research findings must also be questioned, especially when studies from small samples or small universes are generalized to a population. Painting with a broad brush should alert everyone. As in life, when something sounds too good to be true, it probably is.

Institutional ethics committees should prospectively and retrospectively assess the ethical issues raised in competition, marketing, and managed care. They should review the ethical implications of competition as it affects their patients, organization, and the community. Marketing initiatives and their results should be understood from an ethical perspective, especially in terms of creating demand and the honesty and promise keeping involved. Institutional ethics committees can be valuable in monitoring care provided and outcomes to provide assurance that patients in managed care as well as in other payment categories receive the same levels of care.

NOTES

1. Robert M. Cunningham, Jr. (1978). Of snake oil and science. *Trustee, 31*(4), 34–36.
2. Victor Cohn. (1983, October 27). Study says some coronary bypasses are unneeded. *The Washington Post*, p. A5.
3. P.J. Skerrett. (1994, August/September). Screening for prostate cancer. *Technology Review, 97*(6), 16–17.
4. American Hospital Association. (1990). *Guidelines: Advertising by health care facilities*. Chicago: Author.
5. American Medical Association. (1980). *Principles of medical ethics*. Chicago: Author.
6. Sick patients not fond of managed care plans. (1995, October). *Medical Ethics Advisor*, p. 133, citing findings of a study conducted by the Harvard University School of Public Health.
7. David S. Hilzenrath. (1995, August 7). Costly savings: Downside of the new health care. *The Washington Post*, p. A1.
8. E. Haavi Morreim. (1995, November–December). Lifestyles of the risky and infamous: From managed care to managed lives. *Hastings Center Report, 25*, 5–6.
9. Warren L. Holleman, David C. Edwards, & Christine C. Matson. (1994, Summer). Obligations of physicians to patients and third-party payers. *The Journal of Clinical Ethics, 5*(2), 120.
10. Edmund D. Pellegrino. (1994, Fall). Managed care and managed competition: Some ethical reflections. *Calyx, 4*(4), 3.
11. Steven Findlay. (1994, October). The managed care dilemma. *Business and Health*, p. 66.
12. Mary Jane Fisher. (1993, November 1). GAO: Little proof of managed care cost savings. *National Underwriter*, p. 42.
13. Carol Sardinha. (1993, February 12). Doubts about managed care savings stall DOD's CRI plans. *Managed Care Outlook, 6*(3), 2.
14. *Ibid.*
15. Agency for Health Care Policy and Research, U.S. Department of Health and Human Services. (1993, March). *Research Activities*, p. 9.
16. Spencer Rich. (1995, March 19). Study finds savings in some HMOs. *The Washington Post*, p. A5.
17. John J. Hanlon, & George E. Pickett. (1990). *Public health: Administration and practice* (9th ed., p. 4). St. Louis: Times Mirror/Mosby College Publications.

12

Dealing with HIV and AIDS

The human immunosuppressive virus (HIV), which leads to acquired immunodeficiency syndrome (AIDS), has proved to be an elusive foe. A great deal has been learned about HIV since it was identified in the early 1980s. Its spread continues but has slowed since the late 1980s. Both the pessimistic prediction of a major outbreak in the general population and the optimistic prediction that it will be confined to and then eliminated within the homosexual population have proved wrong. Scientific breakthroughs have occurred in understanding HIV and in treating AIDS, but there is neither a vaccine to prevent infection nor a cure once infected. A second strain of HIV was isolated in the late 1980s. A new strain of HIV entered the United States from Africa in the summer of 1996; it is probable there will be others. Work on a vaccine has been tempered by the knowledge that the rapid mutation of HIV makes developing a vaccine with long-term effectiveness difficult, if not impossible. Even if a successful vaccine were developed, it would take several years before testing and clinical trials were completed and the vaccine was made available to the general population. However, there is reason for cautious optimism about a vaccine. Meanwhile, prevention and education have received attention unprecedented in modern public health.

INCIDENCE AND PREVALENCE

At the end of 1995 the cumulative number of AIDS cases reported in the United States since 1981 was 513,486; of this number, 62% have died.[1] Although drugs and improved treatment regimens have increased the life expectancy of persons with AIDS the outlook for long-term survival is not bright.

In 1986 it was estimated that 1–1.5 million Americans were infected with HIV. Ten years later the estimate was 0.6 million, about half of whom have developed frank AIDS. These numbers suggest that the AIDS epidemic in the United States has plateaued and is waning. The incidence rate (number of new cases) of HIV is declining. In 1996 it was reported that since 1993, 10,000–20,000 more persons died of AIDS than became infected with HIV. It is estimated that annually 60,000 Americans die from AIDS; 40,000 are HIV infected. This plateau is believed to have occurred because persons in major risk groups, especially older homosexual caucasian men and intravenous drug users, are protecting themselves. New infections continue to rise among young persons, particularly minorities and heterosexuals, and among minority homosexuals.[2] The incidence of AIDS among African Americans is much higher than among caucasians, and it is estimated that the actual number of AIDS cases among African Americans will surpass those among caucasians.[3] The first national survey of young homosexual and bisexual men found that the prevalence (existing infections) of HIV among those in their teens and early 20s who have homosexual encounters is 7%; more than one third reported engaging in unprotected anal sex in the past 6 months.[4]

The spread of HIV among college students is also troubling. A study of college students showed an average prevalence rate of 0.20%; rates on some campuses were as high as 0.40%.[5] These high rates mean that on average 1–2 in 500 college students is HIV positive. The average prevalence rate for college students is higher than that among military recruits, among whom 0.14% is HIV positive. Undoubtedly, the level of self-selection among military recruits is significant in that persons who know they are HIV positive are less likely to seek military service. The methodology of the study of college students has been challenged and additional research is needed. The data are of great concern, however, because they suggest that college students may not be taking the risk of HIV infection seriously.

In 1996 the World Health Organization estimated that the worldwide prevalence of HIV infection by the year 2000 will be 30 to 40 million, a 50% increase over 1995 estimates, which in turn were a 50% increase over 1994 estimates. The greatest increase in HIV infection is expected in sub-Saharan Africa, north Africa, and the Middle East, where prevalence has doubled since 1994, and in south and southeast Asia, where the increase was 70%.[6] HIV and its progression to AIDS is a pandemic that threatens to destroy the economic and social fabric of whole regions of the developing world.

RESEARCH AND TREATMENT

In 1994 the U.S. government spent 12% of the National Institutes of Health (NIH) budget of $11 billion on AIDS research: "In fact, the NIH budget as a whole is characterized as either AIDS or non-AIDS, a status accorded no other disease."[7] In addition, a great deal of research is being conducted in the private sector. Pharmaceutical companies are working to develop drugs to prevent HIV infection and to treat AIDS. The result will be significant improvement in treating the disease—perhaps at greater cost, perhaps even preventing its spread. New drugs are proving effective in unique ways: blocking the virus's ability to reproduce its genes, blocking the virus from multiplying in the cells, hindering a virus enzyme needed to process key viral proteins, and stimulating the immune system. The sense that combinations of drugs will make AIDS a chronic rather than an acute disease is growing.[8]

Persons with AIDS are living longer as a result of more effective medical management and healthier lifestyles, including better nutrition, and preventive measures that reduce the risk of infection. Zidovudine (formerly known as AZT) was the first drug that slowed progression of the infection, but HIV has shown resistance to it. D4T, in combination with zidovudine, has been used to slow the progression of HIV. Aerosol pentamidine can be used to treat the serious pulmonary infections that afflict AIDS patients in the final phases of the disease. Unfortunately, none of these treatments is a cure.

Political and social pressures from persons with AIDS and their supporters have caused radical changes in the way the U.S. Food and Drug Administration (FDA) approves drugs to treat AIDS. Primarily, the changes mean that clinical trials are less rigorous and that the usual safety concerns receive less attention if preliminary results suggest that a drug is effective. In addition, the FDA has approved "community testing" rather than limiting clinical trials to hospitals, as it has in the past.

A small, countervailing school of thought takes the position that HIV neither causes AIDS nor is it contagious. Instead, they argue, AIDS is caused by malnutrition; recreational drug abuse (especially "poppers" [vials of amyl nitrate], popular among homosexual men); and modern medicines, including zidovudine. These skeptics include an internationally known virologist and a Nobel laureate. They and others note the following:

1. If AIDS were caused by a virus or bacterium it would not strike men more frequently than women.
2. Millions of people are infected with HIV, but do not have AIDS, and there is no convincing proof that HIV is present in everyone who has AIDS.
3. Infectious diseases typically occur soon after infection, not years later as is true of AIDS, and not after the immune system has produced large amounts of antibodies to fight the microbe.[9]

IMPLICATIONS FOR HEALTH SERVICES ORGANIZATIONS

Financial

The lifetime costs of treating persons with AIDS is estimated to range from $35,000 to $91,000, with average monthly costs of nearly $2,300. As would be expected, the cost of care increases dramatically during the last 6 months of life, soaring to an average of $9,098 per month.[10] Even the higher estimates are much lower than estimates made in the mid-1980s, however. Such data are meaningful only when compared with the average cost of treating a person diagnosed with another chronic terminal disease. For example, treatment for multiple sclerosis ranges from $12,769 to $22,875 per year. Costs increase as neurological functioning decreases.[11] It is estimated that the cumulative medical costs of treating all persons with AIDS in the United States from the time of diagnosis until death totaled $15.2 billion by 1995.[12]

The economic and social burdens of treating persons with AIDS are inequitably distributed because a large number of persons with AIDS are concentrated in inner city hospitals in major metropolitan areas.[13] In the early to mid-1980s, when the AIDS pandemic primarily affected middle-class caucasian homosexuals, patients usually carried ample health insurance, although coverage was often lost once the patient was unable to work. Medicaid (or Medicare, if the person is classified as disabled) covered medical expenses once the patient's assets had been depleted. As the demographics of the pandemic have changed, however, the number of uninsured patients has increased dramatically; persons with AIDS are or almost always become uninsured. This dynamic has significant implications for the economic survival of hospitals and other health services organizations, especially nursing facilities and hospices.

AIDS has an impact on medical education. Some commentators have attributed the decline in medical school applications in the late 1980s and early 1990s to concerns about treating persons with AIDS. Patient loads with large numbers of persons with AIDS may also affect medical residency programs. If residents cannot gain experience with a wide range of illnesses, approval for the residency may be withdrawn. Concentrations of persons with AIDS may cause special problems for other types of education as well as for staffing.

The proportion of persons with AIDS in nonurban areas appears to be increasing. Wider dispersion of persons with AIDS means health services organizations nationwide will be affected. In the 1990s providers other than hospitals, including nursing facilities, hospices, and home care, have been shown to be effective in treating persons with AIDS and, increasingly, are sources of care. This effectiveness should result in care delivered in more appropriate settings. Logic suggests this will also reduce costs. However, research findings show that the costs of care for patients who died in the hospital decreased while costs for patients who died at home increased over time. Thus, policies that promote dying at home may improve quality of life (death), but they actually increase costs.[14]

Financing care for persons with AIDS is difficult for the health services organization because so much of what happens lies outside its control. Hospitals must treat persons who present at their emergency rooms, for example. Yet, if it is to carry out its mission of providing health services, the organization must survive. Survival may require setting limits on the amount of uncompensated care the organization will provide. Based on even a limited duty of general beneficence the organization is obliged to provide services that assist all groups and to serve as a community resource. The governing body and the organization's managers should develop a mission statement and policies that reflect this commitment. Some organizations choose to offer services that generate surpluses, which are then used to subsidize uncompensated care and to fund programs for the underserved. Although laudable in their intent and outcome, these efforts may raise other ethical questions, such as creating demand for marginally necessary services.

The dispersion of persons with AIDS to nonurban, low-incidence areas of the United States will spread the social and economic burdens of AIDS and will bring a measure of relief to urban hospitals. These hospitals will likely continue to experience the financial consequences of AIDS disproportionately. No solutions, except to fund treatment through public programs such as Medicare and Medicaid, are obvious. This lack of solutions is fair only if funding is sufficient to give organizations the reimbursement needed to survive. Society cannot escape the heavy economic burdens lying ahead regardless of how the care is funded. In Houston the 1987 bankruptcy of the only dedicated AIDS hospital added to the anxiety felt by all health services managers, even though low occupancy because of few referrals was the apparent cause of that failure.

Legal

The legal dimensions of AIDS are complex. The number of AIDS-related lawsuits is larger than that attributable to any other single disease in U.S. legal history, and there have been predictions that health services organizations will become the most important area of AIDS-related litigation in the 1990s.[15] By mid-1995 one half of the lawsuits filed under the Americans with Disabilities Act (ADA) of 1990 (PL 101-336) have involved AIDS.[16]

The Occupational Safety and Health Act administered by the Occupational Safety and Health Administration (OSHA) requires that employers provide employment and a place of employment that are free from recognized hazards that cause, or are likely to cause, death or serious physical harm. Universal blood and body substance precautions are required by OSHA. Such precautions are likely to be the focus of enforcement that will use a targeted basis (e.g., industry, type of provider) and will respond to employee complaints. Also, OSHA requires employee education programs about hazards and precautions and engages in its own educational activities.

The second legal dimension concerns the risk to patients and staff from employees infected with HIV. Health services organizations are subject to Section 504 of the federal Rehabilitation Act of 1973 (PL 93-112), which requires that employers may not discriminate on the basis of handicap. Complementary state legislation is common. The U.S. Supreme Court has considered a situation that has implications for employees who are HIV positive, *Arline v. School Board of Nassau County, Florida*. In this case a teacher who experienced three recurrences of tuberculosis was discharged because the school board considered her to be a health threat to students. The Court ruled that the teacher's disease was a disability that was protected by the statute. The case was remanded to the trial court to determine whether Arline was otherwise qualified and whether she could have been accommodated in alternative employment.[17]

A footnote in the Arline case stated that the Court was not making a determination as to whether carriers of a contagious disease, such as AIDS, would be considered to have a physical impairment, or whether they would be considered handicapped under the ADA solely on the basis of contagiousness. Several important factors affect the legal rights of an employee with AIDS, including the state of the disease (chronic vs. acute), type of setting in which the employee works, the risk to healthy persons (as in the Arline case) versus the risk to ill non–AIDS patients, and the legal duties health services organizations owe to patients. Employees who are HIV positive may also be treated differently from employees with AIDS. Early cases held that AIDS is a handicap within the meaning of Section 504 of the federal Rehabilitation Act of 1973 and similar state statutes. Additional protection for persons who are HIV positive is found in the Civil Rights Restoration Action of 1988 (PL 100-259).[18]

Cases litigating whether health care staff who are HIV positive are "otherwise qualified" under ADA seem to turn on the potential risk of harm to patients, even when that harm is remote. A state appeals court in Illinois found that by constructively discharging James Davis, a cook with HIV who prepared and distributed food and cleaned the kitchen and storeroom, a nursing facility had violated the ADA by discriminating against him on the basis of his disability. Davis' doctor had written to the nursing facility stating that HIV was not transmitted through preparing and serving food and beverages and that his HIV status did not restrict him from performing his job.[19] Conversely, a federal court case involving William Mauro, a surgical technician with HIV who assisted in exposure-prone invasive procedures, held that the ADA and the Rehabilitation Act of 1973 did not apply because Mauro's HIV status disqualified him from working as a surgical technician and that he was not "otherwise qualified" to perform his job. Mauro acknowledged that his duties occasionally required him to place his hands upon and into surgical incisions and that this placed him at risk for needle sticks and minor lacerations. Mauro's expert witness testified that the risk of transmission of HIV to a patient was very small, but the court agreed with the defendant hospital that a real possibility of transmission of HIV existed and that because the consequence of infection is death, the nature, duration, and severity of the risk outweighed the fact that the chance of transmission was slight.[20]

Ethical and Administrative

Clinical developments in the 1990s allow all health services organizations to treat patients with AIDS more effectively. Generally, staff are better prepared and have developed specialized clinical skills. These advantages, in addition to new drugs, will increase longevity for persons with AIDS. The result will be increased episodes of hospitalization as well as treatment at other types of organizations, especially nursing facilities.

The AIDS pandemic raises significant ethical issues for the organization and its managers. These issues include protecting staff who are providing care to infected patients, protecting patients and staff from infected staff, and maintaining the confidentiality of staff and patients with AIDS. All of these issues are being addressed; some are more easily solved than others. A critical context for analysis is that, for unknown reasons, the probability that care-givers will become infected when exposed to blood and body substances from patients who are HIV positive is several magnitudes greater than that patients will become infected from caregivers who are HIV positive. In addition, with one possible exception, there are no known cases in which a caregiver who is HIV positive, even one with frank AIDS, has infected a patient.

Protecting Staff from Patients The premise for all organizational relationships is that in the presence of a significant infectious disease, it must do all it can to protect staff. This premise is supported by fidelity, part of the principle of respect for persons: Through its managers, the organization has a duty to provide a safe workplace. Rawls's difference principle supports this duty, as does the theory of utility—the greatest good for the greatest number. An effective workforce is achievable only under safe working conditions. Legal obligations reinforce this ethical duty to employees. Having identified the ethical priority of protecting staff, it is necessary to answer the question of how to create and maintain an environment that is compatible with the ob-ligation to provide services to the community as well as to treat persons with AIDS.

In 1987 the Centers for Disease Control and Prevention (CDC) con-firmed that three hospital staff members had tested positive for HIV after occupational exposure to contaminated blood. The risk to caregivers who work with patients who are HIV positive is now well documented and there have been several hundred confirmed cases of transmission of HIV, almost all of which are the result of needle sticks or other direct exposure to contaminated blood. Three large studies have estimated the risk of contracting HIV after accidentally being stuck with a contaminated needle at about 1 in 250.[21] It is estimated that 70,000 health care staff nationwide have tested positive for HIV.[22] Experts have suggested that the incidence of HIV among health care staff is significantly underreported.[23] Despite this suggestion and the estimate that a large number of health care staff are HIV positive, a CDC study of 22,000 patients reported in 1995 showed that no patients who became HIV positive were infected by health care staff.[24]

Although HIV is present in all body substances of people who are HIV positive, AIDS apparently can be spread only by sexual intercourse or intimate contact with body substances, especially blood. The risk for health care staff is low, but the consequences of AIDS make infection a major concern for them and the organization. The CDC and OSHA have developed guidelines for universal precautions. Universal precautions should be used in all health services organizations.

Some physicians and staff are reluctant or unwilling to treat persons with AIDS. Reports have circulated of surgeons who demand preoperative HIV testing of patients and refuse to operate on patients who test positive for the virus. In 1987 the American Medical Association (AMA) Council on Ethical and Judicial Affairs issued a statement that physicians act unethically if they refuse to treat persons with AIDS whose medical conditions are within their competence.[25] Nurses and staff members have been disciplined for refusing to treat persons with AIDS; some have been fired. Given the consequences of AIDS, it is unlikely that statements such as the AMA's or even disciplinary action by the organization will cause all caregivers to agree to treat persons with AIDS.

In mid-1987 the American Hospital Association (AHA) issued recommendations reflecting the growing concern about clinical management of patients with AIDS.[26] These recommendations were consistent with CDC guidelines that universal precautions is the best protection for caregivers. The guidelines suggested that all patients' blood and body substances be considered hazardous and that all patients be subject to the infection-control guidelines originally established for hepatitis and frank AIDS. The impact of these guidelines is that isolation and biohazard precautions should be used for all patients, regardless of HIV status, and that health care staff should protect themselves against body substances and contact with patients. The AHA does not recommend routine HIV testing of all patients. CDC guidelines issued in 1987, which remain in effect, suggest that hospitals must judge whether their patients' characteristics are such that all admissions should be tested. All health services organizations, but especially hospitals, nursing facilities, and hospices, should address this question. In 1991 the CDC issued guidelines stating in part that persons performing exposure-prone procedures should know their HIV status and that those who are HIV positive should inform their patients before engaging in such procedures. Subsequent federal legislation required that states adopt these guidelines by regulation or legislation.

A few hospitals test all admissions for HIV. Patients who refuse to be tested are admitted, but are treated with extra precautions. Using "extra precautions" is at variance with the requirements for universal precautions. In late 1987 the AHA spoke out against routine testing of patients or staff and continues to hold that position.

The risk of caregivers being infected by exposure to blood and body substances from patients who are HIV positive is low. Nevertheless, it is troublesome that one study found high levels of noncompliance with universal precautions. A study conducted at The Johns Hopkins Hospital (Baltimore) emergency department found that physicians complied with universal precautions requirements only 38% of the time. Residents and nurses complied more often (58% and 44%, respectively). Housekeeping staff complied most often (91%). Emergency department personnel blamed their lack of compliance on time pressures and interference of precautions with procedural skills. These low levels of compliance occurred despite ready availability of gloves, gowns, and other protective gear, and despite efforts to educate staff about the known risks of contracting HIV. The study also revealed that the rate of infected patients in The Johns Hopkins Hospital emergency department increased from 5.2% to 6.0% in 1 year.[27] Other research generally confirms compliance problems regarding universal precautions.[28]

Encouraging and achieving compliance pose a special challenge to health services managers; further research on how to meet this goal is needed. Enhanced education can be only a small part of the answer. Caregivers cannot but be aware of the risk of infection with HIV and understand the importance of universal precautions. Management must identify and correct structure and process inhibitors that reduce the staff's willingness or ability to comply with the requirements of universal precautions. Health services organizations that follow CDC and AHA guidelines—the ethically and clinically correct and legally prudent course—treat all patients as if they are HIV positive.

Protecting Patients from Staff   Caregivers who are HIV positive pose a very small but possible risk of infecting patients and staff. This risk comes from both HIV and from the opportunistic diseases that afflict persons with AIDS, including tuberculosis and *Pneumocystis carinii* pneumonia. Immunosuppressed patients are especially at risk.

Also significant are the early but unconfirmed reports that HIV induces neuropsychiatric problems such as impaired coordination and cognitive difficulties, which may occur before physical symptoms are apparent. In normal clinical practice such deficits in performance are likely to be attributed to random error rather than to a medical condition. If they are so attributed, serious problems may occur before a pattern is detected; diminished competence may be apparent only in retrospect, probably after a patient has been harmed. If true, subtle diminutions in competence greatly complicate the question of using staff members who are HIV positive. The ethical (and legal) duty of employers to monitor staff and prevent harm to patients is well established.

The CDC has confirmed that Dr. David Acer, a Florida dentist, infected six of his patients with HIV. It is still unknown how he transmitted the virus to them. Acer was confirmed as the source of transmission after investigators found that the patients' HIV contained genetic material matching his and learned that he did not follow infection-control procedures.[29] The CDC maintains that its investigation was competent and thorough in all respects. However, some evidence suggests that the infected patients had unreported and undetected risk factors for HIV and that the molecular analyses used to determine that Acer and his patients had the same strains of HIV were potentially seriously flawed.[30] The fact that Acer's is the only confirmed case of transmission of infection from a health care provider to a patient suggests that critics might be correct. Suit was brought in 1995 by a patient who was HIV positive against a dentist who was HIV negative. The dentist is alleged to have failed to sterilize his equipment and thus transmitted the virus via this route.

The ethical (and legal) problems for health services organizations are complicated further by the fact that some care providers are HIV positive, but have not yet developed frank AIDS and wish to continue treating patients. The AMA and the American Dental Association (ADA) have taken the position that ethics require practitioners who are infected with HIV to either inform their patients of their HIV status or refrain from performing exposure-prone invasive procedures.[31] Their position holds, despite the CDC's estimates that the risk that an infected surgeon will transmit HIV during an invasive procedure is between 1 in 40,000 and 1 in 400,000 and that the risk of transmission from an infected dentist is between 1 in 200,000 and 1 in 2 million.[32]

The most well-publicized cases of practitioners who tested positive for HIV who wished to continue treating patients have involved physicians. A Cook County (Illinois) Hospital physician was allowed to practice but was barred from performing invasive procedures. He sued, challenging the hospital's definition of invasive as too broad. The hospital board reversed its decision. The physician subsequently died. In the interim the Cook County board, which is also the hospital board, approved a policy that allows patients to refuse to be treated by persons who are HIV positive. It was unclear how the board would put this policy into effect.[33]

Another case occurred at The Johns Hopkins Hospital, where a resident was infected when he was cut by a broken vial containing HIV-infected blood. He sued the hospital because of alleged breaches of confidentiality and defamation. A New York case involved a physician who allegedly became infected with HIV during her residency when she jabbed herself with the needle of a syringe negligently left on a bed after it was used on a patient with AIDS.

Despite the uncertainty of statutory and case law, health services organizations should know the HIV status of all staff who engage in exposure-prone invasive procedures. It is ethically appropriate and legally prudent to prohibit persons who are HIV positive from performing such procedures. This policy is consistent with the positions taken by the CDC, AMA, and ADA. Such a rule meets the principle of nonmaleficence. Implementation is complicated, however, because, except for the disputed case of Dr. Acer, there are no documented cases of transmission from care providers who are HIV positive to patients. This is true even when care providers have frank AIDS. Prominent examples include public reports of surgeons and other physicians performing exposure-prone invasive procedures but with no confirmed cases of transmission of HIV to their patients. These reports suggest the unique aspects of HIV and the likelihood of cofactors in transmissibility as well as infectivity and progression of HIV to frank AIDS, cofactors not present in the general population.

By way of context, hepatitis B virus (HBV) is a much greater threat to patients than is HIV. In early 1996 a thoracic surgeon was found to have transmitted HBV to 19 patients during surgery despite evidence that he used adequate infection-control procedures.[34] This incident, along with that of a Spanish cardiac surgeon who infected five of his patients with hepatitis C (HCV), confirms the importance of mandatory testing for HBV, HCV, and HIV of care providers who perform exposure-prone invasive procedures.[35]

In meeting their ethical duties staff themselves should want to know whether they pose a risk to patients and other staff. Because of the opportunistic diseases they contract as HIV progresses to frank AIDS, infected staff may pose a risk to patients, many of whom are immunosuppressed or physically weakened. Staff members with AIDS may also pose risks to other employees and to visitors. These risks should cause managers to err in favor of caution in assigning staff, at least until legal parameters are established. As staff who are HIV positive become increasingly immunocompromised, infectious diseases common in health services organizations will pose risks to them. If the organization is to discharge its ethical obligations to staff, it must be able to consider such information in job assignment. Given how much is not known about transmissibility of the virus, staff who are HIV positive should be encouraged to accept nonpatient care positions, whether or not they perform exposure-prone invasive procedures. Physicians who wish to continue performing such procedures pose a special problem. Given the unknown but possible risk to patients, it is prudent to prohibit physicians (and other staff) who are HIV positive from performing exposure-prone invasive procedures, as reasonably defined. Protecting staff confidentiality to the greatest extent possible is crucial to the success of any such effort.

Something Must Be Done, but What?

Stunned, Carolyn Aubrey, the CEO of Metropolitan Hospital, sank into her chair and stared out the window for a very long time. She realized that something was afoot when Dr. Midmore's wife had angrily insisted on seeing the CEO. Even in her worst nightmares Aubrey had never imagined that Mrs. Midmore would tell Aubrey that she was suing her husband, an orthopedic surgeon, for divorce because he had given her AIDS. As Mrs. Midmore left Aubrey's office, she had turned back and said, "I was sure you'd want to know. Surely you'll have to do something."

Aubrey thought Mrs. Midmore's statements might be nothing more than the ravings of an angry, vindictive wife, but that was not likely. As she considered what she had just learned, she recalled an incident several years ago involving Dr. Midmore and a male orderly. In retrospect, it suggested that Dr. Midmore might be bisexual. Aubrey also thought about the department of surgery meeting last year when there had been a long discussion about the desirability of knowing the HIV status of all surgical patients. The special risks to surgeons of torn gloves and cuts during orthopedic surgery had been described in detail.

Now it seemed that Dr. Midmore's patients might be at risk. Aubrey called operating room scheduling and learned that Dr. Midmore was maintaining a full surgical load. Aubrey asked her secretary to call the hospital attorney and the medical director and set up an emergency meeting for seven o'clock the following morning. Mrs. Midmore had been right, thought Aubrey. We'll have to do something, but what?

This case suggests several ethical (and legal) issues. Protecting patients is key, and Midmore's surgical privileges must be suspended immediately. Once Midmore no longer poses a risk to patients, further action can follow in a more orderly and deliberate manner. Meeting the principle of justice requires that the investigation be fair to Midmore in terms of process and substance. If Midmore is HIV positive, the hospital may choose from two courses of action: allow Midmore to continue performing surgery if he follows CDC guidelines that physicians who are HIV positive notify their patients before performing exposure-prone procedures, or terminate Midmore's surgical privileges. The first choice maximizes patient autonomy, but the hospital must ensure that Midmore actually informs patients that he is HIV positive and that they understand the implications of this information. As a practical matter, few patients are likely to allow him to perform their surgery if they are informed about his HIV status. The second choice fully meets the principle of nonmaleficence in preventing potential harm to patients, but is paternalistic in terms of Midmore's patients. Prudence suggests choosing the second option. All actions must be consistent with the need to protect patients and meet the requirements in the medical staff bylaws and state and federal law.

Confidentiality regarding Dr. Midmore's HIV status must be safeguarded. Such efforts can never compromise patient safety, however. The issue of confidentiality takes on further complexity if Midmore leaves the staff and applies for surgical privileges elsewhere. Should he do so, the hospital has an ethical obligation to communicate what it has learned in the course of its investigation.

Maintaining Patient Confidentiality Health services organizations must be alert to the special problems of confidentiality when treating patients with AIDS. Within the constraints of state law, however, the first obligation must be to safeguard staff and other patients. Identifying patients who are HIV positive may be an important additional stimulus that will encourage staff to comply with universal precautions.

It has been argued that identifying patients as HIV positive will lead to a two-class medical system. This charge has proved baseless. The potential for this problem has existed since HIV was first identified and patient charts and rooms were marked with biohazard notices as well as with other, less transparent codes. Thus far, there is no evidence that persons with AIDS have received care that is different from that accorded other patients.

Dedicated AIDS Units and Regionalized Care

Dedicated units for persons with AIDS are rare. The vast majority of health services organizations, including hospitals, serve too few persons with AIDS to justify establishing a dedicated unit. Typically, hospitals with large numbers of persons with AIDS admit them to general medical/surgical floors rather than to dedicated units, even for people with advanced cases of the disease.

Managers argue that privacy is better protected; the extra workload is spread among care providers, especially nurses; and staffing and work assignment problems are eased. Dedicated AIDS units may be established as the public becomes more willing to accept persons with AIDS and if the financial effects of AIDS become acute.

Loss of patient confidentiality is a commonly cited problem when dedicated AIDS units or regionalization is discussed. This risk is overstated because staff know (as they should) which patients have AIDS. With the enormous amount of publicity AIDS has received, it is likely that family members and visitors will be aware that AIDS is a possibility, especially in the final stages of the disease. Concentrating persons with AIDS in one unit allows special training and equipment to be used to protect staff and to enhance treatment. Moreover, it allows those staff members who wish to work with persons with AIDS to do so. A dedicated unit also minimizes any drift toward second-class care because the availability of staff and other resources would be readily apparent, whereas such lapses could be more easily overlooked or hidden on a general medical/surgical floor.

Studies done in the early 1990s show sound clinical reasons for regionalizing AIDS treatment. As one would expect by analogy to other medical conditions such as cardiac surgery, these studies show startling differences in mortality for persons with AIDS in low- versus high-experience hospitals. Studies showing the greatest differences were undertaken in California and New York State. The studies found that inpatient mortality for *Pneumocystis carnii* was 10% to 21% higher in low-experience hospitals.[36] All other factors being equal, organizations doing more of something will do it more effectively and efficiently. Regionalization of treatment for persons with AIDS should be considered even though patient inconvenience is likely to increase.

IMPLICATIONS FOR PUBLIC POLICY

Persons infected with HIV have contracted a devastating virus, one that develops into a disease with the highest known case fatality rate. How should persons outside this group view HIV and the consequences of frank AIDS, which are the deadly opportunistic diseases that occur when the immune system is compromised?

Predictions made in the mid- to late 1980s held that HIV would soon spread through the general heterosexual population; the most dire prediction stated that it would sweep over society with consequences similar to those of the Black Death. This outbreak has not occurred, nor is it likely to occur because it has been over 10 years since HIV was identified as the cause of AIDS.

HIV continues to be confined to specific, relatively small populations such as intravenous drug users, male bisexuals and homosexuals, and a relatively small number of heterosexuals. Improved testing has virtually eliminated the transmission of HIV to hemophiliacs and others through contaminated blood and blood products. With an estimated 0.6 million infected and over 300,000 deaths, HIV merits attention, but neither the shrillness nor in the amount thus far accorded it.

Despite clear evidence of the limited numbers of persons and groups affected by HIV, major aspects of the approach to HIV have been and are based on the myth that it is a significant threat to public health, which occurred primarily because HIV became politicized. Instead of being characterized as a public health issue with political and civil rights dimensions, it is seen as a political and civil rights issue with public health dimensions.

Despite Department of Health and Human Services Secretary Donna Shalala's assertion in March 1995 that AIDS had become the leading cause of death for Americans between the ages of 25 and 44, AIDS continues to be relatively insignificant in terms of all causes of death. The emphasis on HIV infection, however, has caused resource allocation decisions that would be considered unconscionable were it not for the fact that HIV/AIDS is politicized. To understand how irrational public policy decisions regarding HIV have been one need only consider the following numbers showing the leading causes of death in the United States in 1993:[37]

1.	Diseases of the heart	739,860
2.	Malignant neoplasms, including neoplasms of lymphatic and hematopoietic tissues	530,870
3.	Cerebrovascular diseases	149,740
4.	Chronic obstructive pulmonary diseases and allied conditions	101,090
5.	Accidents and adverse effects	88,630
6.	Pneumonia and influenza	81,730
7.	Diabetes mellitus	55,110
8.	HIV infection	38,500
9.	Suicide	31,230
10.	Homicide and legal intervention	25,470

Similarly, politicization of HIV/AIDS caused a major shift in research funding from far more common causes of death to HIV/AIDS. In fiscal 1994 over twice as much federal money was spent on HIV/AIDS research than on federally funded research related to heart disease, which afflicted five times as many persons.[38] Another way to understand the disproportionate amount of research on AIDS is to review research expenditures per person with various diseases. In fiscal 1994 federally funded research spent $1,069 per person with HIV/AIDS, $295 per person with cancer, $158 per person with multiple sclerosis, $93 per person with heart disease, $54 per person with Alzheimer's disease, and $30 per person with Parkinson's disease.[39]

Added to the posturing of many public officials, such disproportionate research funding perpetuates the myth of the importance of HIV and blurs its true significance in the general population. The net result is less-than-rational public policy decision making.

PROSPECTS

Early in 1996 the Third Conference on Retroviruses and Opportunistic Infections was held in Washington, D.C. Several promising findings were confirmed by new research reported there, as follows:

- Treatment of HIV infection with a combination of antiviral drugs is generally more successful than treating it with only one drug.
- The amount of virus in the bloodstream is a better predictor of an infected person's future health than any previous laboratory test or calculation used to make a prognosis.
- A few drugs can completely suppress growth of the virus, at least in some patients. Although this does not constitute cure of the infection and may not be sustainable, this finding raises the possibility that HIV's relentless destruction of the immune system could be halted.
- Women with small amounts of virus in their blood are somewhat less likely to transmit HIV to their infants. Researchers have known since 1994 that an infected woman's use of zidovudine can dramatically lower her baby's chance of acquiring the virus. The new finding suggests that, with proper testing and treatment, the mother–infant route of transmission can be controlled further.
- Actively lowering the amount of virus in the bloodstream actually helps patients, making them less likely to develop the unusual infections that are the hallmarks of AIDS. In at least one study this lowering measurably prolonged life.[40]

Other reports delivered at the conference state that laboratories can now measure viral load (viruses in the bloodstream) at about $200 per test. Although not inexpensive, this test allows physicians to monitor HIV and predict the person's future health, which research shows to be a function of viral load. These findings focus on slowing the progression of HIV to AIDS—good news for those infected, both in terms of quality of life and longevity. It is further evidence that HIV is likely to become a chronic affliction.

Work on a vaccine continues. In 1996 about 25 experimental vaccines against HIV were in human testing worldwide, most in phase I, which determines whether the vaccine itself is harmful. Testing that has moved to phase II shows some protective responses, but was not effective for final testing (phase III). Even if a vaccine met specific criteria as to effectiveness, it will take at least until the end of the 1990s to determine whether the vaccine was effective in order to be made available.[41]

CONCLUSION

AIDS has ethical, legal, financial, and managerial dimensions and implications that make it as complex an issue as managers are likely to encounter. Caring for persons with AIDS while protecting staff remains a major ethical and legal challenge, one in which managers will play the leading role.

AIDS continues to represent a threat to society, even though changes in sexual practices and use of preventive measures have proved effective in dramatically slowing the spread of HIV among one high-risk group, homosexual men. The challenge is to find ways to encourage other high-risk groups, including intravenous drug users, minority populations, and college students (a new group)—to protect themselves.

Hospitals must find ways to provide effective acute, episodic treatment and to assist health services organizations, especially nursing facilities and hospices, that provide alternative sources of care. Financing care will remain problematic for all providers.

Encouraging in the effort to solve the health problems associated with HIV is the fact that the debate has become less shrill. Increasingly, there is a willingness to treat HIV as primarily a public health problem with political and civil rights dimensions, rather than as primarily a political and civil rights problem with public health dimensions.

Most disconcerting in both the short and long term is that the public has turned its attention elsewhere. The major reason for this loss of interest is that the pandemic has been milder than predicted in the mid-1980s. Psychologically, it is "yesterday's news." Health services organizations are seeking a just solution to financing care for the underserved and uninsured with HIV and AIDS; lack of public attention, however, will make this task more difficult, if not impossible.

NOTES

1. Karen Hill. (1996, April 23). AIDS rate declined last year, CDC says. *The Washington Post*, Health Supplement, p. 15.
2. Joyce Price. (1996, February 1). Deaths from AIDS in U.S. outpace new HIV infections. *The Washington Times*, p. A3.
3. Hill, p. 15.
4. The scourge of AIDS marches on. (1996, May 4). *The Washington Post*, p. A17.
5. Susan Okie. (1989, May 23). HIV infection found in 1 of 500 college students. *The Washington Post*, p. A5. (The study reported in this article has not been replicated, but the data are believed to reflect the situation in 1996. [Personal communication, American College Health Association, Baltimore, May 21, 1996.])
6. (1996, February 11). HIV found in 7% of gay young men: Education fails to halt spread. *The Washington Times*, p. A3. (Reporting results from the first national survey of young homosexual and bisexual men.)
7. William E. Paul. (1994, September 15). A turning point in AIDS research: Building on firmer foundations. *Vital Speeches of the Day*, 60(23), 709.
8. Larry Thompson. (1990, April 3). New treatments: Drug combinations might hobble AIDS virus. *The Washington Post*, Health Supplement, p. 7.
9. Rick Weiss. (1994, November 1). And now for something completely different. *The Washington Post*, Health Supplement, p. 7.

10. Home care for terminally-ill AIDS patients may not lower costs. (1995, July/ August). *Research Activities, 186*, 11.

11. Personal communication. (1995, June 25). New York: National Multiple Sclerosis Society.

12. Personal communication. (1995, June 24). Atlanta: Centers for Disease Control and Prevention.

13. Sandra G. Boodman. (1989, September 5). Up against it: In Newark, a public hospital fights the twin plagues of AIDS and drugs. *The Washington Post*, Health Section, p. 12. (1990, May 5). AIDS update: An executive report. *Hospitals*, 26–34.

14. Home care for terminally-ill AIDS patients may not lower costs. (1995, July/ August). *Research Activities, 186*, 11.

15. (1990, April 16). AIDS-related lawsuits will continue to rise, report shows. *AHA News*, p. 3.

16. Sibyl C. Pranschke, & Barbara M. Wright. (1995, Third Quarter). HIV and AIDS—Employers grapple with difficult issues. *Benefits Quarterly, 11*(3), 41.

17. Arline v. School Board of Nassau County, Florida, 481 U.S. 1024, 107 S.Ct. 1913, 95 L.Ed. 2d 519.

18. Lawrence Gostin. (1989, January/February). HIV-infected physicians and the practice of seriously invasive procedures. *Hastings Center Report, 19*(1), 37.

19. Raintree Health Care Center v. Human Rights Commission, Ill. App. Ct., 1st Dist., Aug. 25, 1995. p. 899.

20. Mauro v. Borgess Medical Center, W.D. Mich., S. Div., May 4, 1995. p. 1025.

21. Okie, p. A5.

22. Joanne Wojcik. (1992, August 24). Health care workers with HIV. *Business Insurance, 26*(34), A11.

23. Okie, p. A5.

24. Bruce Japsen. (1995, May 8). Study casts doubt on need to test healthcare workers for HIV. *Modern Healthcare, 25*(19), 26.

25. American Medical Association. (1987, December). Ethical issues involved in the growing AIDS crisis. In *Reports of the Council on Ethical and Judicial Affairs*. Chicago: Author. (The report states that "A physician who knows that he or she has an infectious disease should not engage in any activity that creates a risk of transmission of the disease to others. . . . disclosure of that risk to patients is not enough; patients are entitled to expect that their physicians will not increase their exposure to the risk of contracting an infectious disease, even minimally." [p. 169])

26. American Hospital Association. (1987–1988). *AIDS/HIV infection: recommendations for health care practices and public policy, report and recommendations of the special committee on AIDS/HIV infection policy*. Chicago: Author.

27. Mary Koska. (1989, September 5). AIDS precautions: Compliance difficult to enforce. *Hospitals*, p. 58.

28. Cynthia Carter Haddock, Gail W. McGee, Hala Fawal, & Michael S. Saag. (1994, Fall). Knowledge and self-reported use of universal precautions in a university teaching hospital. *Hospital & Health Services Administration, 39*(3), 295–307.

29. Joyce Price. (1996, February 9). 2 of 6 who got HIV from dentist are alive. *The Washington Times*, p. A7.

30. Stephen Barr. (1996, January 15). The 1990 Florida dental investigation: Is the case really closed? *Annals of Internal Medicine, 124*(2), 250–254.

31. Ronald Bayer. (1991, May). The HIV-infected clinician: To exclude or not exclude? *Trustee, 44*(5), 16.

32. *Ibid.*, p. 17.

33. Chicago patients gain curb on AIDS carriers. (1988, September 22). *The New York Times*, p. A10.

34. Rafael Harpaz, Lorenz von Seidlein, Francisco M. Averhoff, Michael P. Tormey, Saswati D. Sinha, Konstantina Kotsopoulou, Stephen B. Lambert, Betty H. Robertson, James D. Cherry, & Craig N. Shapiro. (1996, February 29). Transmission of hepatitis B virus to multiple patients from a surgeon without evidence of inadequate infection control. *New England Journal of Medicine, 334*(9), 549–554.

35. Juan I. Esteban, Jordi Gomez, Maria Martell, Beatriz Cabot, Josep Quer, Joan Camps, Antonio Gonzalez, Teresa Otero, Andres Moya, Rafael Esteban, & Jaime Guardia. (1996, February 29). Transmission of hepatitis C virus by a cardiac surgeon. *New England Journal of Medicine, 334*(9), 555–559.

36. Karen Sandrick. (1993, April 5). Learning from experience: In AIDS treatment, knowledge means quality. *Hospitals, 67*(7), 32–35.

37. U.S. Department of Health and Human Services and provisional data from the Centers for Disease Control and Prevention/National Center for Health Statistics. (1994, October 11). *Monthly vital statistics report, 42*(13). (Table H. Estimated deaths, death rates, and percent of total deaths for the 15 leading causes of death, United States, 1993. Data are provisional; estimated from a 10% sample of deaths.)

38. Parkinson's Action Network. *Federally-funded research per afflicted, by disease, FY 1994*. Santa Rosa, CA: Author (citing various original sources).

39. *Ibid.*

40. David Brown. (1996, February 6). AIDS conference offers reasons for hope. *The Washington Post*, Health Supplement, p. 7.

41. U.S. joins drug firms in fight against AIDS. (1996, February 13). *The Washington Times*, p. A3.

13

Resource Allocation and Social Responsibility

RESOURCE ALLOCATION

Ethical issues are raised as managers make resource allocation decisions. Whether resource allocation affects populations or groups (*macroallocation*) or individuals (*microallocation*), allocation involves making choices. Decisions are based on explicit or implicit criteria. Some managers use subjective criteria such as social worth, usefulness to society, and need; others use more objective criteria such as selection through a lottery or queue or ability to pay once medical need has been determined. Values and philosophical statements about individuals and society underlie both, although these are usually implicit and may be only vaguely understood by decision makers.

Various methods and guidelines are used by decision makers in allocating resources. Often, decisions made by governments are based on economic motives or political effect. Like governments, health services organizations involve managers and clinicians in making macroallocation decisions. Microallocation in health services means making decisions about clinical treatment for individuals and involves nonclinician managers to a lesser extent. Important aspects of microallocation decision making are a physician's willingness to refer, patient geographic and economic access to services and technologies, and patient desire for treatment. Decisions at the microlevel are often guided (in a sense, prejudged) by macroallocation decisions that the organization (or government) has made.

As discussed in Chapter 1, utilitarians judge the morality of an act by assessing the results produced and determining whether the greatest good for the greatest number is achieved. Economists and managers use this approach in their cost-benefit analyses. Applying criteria of utility is only a partial answer, however. This narrow approach ignores considerations of human need, fairness, and justice, all of which health services managers find important.

Macroallocation

Specific theories have been developed to suggest how macroallocation does or should occur. The concept of a right to health care is prominent in several theories. One extreme is hyperegalitarianism, which asserts that all technologies should be available to all persons. Its corollary is that if technology is not available to all, it should be available to none. This theory is an extreme expression of respect for persons and mandates that society recognize every person's inherent right to receive equal health services. To some, providing different levels of treatment implies that some persons are, in effect, given less respect than others. To these persons, equal respect means receiving equal levels of services. Absent this criterion, the service should not be available to any.

At the other end of the continuum are the people who argue that access to health services is not a right to be guaranteed by society but a privilege. This hyperindividualistic position holds that health services providers, such as physicians, have no moral obligation to render services. In providing services, they act out of free will and humanitarian instinct. The hyperindividualists argue that, were there a right to health care, providers would have an obligation to render services. A duty to render services would diminish the freedom and dignity of providers and fails to recognize their inherent value and worth as human beings, thus violating the respect they are owed.

Between these extremes is the position that society has a duty to assist in developing, encouraging, and even providing health services. Fried[1] has suggested that routine basic services ought to be available to all, a position he calls the "decent minimum." More exotic high technology services are limited in ways such as location, cost, and referrals and must be available on a different basis. Where to draw this line is a political decision and depends on society's willingness to provide the resources needed.

Health services managers face similar macroallocation questions; the principles are almost identical to those applied by government decision makers.* Questions of who gets what, when, where, and how are found in many issues, such as whether to build a new outpatient department, when to purchase a magnetic resonance imager, and how to allocate staff. Answering these questions requires careful attention to economic considerations. Financial well-being is critical because it enables the organization to engage in its mission, one aspect of which is service to people who are socially and economically disadvantaged.

---

*The Oregon Health Plan, for example, prioritizes and rations health services for its Medicaid beneficiaries. It implicitly uses a hyperegalitarian philosophy, which, its proponents argue, means sacrifice for some Medicaid recipients, but greater equality for all.

The Feasibility of Brain Electrical Activity Mapping

Brain electrical activity mapping (BEAM) is a relatively new technology used to image the brain. It significantly improves the ability to localize an abnormality. Responding to demands for the procedure from staff radiologists and local neurologists and to reports in the literature on its usefulness, City Hospital decided to investigate the possibility of acquiring access to BEAM. Options included leasing, purchasing, and approaching nearby County Hospital about sharing its recently acquired BEAM machine.

A factor in the decision was uncertainty as to how changes in reimbursement would affect hospital revenues. Questions about reimbursement and a potential major expenditure of capital funds caused the chairman of the board to ask the chief executive officer (CEO) to form a committee to evaluate options, including forgoing access to BEAM. This assessment would be used to make a final decision between BEAM and a proposed addition to the intensive care unit (ICU), a project that is strongly supported by the surgical staff and that has already been delayed twice.

The board wanted to delay this decision until the reimbursement implications were understood, but several attending physicians stated that BEAM testing is critical to their practices. They said they prefer the nursing staff at City, but felt that they will be forced to admit certain patients to County in order to use BEAM. A rumor surfaced among the medical staff that several prominent members were considering forming a consortium to purchase and operate BEAM and other diagnostic equipment in a professional office complex under construction.[2]

What are the important aspects of this case? First, the new technology will improve the quality of care. Second, its availability will affect the organization's financial situation—operating costs for BEAM are high, typically exceeding capital costs in a few years. Financial considerations are complicated by reimbursement issues. Third, the physicians are divided about the expenditure and this adds to the complexity of medical staff politics. Fourth, BEAM is expensive technology, which makes the decision even more important and difficult.

The obvious starting point in solving this problem is to review the organizational philosophy and vision and mission statements. If City Hospital's mission is to serve special populations or needs, both BEAM and an ICU addition may use resources in a manner consistent with that mission. Are there even better uses for the resources? The various issues are not easily resolved, but internal decision processes, such as an ethics committee, can be of assistance. The expected context for decision making will be the organizational philosophy, as reflected in the strategic plan, which was described in Chapter 3. The technological imperative is present not only in delivering services to individual patients but in macroallocation decisions as well.

Microallocation

One usually thinks of microallocation decisions in terms of exotic lifesaving treatment. All scarce resources require allocation, however, and scarcity may be a function of time and circumstances, as in the following example.

Who Gets the Penicillin?

In 1943 penicillin was in short supply among U.S. armed forces in North Africa. Competitors for its use were two groups of soldiers suffering from infections that would respond to it: those with venereal disease and those with battle wounds. The chief surgical consultant advised that priority be given to the wounded; the theatre medical commander directed that priority be given to soldiers with venereal disease, arguing that soldiers cured of venereal disease could be restored to fighting trim more rapidly, and that left untreated, such men represented a threat of spreading the infection. The decision to use the penicillin on soldiers with venereal disease was a pragmatic judgment consistent with the morality of utility in a situation where objectives—achieving maximum fighting power as rapidly as possible—were narrowly defined.[3]

Treating solely the men infected with venereal disease is the morally correct choice only if the utilitarian criterion of returning the greatest number of men to the line as quickly as possible is applied. This decision is made without judging either the relative worth of the soldiers in need of treatment or the way in which they came to require it.

Foreign transplant recipients obtaining human organs from American donors suggest another dimension of microallocation decisions. These patients tend to come from countries in which technological impediments or religious customs prevent organ harvesting. They are health services consumers who pay out of pocket rather than out of insurance or government programs, and thus are highly favored by transplant centers. In addition, they are generally willing to accept organs that may be somewhat older or are not optimal tissue matches. Transplanting American organs into non-Americans raises legitimate concerns about priorities in a system in which American patients wait for organs while non-Americans receive them.

Theories of allocating exotic lifesaving treatment to individual patients have been developed by James Childress and Nicholas Rescher.[4] They address the problem of how decisions about who gets what should be made. Childress rejects the use of subjective criteria, such as worth to society, because such comparisons demean the potential recipient and run counter to a belief in the inherent dignity of each human being. His position is Kantian because it stresses respect for persons and its derivative, autonomy. He argues that a system that views all persons requiring treatment as equals recognizes inherent human worth. According to Childress, once medical criteria determine the need for and the appropriateness of therapy, opportunities for exotic lifesaving treatment should be available on a first-come, first-served basis, or alternatively, through some random selection process, such as a lottery.

A world-class ethicist, the late Paul Ramsey, agreed with Childress as to the desirability of a lottery or a policy of first-come, first-served that ignores the subjective judgments one finds in other, criteria-oriented schemes. At the same time, Ramsey found nondiscriminatory, predetermined, and announced rules based on statistical medical probabilities acceptable. This view would, for example, permit groups such as the very young and the very old to be excluded from kidney dialysis programs.[5]

Rescher's schema has two tiers. The first tier is devoted to basic screening and applies to groups of potential patients. It consists of factors such as constituency served, benefit to science, and likelihood of success by type of treatment or recipient. The second tier deals with individuals. It judges medical factors (e.g., relative likelihood of success, life expectancy) and social aspects, such as family role, potential future contributions, and past services rendered. Rescher states that if all factors are equal, a random selection process should be used for the final choice. For Rescher, the social aspects cause the most difficulty because they are heavily dependent on value judgments. However, he considers it irrational to make choices subject to chance, even if medical criteria are objective.

Each of these microallocation theories has advantages and disadvantages, both moral and pragmatic. Each theory develops a formal or semiformal process that permits users to address issues and problems in an organized manner. Although these approaches may not make possible a decision that satisfies everyone, the theories offer the advantage of an identified system that at least provides frameworks within which to make decisions. Given that medical criteria are met, a person's chances of being selected for exotic lifesaving treatment may be unpredictable (Childress), partially predictable (Ramsey), or almost totally predictable (Rescher). The basis for selection may hinge on largely subjective criteria (Rescher) or may be solely a matter of chance, and in that sense eminently fair to all who need the treatment (Childress) or all who meet the criteria for medical statistical probabilities (Ramsey).

Choices

Randy Glenn had just fallen asleep when the phone rang. It was the night supervisor at the comprehensive care center and hospital of which Glenn was the CEO. The supervisor was quite agitated and had trouble getting her words out. It took a few minutes for the message to become clear. One of Glenn's nightmares had come true: The four-bed ICU was full and an emergency case had just arrived.

The night supervisor explained that the new patient had been injured in a car accident. She had been stabilized in the emergency department, but neither air medivac nor mobile ICU ambulance services were available. It was certain that she would not survive transfer by any other means. She needed to be admitted to the ICU within 2 hours.

The night supervisor then quickly described the patients currently occupying ICU beds:

- Patient A: 60-year-old woman, comatose, stroke victim who required respirator support; 27 days in the ICU; uncertain prognosis; retired; no family; city resident
- Patient B: 9-year-old boy with Down syndrome, acute respiratory infection; 4 days in ICU; family in adjacent city
- Patient C: 36-year-old man who had undergone an emergency appendectomy, developed severe wound infection and probable septicemia; source of infection unknown; requires ICU care for blood pressure instability secondary to sepsis; bachelor; mother lives in city
- Patient D: 12-year-old girl undergoing chemotherapy for leukemia with an experimental drug; had been in remission three times; monitoring of experimental protocol and potential reaction to drug requires ICU care; family in city
- New Patient: 24-year-old woman; college honor student in physics, scholarship winner; pregnant; engaged; no family known

The supervisor ended the phone call by asking Glenn, "What should I do?" Indeed, what to do, thought Glenn, who wished the institutional ethics committee had been more active. Glenn pondered the alternatives as the garage door opened and the 10-minute trip to the hospital began.[6]

This example is the classic "last bed in the ICU" dilemma. Under Childress's and Ramsey's criteria, if all patients meet the medical criteria for ICU care, the new patient would be left to receive the best care she could obtain outside of the ICU. Applying Rescher's criteria, the prognosis (likelihood of success) for one of the current patients is not as good as the prognosis for the new patient. Thus, one of the current patients should be removed from the ICU. None of the models permits patients unable to obtain ICU care to be abandoned and left to fend for themselves. In all models they would receive the best alternative care the facility could offer.

Public awareness of how choices are made may or may not enhance the public's view that health services organizations and the system act justly. However, public scrutiny will focus greater attention on decision criteria, the decision process, and the fairness of their application. Kantian principles of respect for persons and of not using persons as ends are reflected in Childress's approach, which stresses autonomy. Rescher includes a mix of Kantian and utilitarian views and, most important, emphasizes justice, as described in Chapter 1. Few health services organizations determine resource allocation within the context of formally recognized ethical criteria. As with macroallocation decisions, these criteria must be developed within the context of the organizational philosophy and vision and mission statements.

SOCIAL RESPONSIBILITY

Two dimensions of the social responsibility of health services organizations are examined in this section; they are framed in terms of service versus profitability. One dimension is protecting and enhancing organization assets while maximizing community benefit. The second dimension is the organization's obligation to protect the commonweal—public expenditures for programs such as Medicare and Medicaid.

Community Benefit

Controlling costs and improving efficiency are matters of great concern to administrative staff. They ultimately benefit the community and also should be a focus for clinicians.

Different Settings, Different Costs

In late 1991 Metropolitan Hospital undertook successful negotiations for a 50–50 joint venture with a six-physician group of gastroenterologists to establish a freestanding endoscopy center. This agreement was a natural outgrowth of a long-term affiliation with the same single-specialty group whose members had been on the active staff at Metropolitan for over 10 years. Two thirds of the endoscopies at Metropolitan are performed by these six physicians.

Alice Macalin, a memeber of Metropolitan's staff, manages the center as well as in-patient endoscopy services at Metropolitan. Cost data were collected from the time the center became operational. These data showed that supply costs at the center were almost 35% lower than for endoscopies performed in the hospital. Initially, it was thought that the higher acuity level of patients undergoing endoscopy at the hospital increased costs significantly, but investigation showed this had only a marginal effect.

Macalin noted significant differences in attitudes among the physicians, depending on where they worked. When wearing her center director hat, Macalin is often approached by the physicians with cost-savings ideas, such as switching to reusables for certain supplies. The physicians took it upon themselves to ask technologists to remind them of the cost of expensive disposables before they opened the package. In addition, they track one another to determine who might be overusing supplies or using expensive supplies when less expensive alternatives could have been used. On their own the physicians discuss what might be done to increase operational efficiency at the center, and they recently devised a scheduling change to better fill down time.

Regrettably, little of this interest in cost reduction has transferred to the hospital. When practicing at Metropolitan the physicians are not deliberately wasteful, but there is a noticeably lessened interest in developing or initiating cost savings. Macalin had hoped that the patterns from the center would transfer automatically to the hospital, but after almost a year it had occurred only marginally and cost differences continued to be significant. She knew something should be done, but what?

Waste is an ethical issue. Obviously, the financial implications of ownership make the physicians much more interested in improving efficiency at the center. Changing physicians' attitudes about the use of resources is a major challenge for managers and is reflected in efforts to tie physicians into the economic health of the organization through such arrangements as physician–hospital organizations. Macalin could attempt to force changes, but doing so would risk both physician antipathy and apathy. Gross transfers of expectations and patterns from the center to the hospital may be interpreted by physicians as interfering with professional judgment and decision making because the patients are hospitalized when endoscopies are performed in Metropolitan. Education and working patiently with the physicians to gain their understanding of the applicability and transferability of efficiency from the center to the hospital are essential activities for Macalin.

Improving efficiency benefits the community by reducing costs, thus making health services affordable and accessible. Some health services organizations find themselves in the enviable position of having a very positive financial picture, and this raises other ethical issues.

We've Earned It, We'll Keep It!

Freeland Hospital is a not-for-profit, general acute care hospital located in an affluent suburban neighborhood. Its Medicare census is less than 20% and it receives less than 1% of its revenues from Medicaid. Uncollectibles are under 3%. Freeland Hospital's current financial situation is solid.

Sherwood Shurman had been the CEO of Freeland for almost 20 years and is justifiably proud of the changes and improvements that he has achieved during his tenure. One improvement has been to establish the Freeland Hospital Foundation, Inc., which receives charitable donations as well as profit from the operations of Freeland Hospital. In only 10 years the Foundation has accumulated $12 million; $2 million were used to acquire equipment.

Occasionally, board members question whether the hospital is sufficiently socially conscious. The most common suggestion is that Freeland ought to establish an outpatient clinic in the adjacent city, where access to primary care is very limited. Shurman has assiduously avoided acting on these informal recommendations.

Shurman recently hired a marketing director, Maureen O'Riley, and asked her to identify new initiatives for Freeland. O'Riley's market research resulted in a plan that included programs for respite care, addiction treatment, and rehabilitation medicine. O'Riley noted that there are no competing programs in the service area and that expected demand will be covered by private pay or nongovernmental third-party payers, both of whom are likely to pay charges. Shurman is enthusiastic about the suggestions and asked the board to review the proposals.

Shurman was shocked when his proposal met significant resistance. No member of the board disputed the well-documented need and the potential demand for the proposed programs. Instead, they were troubled by the prospect of generating additional revenues and adding them to the endowment. Several members indicated that they would support the new programs only if a large part of any surplus was used to assist the city's underserved areas. Others mentioned social consciousness; one even used "guilt" to describe her feelings about having so much while others had so little. The issue was unresolved.

Shurman was angry as he left the board meeting, but took care not to allow others to see his state of mind. After a few minutes' reflection on the meeting, he asked to meet with his chief operating officer (COO). Shurman told the COO what had happened and asked her to solicit any equipment requests submitted by the medical staff and to ensure that they were in his office by week's end. He told the COO to dust off the plans that had been developed several years earlier to build a staff education wing and the more recent request from the oncology department for an expanded unit. As the COO left, Shurman thought to himself that he'd be damned if he'd see his hard work and fiscal success wasted on a harebrained scheme to provide primary care to a population that should be the city's concern.

Freeland Hospital is wealthy and likely to become wealthier. Some members of the board recognize a broader social responsibility for the hospital, while Shurman sees Freeland's role as narrower. The questions raised by the board should have been addressed in the hospital's philosophy and vision and mission statements and these documents should be reviewed for guidance. If no attention has been given to Freeland's broader social responsibility, this fundamental question must be addressed before decisions are made on the marketing plan and the programs that have been recommended. To proceed without a clear direction and a consensus that it be pursued is folly.

"Service area" is the strongest reason for opposing the board's interest in aiding the city's underserved. The facts suggest that the city is out of Freeland's service area. Is it just to take resources from Freeland's service area and redirect them to individuals elsewhere, however compelling the reason? This view suggests that Freeland should reduce its surpluses and simultaneously benefit its service area by reducing charges. This action would directly benefit those whom it serves. Alternatively, Freeland could identify health needs that are not adequately insured or are not likely to be highly sought by private payers but are important nonetheless. Examples of such needs include mental health programs and various types of counseling services.

Shurman's attitude seems extraordinarily parochial, while the board's attitude may be too altruistic. A wide middle ground exists that could accommodate both. It is reasonable to study what role Freeland could play in meeting the health needs of the wider community, whether or not it is in Freeland's service area. Additional information may make the answer apparent.

Historical attitudes about competition, lack of profit motive, and not-for-profit status have both helped and hindered the health services system. The absence of economic incentives has contributed to health services organizations feeling good about themselves because they were doing good rather than concentrating on performing well and efficiently. An important contributing factor has been that the social welfare programs (primarily Medicare) introduced in the 1960s have reimbursed providers for their costs, thus rewarding the inefficient.

The health services organization loses community confidence if it appears not to have the community's best interests in mind. The conflict is between protecting its financial integrity—an ethical obligation of the organization linked to its role of providing services to the community—and serving an individual patient.

How Can We Afford This?

A 63-year-old woman slipped into an irreversible coma after two heart attacks. Three years later she was still a patient in an acute care hospital. Her aggregate unpaid bill totaled $750,000 after private insurance coverage lapsed. The insurer argued that the patient was receiving only custodial care, and therefore it would not pay for acute care. According to state law, the patient could be transferred to another facility only if she were declared mentally incompetent. Hospital efforts to achieve this through court action caused much adverse publicity in the community. Ultimately, the hospital failed to achieve its goal of moving the woman out of the facility and she died there.

The organization and its managers faced an ethical dilemma—their ongoing relationship with a patient no longer needing acute care. The principles of beneficence and nonmaleficence prevented them from abandoning the patient, but the uncompensated costs of her care increasingly conflicted with the hospital's obligation to maintain its financial integrity, which was necessary to serving the community. This large, financially healthy hospital could absorb the losses attributable to this patient, but there remains nonetheless the issue of resource allocation. For other hospitals, however, the cost of a microallocation decision—continued treatment for someone unable to benefit from hospital care—could have been so great as to affect other hospital services to the community (macroallocation).

It seems trite to characterize this case as a public relations failure, but the hospital might have gained community understanding had it been more forthright and communicative in describing the problem and the dilemma it faced as it sought to move the woman into a suitable alternative facility. Working to change the law so that mental status is but one criterion used in making such decisions is important for the future and should be undertaken by the trade association.

The Commonweal

In 1995 American Hospital Association (AHA) national data developed from a survey of 5,300 acute care hospitals showed that acute care hospitals in 1993 incurred $16 billion in uncompensated care costs, an 8.8% increase from 1992.[7] Uncompensated care was defined as the total of charity care and bad debt expense. Despite the increase in current dollars, hospitals' level of uncompensated care remained stable as a percentage of total expenses, which suggests that hospitals' commitment to treating those unable to pay has not wavered. "(This) information casts doubt on the conclusion of the new Rand study, which suggests that hospitals will reduce their levels of uncompensated care to counter payment shortfalls from Medicare and Medicaid and price discounts negotiated by managed care plans." [8]

Comparisons of not-for-profit and for-profit hospitals also provide useful insights into uncompensated care. Using 1993 data, a study of 116 Tennessee hospitals, about one third of which are for-profit, showed that, as a percentage of expenses, not-for-profit hospitals provided more uncompensated care than did for-profit hospitals. The difference was not as large on average as one might expect, however. The statewide median for all hospitals was 8.4%; the median for not-for-profit and for-profit hospitals was 8.9% and 8.1%, respectively. It is important to note that the value of taxes paid by for-profit hospitals is not included in calculating their direct and indirect contribution to programs such as Medicare and Medicaid. These taxes would include federal and state income taxes and sales, property, and local business taxes. [9]

The tax variable was considered in a study undertaken by the Virginia Health Services Cost Review Council, an independent state data commission. Using 1993 data, it ranked 88 acute care hospitals in Virginia via 18 productivity and efficiency variables. A variable that attempted to measure community benefits provided by each hospital proved controversial. "Community support" was defined as the percentage of a hospital's total expenses spent on charity care, bad debt, and all taxes. Including taxes moved the for-profit hospitals ahead of most not-for-profit hospitals. A Virginia Hospital Association analysis, which excluded two state-supported university hospitals, found that 13 for-profit hospitals used 14% of their operating expenses for community support as compared to the 73 not-for-profit hospitals, which spent 7.7%. In commenting on the data, representatives of the for-profit sector argued that taxes should be included because the money is used to support local communities as well as Medicaid and Medicare. Conversely, representatives of the not-for-profit sector argued that including taxes is misleading because most taxes are state and federal income taxes, which may or may not be used for local health care programs. [10]

Such studies are often marred by methodological problems; the definitive study remains to be done. It is clear that one must be cautious about attributing motives and results solely to ownership. A study reported in 1990 found that not-for-profit hospitals appear more likely to be accessible to the uninsured and medically indigent than would be for-profit hospitals. Moreover, not-for-profit hospitals appear more likely to carry a heavier indigent load and for-profit hospitals appear to serve relatively more patients with "good" insurance. The same study found that for-profit hospitals appear to be more efficient than not-for-profits. [11] Since 1983 the AHA has not provided data on uncompensated care that distinguish not-for-profit and for-profit hospitals.

Baby K

Background Few events are as joyful as the birth of a healthy baby. If the baby is profoundly impaired, the heartbreak is unequalled. The legal case, entitled *In the Matter of Baby K,** began in 1992, when an anencephalic baby girl was born at Fairfax Hospital in northern Virginia. This case raises several ethical issues; the focus here is on resource allocation and the organization's responsibility when futile treatment is demanded.

Distinguishing this case from others involving anencephalics is that the mother demanded that everything be done for Baby K. In the realm of ethics decisions about anencephalics raise questions of futile care. In the realm of politics such emotionally charged situations are almost beyond public debate and politicians will undoubtedly flee from any discussion of them.

Anencephaly is a rare congenital anomaly in which the cerebral cortex of the brain has not developed and the top of the skull and scalp are absent. It is estimated that 1,000–2,000 anencephalics are born annually in the United States. Most die within hours or days of birth, with or without intervention. Some anencephalics are born with better-developed brain stems and live weeks or months. Rarely do anencephalics live more than a few months. Baby K was an exception and lived $2\frac{1}{2}$ years, with a need for intermittent aggressive intervention.

Clinical Aspects   Baby K's anencephaly had been diagnosed prenatally. The mother, Ms. H, continued the pregnancy despite the recommendations of her obstetrician and a neonatologist that terminating the pregnancy was best. Baby K's father was not married to her mother and was not involved in her care nor in decision making regarding her. He did, however, support the efforts to write a do-not-resuscitate (DNR) order.

Baby K was delivered by cesarean section. She was born permanently unconscious and could not see, hear, or otherwise interact with her environment. Brain stem functions were limited to feeding and respiratory reflexes and she reflexively responded to sound or touch. Mechanical ventilation was begun at birth, but it served no therapeutic or palliative purpose because the underlying anencephaly was untreatable.

Ethical and Legal Aspects   The physicians urged the mother to authorize a DNR order, but she refused and would not authorize discontinuation of the ventilator. Ms. H and Baby K's physicians met with a specially appointed three-person panel of the hospital ethics committee, two of whom were physicians (a family practitioner and a psychiatrist). The third member was a minister. "The(y) [the three-person panel] . . . concluded that Baby K's ventilator treatment should end because 'such care was futile' and decided to 'wait a reasonable time for the family to help the caregiver terminate aggressive therapy.' " [12] If the mother refused to follow the advice, the panel recommended that the hospital seek a legal solution. Ms. H subsequently rejected the panel's recommendation. The extent to which ethical issues were ad-

---

*The identities of mother and child were sealed and not revealed until after the U.S. Supreme Court refused to review the appeals court decision.

dressed or discussed is unclear. The panel met multiple times, and the ethics committee as a whole discussed the case on more than one occasion. The roles of both entities were seen as advisory, not as achieving a certain result or acting as an advocate for any position.

Baby K was successfully weaned from the ventilator. After disagreement about treatment, Fairfax Hospital sought to move her to another hospital, but hospitals with pediatric intensive care units declined. Six weeks after the birth, the mother allowed Baby K to be transferred to a nursing facility on the condition that Baby K could be readmitted to the hospital if respiratory problems recurred. Baby K was brought to the hospital in respiratory distress several times after the transfer. Between acute episodes Baby K remained at the nursing facility and did not require life-sustaining treatment except for the occasional use of a ventilator.

Trial Court   To protect itself legally, Fairfax Hospital sought a declaratory judgment in federal district court that it would not violate the Emergency Medical Treatment and Active Labor Act of 1986 (EMTALA; PL 99-272), the Rehabilitation Act of 1973 (PL 93-112), or the Americans with Disabilities Act (ADA; PL 101-336) of 1990 by refusing to administer life-sustaining treatment to an infant with anencephaly. The EMTALA requires that emergency departments in hospitals that receive Medicare funds must treat all who arrive with an emergency medical condition and must continue treatment until the person can be transferred safely. PL 93-112 and PL 101-336 prohibit discrimination because of handicap or disability, respectively.

The hospital conceded that respiratory distress is an emergency condition, but argued that the EMTALA should be interpreted to include an exception for treatment deemed "futile" or "inhumane" by hospital physicians. The trial judge found no such exception in the EMTALA; regardless, he reasoned, the exception would not apply to Baby K because her breathing could be restored, and therefore mechanical ventilation could not be considered futile or inhumane. The trial court also found Baby K's condition was a handicap and a disability and that the hospital could not legally refuse treatment (per Section 504 of PL 93-112 and PL 101-336, respectively). Denying care to Baby K would constitute discrimination. The trial court ruled further that as a general matter of law, absent a finding of neglect or abuse, parents have a constitutionally protected right under the 14th Amendment's due process clause to raise children as they see fit and to make decisions about medical treatment for them. The judge concluded that when parents disagree the courts should support the parent who decides in favor of life. The attorney appointed by the court as guardian *ad litem* for Baby K agreed with the hospital. Fairfax Hospital appealed the trial court decision.

Appeals Court   In a 2 to 1 decision the 4th U.S. Circuit Court of Appeals affirmed the trial court decision. It ruled that the EMTALA requires hospitals receiving Medicare funds to provide care in life-threatening situations, regardless of the patients' conditions. The appeals court determined that because the hospital has a duty to render medically stabilizing treatment under the EMTALA there was no need to address the hospital's obligations under other federal statutes or the laws of the state of Virginia.

The majority agreed with the hospital that the standard of care for infants with anencephaly is to provide only warmth, nutrition, and hydration. Nevertheless, it held that the statutory language was unambiguous and included no such limitation. The majority declined to legislate from the bench: "It is beyond the limits of our judicial function to address the moral or ethical propriety of providing emergency stabilizing medical treatment to anencephalic infants. We are bound to interpret federal statutes in accordance with their language and any expressed congressional intent." [13]

The dissenting judge argued that the EMTALA was enacted to prevent patients from being dumped for economic reasons, that dumping was not an issue for Baby K, and that therefore the statute should not apply. Baby K's respiratory failures related to anencephaly; her necessary care should be viewed as a continuum in which no medical treatment can improve her condition of permanent unconsciousness.

Various groups filed *amici curiae* briefs in the appeal. The American Academy of Pediatrics and the Society of Critical Care Medicine supported the hospital. The Virginia Department for Rights of Virginians with Disabilities provided legal assistance to Ms. H and argued that Baby K had a right to treatment. In 1994 the U.S. Supreme Court refused to review the case and the appeals court decision was allowed to stand.

A statement released by Fairfax Hospital in 1993 before the appeals court decision stated, "We believe that continuing to provide extraordinary measures to prolong the dying process is medically and ethically inappropriate, and not in the best interests of this infant. . . . The hospital and its physicians remain ready to provide appropriate medical care, which in this case includes nutrition, hydration, and warmth." [14]

Analysis Anencephaly had been diagnosed months before birth. If the physicians believed mechanical ventilation was medically inappropriate, this should have been made clear to Ms. H at that time. She should have been encouraged to find alternative sources of physician and hospital care, which may have been impossible because of her enrollment in the Kaiser health plan. It is certain, however, that had Ms. H refused to follow the physicians' recommendation, or had she been unable to find a physician and a hospital to provide the care she wanted, Fairfax Hospital and its physicians would have had little choice but to continue treating her and Baby K after her birth. Further efforts should have been made to convince Ms. H of the inappropriateness of her position.

If mechanical ventilation were to be used, the goal of the intervention (e.g., confirmation of the diagnosis) should have been specified and respiratory support should have continued only until that goal was reached or found to be unattainable. Ms. H might have reneged on an agreement to discontinue respiratory support, however, which would have put the physicians and hospital back where they started.

Hospital administration and legal counsel seem to have overreacted. They should have supported the physicians in their application of existing medical standards and encouraged further discussions with Ms. H through the ethics committee and its special panel. Such efforts could have continued even after Baby K was discharged to the nursing facility.

By going to court they turned an issue of medical practice and medical ethics into a legal issue. Having once undertaken legal proceedings the hospital effectively lost control of the situation—highly undesirable by any measure. Court proceedings are always difficult, expensive, and energy and emotionally intensive. The publicity surrounding such cases is often a public relations nightmare, regardless of the result.

The appeals court decision rejected the argument that the standard of care should be used implicitly to guide interpretation of the EMTALA. This substantially limits the discretion of providers in terms of the circumstances that justify withholding or withdrawing care where patients have not or cannot express their wishes regarding life-sustaining treatment. Meeting the standard of care may protect physicians and hospitals from malpractice actions, which are governed by state law, but it does not protect them from liability under federal law.

The extent to which the ethics committee or its special panel sought to solve the problem from an ethical standpoint is unclear. Apparently, the focus was advising as to medical practice and legal strategy. The result confirms this focus, which runs counter to good practice. Organizations and their ethics committees must meet the value system reflected in their organizational philosophy to prospectively address ethical issues such as futile care. Specific cases are analyzed in this context. This analysis provides the basis for advising participants and maintaining the integrity of the hospital's philosophy.

Ethics committees do not make decisions, but their evaluative, educative, and consultative roles are well known. In terms of the educative and consultative roles, all efforts should have been made to continue a dialogue with Ms. H until a resolution acceptable to both was reached. Here, however, they advised only on the elements of futility and how clinical decisions should be addressed. This role is too passive.

In addition, one must question whether it was wise to focus on the medical dimensions of the case by appointing physicians as two of the three members of the special panel. Ms. H must have been knowledgeable about the clinical (scientific) aspects of anencephaly, but she chose to ignore them. This decision suggests the need to focus on the psychosocial dimensions, a task likely best undertaken by nonphysicians. The role of the member of the clergy and whether he was a member of her faith are unclear.

Because the ethics subcommittee and Baby K's mother were at loggerheads, mediation should have been used to resolve the dispute. The mediator is a neutral person who works with the parties to develop an acceptable solution, which may be a compromise. In such situations keeping the parties talking is essential to success.

Conclusion   The U.S. Supreme Court may consider a similar case in the future and reverse the decision in Baby K. In the meantime Congress can amend the EMTALA as well as other federal legislation to allow care to be withheld or withdrawn when treatment is deemed futile or inhumane by caregivers. Such exceptions are found in the Child Abuse Amendments of 1984 (PL 98-457), which was enacted to prevent denial of care to infants with disabilities. The problem for Congress is that in terms of politics it will be virtually impossible to deny parents the right to demand treatment even when deemed by caregivers to be futile or inhumane.

Baby K had a grim prognosis, but lived far longer than other infants with her condition. She died in April 1995, $2\frac{1}{2}$ years after her birth. Private insurance (Kaiser health plan) and Medicaid covered her medical bills of almost $500,000; approximately one half of the cost was for hospital services. Hospital officials' denial that economics motivated their legal action is supported by the fact that all hospital services had been paid.[15] The challenge for health services organizations in cases such as Baby K will be to meld the concerns of family, caregivers, and organization in a way that eliminates or minimizes futile and inhumane treatment while meeting federal and state law, organizational values, and the personal ethic of the persons involved.

Futile Treatment

As suggested by the case of Baby K, increased attention is being paid to continuing to treat a patient when doing so is considered futile. The definitions of *futile* are lengthy, but at its root futility theory focuses on the absence of possible benefit from continued treatment.

Futility theory has quantitative and qualitative aspects. *Quantitative* is concerned with the probability of success if a treatment were attempted or continued. *Qualitative* assumes a successful treatment, but asks whether the resulting quality of life is such that the treatment ought to be undertaken. The quantitative determination is made by caregivers. The qualitative determination can be made only by the patient or someone speaking for the patient. A question arises as to the limits of decisions about the qualitative dimensions.

Background   In many ways futility theory is old wine in new bottles. Its origins lie in the distinction between ordinary and extraordinary care, which is repeated here for ease of reading. *Ordinary care* is all medicines, treatments, and operations that offer reasonable hope of benefit and that can be obtained without excessive expense, pain, or other inconvenience. *Extraordinary care* is all medicines, treatments, and operations that cannot be obtained or used without excessive expense, pain, or inconvenience, or that, if used, would not offer a reasonable hope of benefit. "Hope of benefit" and "excessive expense, pain, or other inconvenience" are key elements. This definition makes it ethical to withhold any medicine, treatment, or operation that offers no reasonable hope of benefit or that cannot be obtained or used without excessive expense, pain, or inconvenience. A common mistake is to define ordinary as usual or customary treatment; this results in statements such as "Ill persons must always be given food and water because this is ordinary (usual and customary) care for them."

These concepts provide only general guidelines to assist decision making and do not distinguish the roles of patient and physician. In addition, it is argued that the definitions are imprecise. Most important, however, these historical concepts do not determine whether patients (or surrogate decision makers) can demand care that clinicians consider futile. It is asserted that the net result is many "Hollywood" codes, so called because staff halfheartedly go through the motions because performing a real, effective code is considered futile in terms of hope of benefit or quality of life.

It is the issue of patients and/or surrogates demanding care that clinicians consider futile that a futility policy most aggressively seeks to remedy. This has occurred despite few reported cases in which surrogates demanded care that clinicians determined was futile. Two such cases are Helga Wanglie, the Minneapolis woman in a persistent vegetative state (PVS) whose husband demanded that all efforts be made to keep her alive, despite a prognosis that doing so offered no hope of benefit; and the case of Baby K, the anencephalic infant whose mother refused to authorize a DNR order and insisted that all treatment continue. Apparently, even less common are situations in which it is the patients who request futile care. In fact, prominent cases such as the Quinlan and Cruzan cases occurred because organizations insisted on providing care that patients and/or surrogates determined was futile and should not be provided. Cases such as this of course suggest that futility policies are better aimed at organizations and staff than at patients and families. Nevertheless, there is a perception and some anecdotal evidence that patient- and surrogate-demanded futile treatment is a problem common enough to warrant a policy.

Definition Applying the futility concept has been described as a unilateral DNR order, a decision made by the physician using a physiologic definition.[16] The futility policy of Santa Monica Hospital Medical Center defines futile care as

> Any clinical circumstance in which the doctor and his consultants, consistent with the available medical literature, conclude that further treatment (except comfort care) cannot, within a reasonable possibility, cure, ameliorate, improve or restore a quality of life that would be satisfactory to the patient.[17]

The first two thirds of this policy is clinical and seeks to quantify the futility of continued care. The final third is patient focused and adds a subjective criterion, a value judgment: "a quality of life that *would be satisfactory to the patient*"(emphasis added). A plain-language reading of the policy shows these two portions to be in conflict. If the quality of life is satisfactory to the patient, regardless of how poor others might consider it to be, clinical judgments about futility are irrelevant. These two elements of the policy can be reconciled only if physicians act paternalistically and decide that a certain quality of life would be unsatisfactory to the patient.

Implementation of the policy includes several steps: informing the competent patient and family about the ailment, options, and prognosis; emphasizing that the patient will be given all other support; providing names of consultants to render an independent opinion; providing assistance of nurses, chaplain, and others; involving the ethics committee, as appropriate; and allowing sufficient time for the patient and family to consider the information. If, after taking these steps, the family is unconvinced, "neither the doctor nor the hospital is required to provide care that is not medically indicated, and the family may be offered a substitute physician . . . and another hospital."[18] Most significant is the final step: "If it is determined that the patient can no longer benefit from an acute hospital stay and the patient insists on staying, or the family insists that the patient should remain, the mechanism for personal payment can be invoked." [19] The policy concludes with examples of futile care, such as irreversible coma or PVS; a terminally ill patient, for whom applying life-sustaining procedures would only artificially delay the moment of death; and permanent dependence on ICU care.

The final step in the policy focuses on economics by stating that the hospital can bill the patient for care that is not medically indicated. This harsh result is likely to be employed infrequently because third parties pay for most hospital services, especially Medicare for older adults and people with disabilities, in which cases of futile care are likely to occur. In addition, the legal implications of such a policy are complex and unresolved.

Knowing Whether or When to Stop

An 18-year-old woman suffered severe head injuries in a car accident in 1987. After a few weeks in a coma, she opened her eyes, but was totally nonresponsive for 15 months. Then, nurses noticed a hopeful sign when she twice seemed to obey their orders to move her leg or to close her eyes. These responses were rare, but 2 months later her physicians administered drugs to improve alertness and her condition improved slowly. Over time, she learned to answer multiple-choice questions and calculate simple math problems using eye blinks. At one point, she wrote, "Mom, I love you."

Three years after the accident, she was communicating regularly with eye blinks and could move her arms somewhat. After 5 years, she could mouth words and short phrases. Although her attention span was limited to 15 minutes, she liked to be pampered and took pleasure in teasing her nurses. Her favorite joke was pretending not to know their identities.

Her mother was overjoyed. She reveled in each small bit of progress. She was sent home 5 years and 2 months after the injury, totally dependent on others. Her rehabilitation had cost well over $1 million.[20]

This tragic case raises squarely the issue of futile care. By emerging from PVS this patient has had a rare, almost miraculous outcome. Her family demanded that care be continued; the result is that care must be continued.

Implications Futility theory extends well beyond the contemporary concept of autonomy. Patient autonomy is a negative right, the right to be free from unwanted treatment—to be able to say no, thank you. Futility theory limits what is seen as a positive right, a right to demand care when it is claimed there is no medical benefit to receiving it. From an ethical standpoint it is arguable no such right exists.

Futility theory is an aggressive approach to issues of extraordinary, disproportionate, and burdensome care. The decision maker is the physician. The sample policy states that there is a need to educate and inform the patient. The patient and/or family need not concur with the decision. Futility theory is very different from the shared decision making in what is considered the ideal, a nonpaternalistic physician–patient relationship. In fact, the problem that futility theory purports to address may be only partly attributable to patient demands. Research documents many shortcomings in the care of seriously ill, dying patients, especially the effectiveness of patient–physician communication.

The findings of the Study to Understand Prognoses and Preferences for Outcomes and Risks of Treatments (SUPPORT) research are compelling:

> (The) Study to Understand Prognoses and Preferences for Outcomes and Risks of Treatments patients were seriously ill, and their dying proved to be predictable, yet discussion and decisions substantially in advance of death were uncommon. Nearly half of all DNR orders were written in the last 2 days of life. The final hospitalization for half of patients included more than 8 days in generally undesirable states: in an ICU, receiving mechanical ventilation, or comatose. Families reported that half of the patients who were able to communicate in their last few days spent most of the time in moderate or severe pain.[21]

These results occurred in the intervention phase of the SUPPORT study despite the presence of nurses whose tasks were to improve communication and encourage the patient and family to engage in an informed and collaborative decision-making process with a well-informed physician. The authors concluded that additional proactive and forceful measures may be needed. It was estimated that patients meeting SUPPORT criteria account for approximately 400,000 admissions per year in the United States. Such findings seem to support the rather harsh approach in the futility policy noted above, but there is reason for caution.

In a corollary to the first phase of SUPPORT, investigators examined the impact of prognosis-based futility guidelines on survival and hospital length of stay on a cohort of adults with serious illness. They calculated the hospital days that would not be used if, on the third day, life-sustaining treatment had been stopped or not initiated for patients with an estimated 2-month survival of 1% or less. They found that only 10.8% of hospital days would have been forgone and concluded that only modest savings would have resulted.[22]

If large numbers of patients demand futile care, such guidelines will have several important effects: Voluntary (patient and/or surrogates have consented) passive euthanasia will exist in theory, but will be necessary rarely. Involuntary (patient and/or surrogates have not consented) passive euthanasia will increase dramatically. Futile care policies and guidelines may become a means by which physicians are permitted to feel that they are relieved of the obligation to talk to their patients and/or surrogates. The system requires physicians to obtain consent before withdrawing life-sustaining treatment, but this action would be subject to reconsideration.

An apparent contradiction exists between science and the quality of life suggested in the definition of futile care noted earlier. This contradiction raises the question of whether a paternalistic quality of life decision is masquerading as scientific, objective decision making. If so, futile care policies are more than a step back for patient autonomy—they are a return to the physician paternalism of the Hippocratic tradition.

Another result is that the right to die may become a duty to die. Do futile care policies put health services organizations and providers on a slippery slope? Will the policies become broader and increasingly focused on the quality of life that clinicians determine would be acceptable to the patient? These questions can be answered only in retrospect, in itself not a cheery prospect.

Alternatives to Futile Care Policies   Absent data showing that it is common for patients and/or surrogates to demand care considered by caregivers to be futile, it is possible that futility policies are solving a nonproblem, especially true in light of published cases of patients being forced to accept care. In addition, the SUPPORT investigators' findings as to economic impact should be explored further.

Assuming, however, that a problem exists, the first alternative solution is the status quo—patients and/or surrogates must agree to discontinue care after physicians have diagnosed it is futile. An adjunct to this alternative is to enhance the communication skills of physicians and other caregivers. It may be that patients and/or surrogates inadequately understand the prognosis. Health professionals such as nurses and social services staff may be used more effectively, for example. The task should not be left only to physicians and ethics committees: Both are likely to be much more daunting to patients and surrogates. Increasing availability of objective predictions of survival or probability of good result, such as the Acute Physiological and Chronic Health Evaluation (APACHE) system, can be used to assist decision makers (patients and/or surrogates) in understanding the best course of action. APACHE predicts probable outcomes of treatment based on various physiological variables, and the resulting data are useful to patients and other decision makers as well as to physicians.

A second alternative (more long range) solution is to change the presumption about care. The presumption in clinical interactions is that care is to be provided absent express directives to the contrary from patients or surrogates. This presumption, reflecting Baconian theory about science conquering nature, has been reinforced by the law. Recognizing that medicine has limits requires a return to the Hippocratic tradition.[23] Although usually desirable, the presumption should be changed where terminal illness or PVS have been diagnosed. The presumption should be that care will be provided if there is a probability it will benefit the patient (i.e., the care contemplated is not futile). Under this new presumption certain cases simply will not receive care.

A third alternative solution is to develop and apply a community standard. Although not easily done, the operational aspects of this approach are within every health services organization's ability to develop. This is the idea of protecting the commons or, its contemporary manifestation, communitarianism, a concept developed by Amitai Etzioni. Communitarianism involves recognizing resource limits and cooperatively working within them.

Futility theory is growing in popularity. Implicit in the theory, however, are several issues that every health services organization should address before developing a futile care policy. The first step should be to determine the extent of the problem. Perhaps other remedies are more appropriate, such as making education on advance directives more effective and increasing the likelihood that they will appear on the medical record. Such obvious first steps may obviate the need for a futile care policy.

The most important use for a futile care policy may be to provide administrative guidelines and support for physicians, whose clinical practice will benefit from defining and understanding futile care. In turn, the policy is available to convince patients and/or surrogates that nonbeneficial treatment should be discontinued.

CONCLUSION

This chapter addressed issues of macro- and microallocation of resources. Questions related to the allocation of resources are common to all types of health services organizations, but often go unrecognized. Both macro- and microallocation issues are becoming more important as economic constraints increase, and it is crucial that the organizational philosophy and vision and mission statements guide these decisions. This guidance requires a level of precision and specificity that many health services organizations lack. This deficit must be overcome.

Cases such as that of Baby K suggest primary issues of resource allocation that may be remedied only through federal legislation. Futility theory is in the early phases of development and as it matures may come to be a primary guideline in resource allocation decisions. The ethical dilemma for the organization is husbanding resources, whether they are exclusive to it or are part of the commonweal.

Hospitals with large amounts of uncompensated care may see offering better reimbursed services, such as rehabilitation and cosmetic surgery, as

ways to offset these losses. "No margin, no mission" is an oft-repeated justification for such actions, if one were needed. Fiscally sound health services
organizations must ask whether they are meeting their obligations under the
principle of justice to offer unprofitable but needed services that benefit the
wider community, as well as whether they are meeting a duty of general
beneficence to the community to use surpluses to assist persons requiring
health services.

NOTES

1. Charles Fried. (1976, February). Equality and rights in medical care. *Hastings Center Report, 6,* 29–34.
2. Adapted from Jonathon S. Rakich, Beaufort B. Longest, Jr., & Kurt Darr. (1992). *Managing health services organizations* (3rd ed., p. 198). Baltimore: Health Professions Press. Used with permission.
3. *Ibid.,* pp. 139–140.
4. James F. Childress. (1970, Winter). Who shall live when not all can live? *Soundings, An Interdisciplinary Journal, 53*(4), 339–355; Nicholas Rescher. (1969, April). The allocation of exotic medical lifesaving therapy. *Ethics, 79*(3), 173–186.
5. Paul Ramsey. (1970). *The patient as person* (p. 252). New Haven, CT: Yale University Press.
6. Adapted from Jonathon S. Rakich, Beaufort B. Longest, Jr., & Kurt Darr. (1992). *Managing health services organizations* (3rd ed., p. 142). Baltimore: Health Professions Press. Used with permission.
7. David Burda. (1995, May 8). Hospitals' care for poor rises slowly. *Modern Healthcare, 25*(19), 30.
8. *Ibid.*
9. David Burda. (1995, April 24). Tennessee for-profits lag in care for poor. *Modern Healthcare, 25*(17), 70, 72, 74.
10. David Burda. (1995, May 8). For-profits, not-for-profits reignite battle. *Modern Healthcare, 25*(19), 28, 30.
11. Barbara Arrington, & Cynthia Carter Haddock. (1990, June). Who *really* profits from not-for-profits? *Health Services Research, 25*(2), 291–304.
12. In the Matter of BABY "K" (E.D. Va. July 1, 1993), 832 F. Supp. 1025.
13. In the Matter of BABY "K", 16 F. 3d 598 (4th Cir. February 10, 1994).
14. Bill Miller, & Marylou Tousignant. (1993, September 25). Mother fights hospital to keep infant alive. *The Washington Post,* p. A14.
15. Marylou Tousignant, & Bill Miller. (1995, April 7). Death of "Baby K" leaves a legacy of legal precedents. *The Washington Post,* p. B3.
16. David B. Waisel, & Robert D. Truog. (1995, February 15). The cardiopulmonary resuscitation-not-indicated order: Futility revisited. *Annals of Internal Medicine, 122*(4), 304–308.
17. Terese Hudson. (1994, February 20). Are futile-care policies the answer? *Hospitals & Health Services Networks,* pp. 26–32.
18. *Ibid.,* p. 28.
19. *Ibid.*

20. Nancy L. Childs, & Walt N. Mercer. (1996). Brief report: Late improvement in consciousness after post-traumatic vegetative state. *New England Journal of Medicine, 334*(1), 24–25. "Permanent" coma can be misnomer, Texas case shows. (1996, January 4). *The Washington Post*, p. A16.
21. The SUPPORT Principal Investigators. (1995, November 22/29). A controlled trial to improve care for seriously-ill hospitalized patients: The study to understand prognoses and preferences for outcomes and risks of treatments (SUPPORT). *Journal of the American Medical Association, 274*(20), 1595.
22. Joan M. Teno, Donald Murphy, Joanne Lynn, Anna Tosteson, Norman Desbiens, Alfred F. Connors, Jr., Mary Beth Hamel, Albert Wu, Russell Phillips, Neil Wenger, Frank Harrell, Jr., & William A. Knaus for the SUPPORT Investigators. (1994, November). Prognosis-based guidelines: Does anyone win? *Journal of the American Gerontological Society, 42*, 1202–1207.
23. Nancy S. Jecker. (1991, May–June). Knowing when to stop: The limits of medicine. *Hastings Center Report*, pp. 5–8.

Appendixes

Appendix A

Organizational Philosophies and Mission Statements

VALUES, MISSION, AND VISION STATEMENTS OF SIBLEY MEMORIAL HOSPITAL

Values

Our values provide guidelines and parameters for the decisions that we make as we work to improve our processes and respond to our patients' and other customers' needs.

- Personalized and compassionate service
- Excellence and continually improving quality
- Teamwork
- Job satisfaction
- Professionalism
- Using resources wisely and providing value
- Innovation
- Trust and respect
- Up-to-date technology
- A clean, attractive, quiet, and safe environment
- Honesty, integrity, flexibility, and selflessness

Mission

Our mission is to provide quality health services and facilities for the community, to promote wellness, to relieve suffering, and to restore health as swiftly, safely, and humanely as it can be done, consistent with the best services we can give at the highest value for all concerned.

Vision

Our vision is to provide superior healthcare service and value, with the goal of improving the health and well-being of our community. We plan to continuously improve that service by using scientific methods, teamwork, and knowledge of best practices and customer expectations. Our vision guides us to work continuously to improve our services.

From Sibley Memorial Hospital, Washington, D.C. (1996). Reprinted with permission.

MISSION STATEMENT OF ST. MARY MEDICAL CENTER

Empowered by the Spirit of JESUS CHRIST and inspired by the examples of Saint Francis of Assisi, Saint John Neumann, Mother Francis Bachmann, and the Sisters of Saint Francis of Philadelphia, we manifest our participation in the healing ministry of the Roman Catholic Church through our commitment to provide, within the limits of our resources, compassionate and quality holistic care to all in our community, within which we especially cherish the poor. We envision that the scope of the healing ministry will become more expansive and varied. Therefore, we will endeavor to accept, discover and create new structures, models and services to enhance health care at St. Mary Medical Center of Langhorne.

From St. Mary Medical Center, Langhorne, Pennsylvania. (1996). Reprinted with permission.

Values, Mission, and Vision Statements of Suburban Hospital

Shared Values

Accountability
We know what our community and co-workers expect of us, and we are committed to meet and exceed those expectations. What we say and do shows we care about the immediate results of our work, the well-being of our patients, and the health of our community.

Flexibility
We embrace change and know it is not only an unending process but also the arena of creativity, productivity, and success. We take satisfaction in the process, not in a false sense of arriving at some destination.

Innovation
We seek out and build upon the best ideas—anyone's, at any time. We continuously measure and improve the quality of our work in the eyes of those we serve.

Integrity
We do what we say we will do. Our actions and our words are one and the same.

Respect
We foster an environment where care and consideration for others is obvious, where each person has the freedom and confidence to express any view in a constructive way, and where conflict is treated fairly.

Teamwork
Employees in our organization are empowered to exercise their judgment and creativity within their area of competence, to take the initiative, to accept responsibility, to deliver results. We take pride and share in everyone's accomplishments.

Viability
We act with common sense and good judgment in the best interest of our patients and community. By keeping our promises, creating value and satis-

faction in everything we do, we will ensure the viability of the institution and make our vision a reality.

Mission

Suburban Hospital is a community-owned not-for-profit organization dedicated to maintaining and improving the physical and mental health status of the citizens of Montgomery County and northwest Washington, D.C.

Through the efforts of our medical staff, employees, volunteers, and Board of Trustees, the hospital strives to meet the needs of our community by providing a comprehensive range of high-quality, compassionate, and cost-effective services, including acute and subacute inpatient care, emergency and trauma services, ambulatory care, and community health education and prevention programs.

Vision

Forging an Integrated
Partnership for Health

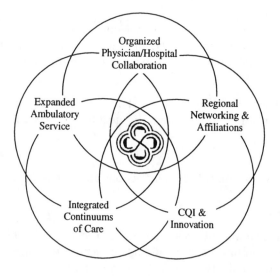

From Suburban Hospital, Bethesda, Maryland. (1996). Reprinted with permission.

MISSION AND VISION STATEMENTS AND QUALITY POLICY OF THE GEORGE WASHINGTON UNIVERSITY MEDICAL CENTER

Guiding Principles

1. **Quality:** The organization will be oriented to improve continuously every aspect of its work. All those who interact with the Medical Center will be pleased by their experiences.
2. **Innovations:** Our innovative teaching and research programs, management systems, and sophisticated medical care will be models for emulation.
3. **Service:** Service will be the cornerstone of the organization. Customers will believe that our services will be worth their cost.
4. **Humanity:** We will demonstrate compassion and empathy.
5. **Integrity:** The organization will be honest and forthright.
6. **Loyalty:** There will be loyalty among students, patients, employees, faculty, and alumni. There will be a strong sense of tradition and pride centered around our achievements. We will appropriately balance institutional, departmental, and personal priorities.
7. **Advocacy:** The Medical Center will be active nationally and locally advocating for the promotion of health and the advancement of knowledge. The institution will be recognized as a partner with the community.

Mission Statement

The mission of The George Washington University Medical Center is innovation and excellence in medicine and health sciences. Since 1821, this mission has been carried out by providing superior patient care and health promotion, by excellence in the education of health professionals, and by advancing medical knowledge through basic and applied research. Our core values are compassion and integrity supported by the constant improvement of every aspect of our work and the wise allocation of resources.

Vision Statement

It is the vision of The George Washington University Medical Center to be a preeminent academic health center where excellence is pervasive.

Quality Policy

Quality means the continuous improvement of services in order to meet the needs and exceed the expectations of all those who interact with the Medical Center. This group includes, but is not limited to, patients, employees, trainees and students, physicians, faculty, payors, grantors, philanthropic donors, affiliated hospitals, and the community.

MISSION AND CUSTOMER SERVICE MISSION STATEMENTS OF THE LEVINDALE HEBREW GERIATRIC CENTER AND HOSPITAL

Mission Statement

Levindale is a geriatric center and hospital dedicated to providing superior service in a cost-effective manner for the aged, frail, and ill in institutional, community, and home settings. As an advocate for the elderly, Levindale accepts a leadership role in defining and developing, in collaboration with other agencies, a comprehensive continuum of nursing, medical, and social services within the Jewish community of the Baltimore metropolitan area. Programs are operated within the values inherent in Judaism pursuant to Levindale's charter.

Customer Service Mission Statement

Levindale's mission is to provide superior service in a cost-effective manner for the aged, frail, and ill in institutional, community, and home settings.

Empowerment is given to all staff in demonstrating initiative and positive changes to guarantee patients' and residents' fulfillment.

Visitors' concerns and problems will be addressed courteously, and followed through to harmonious solution.

Information provided to families will be current, factual, and accurate.

New requests for information and services by families will be addressed appropriately so that satisfaction is achieved.

Department in-service training and new employee orientation will keep staff well-informed as to all pertinent policies, procedures, and guidelines.

Acknowledgment and support will be shown by all staff regarding the Patients' and Residents' Bill of Rights and Responsibilities.

Levindale believes that customer satisfaction is every staff member's number-one priority.

Etiquette in communication will be exhibited at all times when greeting visitors by telephone or in person.

From Levindale Hebrew Geriatric Center and Hospital, Baltimore, Maryland. (1996). Reprinted with permission.

Vision and Mission Statements of Baltimore Medical System, Inc.

Vision Statement

BMSI shall become the provider of choice for primary care services in East Baltimore.

Mission Statement

It shall be the mission of Baltimore Medical System, Inc., to:

Provide quality health care for the residents of the communities we serve, regardless of age, sex, race, creed, disability, or ability to pay for services.

Promote awareness and appreciation of diversity through ongoing staff education and an organizational commitment to achieve a diverse workforce and patient population.

Provide services with respect and compassion in a healthy, comfortable environment.

Provide ready access to needed acute and preventive health care, reaching those who traditionally experience limited access to services.

Provide additional services beyond primary health care and serve as an educational resource to benefit our patients, their families, and the community.

Administer services efficiently and manage the organization's resources prudently.

Improve the quality of our services continuously through staff education, organizational accreditation, and feedback from our patients, staff, and community.

Respond to changes in the health care system and the community with flexibility, creativity, and assertiveness.

From Baltimore Medical System, Inc., Baltimore, Maryland. (1996). Reprinted with permission.

MISSION STATEMENT OF THE GEORGE WASHINGTON UNIVERSITY HEALTH PLAN

Through innovation and commitment to excellence, The George Washington University Health Plan strives to provide the highest quality patient care supported by a preeminent medical center, community hospitals, and physicians. We are committed to improving the quality of our members' health and their lives.

From the 1995 *Annual Report to Our Members*, The George Washington University Health Plan, Washington, D.C. (1995). Reprinted with permission.

273

Appendix B

Ethical Codes

American College of Healthcare Executives (ACHE) Code of Ethics[1,2]

Preface

The *Code of Ethics* is administered by the Ethics Committee, which is appointed by the Board of Governors upon nomination by the Chairman. It is composed of at least nine Fellows of the College, each of whom serves a three-year term on a staggered basis, with three members retiring each year.

The Ethics Committee shall:

- Review and evaluate annually the Code of Ethics, and make any necessary recommendations for updating the Code.
- Review and recommend action to the Board of Governors on allegations brought forth regarding breaches of the Code of Ethics.
- Develop ethical policy statements to serve as guidelines of ethical conduct for healthcare executives and their professional relationships.
- Prepare an annual report of observations, accomplishments, and recommendations to the Board of Governors, and such other periodic reports as required.

The Ethics Committee invoked the Code of Ethics under authority of the ACHE *Bylaws*, Article II, Membership, Section 6, Resignation and Termination of Membership; Transfer to Inactive Status, subsection (b), as follows:

> Membership may be terminated or rendered inactive by action of the Board of Governors as a result of violation of the Code of Ethics; nonconformity with the Bylaws or Regulations Governing Admission, Advancement, Recertification, and Reappointment; conviction of a felony; or conviction of a crime of moral turpitude or a crime relating to the healthcare management profession. No such termination of membership or imposition of inactive status shall be effected without affording a reasonable opportunity for

---

[1]As amended by the Council of Regents at its annual meeting on August 22, 1995.

[2]Appendixes I and II, entitled "American College of Healthcare Executives Grievance Procedure" and "Ethics Committee Action," respectively, are a material part of this Code of Ethics and are incorporated herein by reference.

the member to consider the charges and to appear in his or her own defense before the Board of Governors or its designated hearing committee, as outlined in the "Grievance Procedure," Appendix I of the College's Code of Ethics.

Preamble

The purpose of the Code of Ethics of the American College of Healthcare Executives is to serve as a guide to conduct for members. It contains standards of ethical behavior for healthcare executives in their professional relationships. These relationships include members of the healthcare executive's organization and other organizations. Also included are patients or others served, colleagues, the community and society as a whole. The Code of Ethics also incorporates standards of ethical behavior governing personal behavior, particularly when that conduct directly relates to the role and identity of the healthcare executive.

The fundamental objectives of the healthcare management profession are to enhance overall quality of life, dignity, and well-being of every individual needing healthcare services; and to create a more equitable, accessible, effective, and efficient healthcare system.

Healthcare executives have an obligation to act in ways that will merit the trust, confidence, and respect of healthcare professionals and the general public. Therefore, healthcare executives should lead lives that embody an exemplary system of values and ethics.

In fulfilling their commitments and obligations to patients or others served, healthcare executives function as moral advocates. Since every management decision affects the health and well-being of both individuals and communities, healthcare executives must carefully evaluate the possible outcomes of their decisions. In organizations that deliver healthcare services, they must work to safeguard and foster the rights, interests, and prerogatives of patients or others served. The role of moral advocate requires that healthcare executives speak out and take actions necessary to promote such rights, interests, and prerogatives if they are threatened.

I. The healthcare executive's responsibilities to the profession of healthcare management

The healthcare executive shall:

A. Uphold the values, ethics and mission of the healthcare management profession;

B. Conduct all personal and professional activities with honesty, integrity, respect, fairness, and good faith in a manner that will reflect well upon the profession;

C. Comply with all laws pertaining to healthcare management in the jurisdictions in which the healthcare executive is located, or conducts professional activities;

D. Maintain competence and proficiency in healthcare management by implementing a personal program of assessment and continuing professional education;

E. Avoid the exploitation of professional relationships for personal gain;

F. Use this Code to further the interests of the profession and not for selfish reasons;

G. Respect professional confidences;

H. Enhance the dignity and image of the healthcare management profession through positive public information programs; and

I. Refrain from participating in any activity that demeans the credibility and dignity of the healthcare management profession.

II. The healthcare executive's responsibilities to patients or others served, to the organization, and to employees

A. Responsibilities to patients or others served

The healthcare executive shall, within the scope of his or her authority:

1. Work to ensure the existence of a process to evaluate the quality of care or service rendered;

2. Avoid practicing or facilitating discrimination and institute safeguards to prevent discriminatory organizational practices;

3. Work to ensure the existence of a process that will advise patients or others served of the rights, opportunities, responsibilities, and risks regarding available healthcare services;

4. Work to provide a process that ensures the autonomy and self-determination of patients or others served; and

5. Work to ensure the existence of procedures that will safeguard the confidentiality and privacy of patients or others served.

B. Responsibilities to the organization

The healthcare executive shall, within the scope of his or her authority:

1. Provide healthcare services consistent with available resources and work to ensure the existence of a resource allocation process that considers ethical ramifications;

2. Conduct both competitive and cooperative activities in ways that improve community healthcare services;

3. Lead the organization in the use and improvement of standards of management and sound business practices;

4. Respect the customs and practices of patients or others served, consistent with the organization's philosophy; and

5. Be truthful in all forms of professional and organizational communication, and avoid disseminating information that is false, misleading, or deceptive.

C. Responsibilities to employees

Healthcare executives have ethical and professional obligations to employees of the organizations they manage that encompass but are not limited to:

1. Working to create a working environment conducive for underscoring employee ethical conduct and behavior.
2. Working to ensure that individuals may freely express ethical concerns and providing mechanisms for discussing and addressing such concerns.
3. Working to ensure a working environment that is free from harassment, sexual and other; coercion of any kind, especially to perform illegal or unethical acts; and discrimination on the basis of race, creed, color, sex, ethnic origin, age or disability.
4. Working to ensure a working environment that is conducive to proper utilization of employees' skills and abilities.
5. Paying particular attention to the employee's work environment and job safety.
6. Working to establish appropriate grievance and appeals mechanisms.

III. Conflicts of interest

A conflict of interest may be only a matter of degree, but exists when the healthcare executive:

A. Acts to benefit directly or indirectly by using authority or inside information, or allow a friend, relative, or associate to benefit from such authority or information.
B. Uses authority or information to make a decision to intentionally affect the organization in an adverse manner.

The healthcare executive shall:

A. Conduct all personal and professional relationships in such a way that all those affected are assured that management decisions are made in the best interests of the organization and the individuals served by it;
B. Disclose to the appropriate authority any direct or indirect financial or personal interests that pose potential or actual conflicts of interest;
C. Accept no gifts or benefits offered with the express or implied expectation of influencing a management decision; and
D. Inform the appropriate authority and other involved parties of potential or actual conflicts of interest related to appointments or

elections to boards or committees inside or outside the healthcare executive's organization.

IV. The healthcare executive's responsibilities to community and society

The healthcare executive shall:

A. Work to identify and meet the healthcare needs of the community;
B. Work to ensure that all people have reasonable access to healthcare services;
C. Participate in public dialogue on healthcare policy issues and advocate solutions that will improve health status and promote quality healthcare;
D. Consider the short-term and long-term impact of management decisions on both the community and on society; and
E. Provide prospective consumers with adequate and accurate information, enabling them to make enlightened judgments and decisions regarding services.

V. The healthcare executive's responsibility to report violations of the code

A member of the College who has reasonable grounds to believe that another member has violated this Code has a duty to communicate such facts to the Ethics Committee.

From the American College of Healthcare Executives, Chicago. (1995). Reprinted with permission.

American College of Health Care Administrators (ACHCA) Code of Ethics

Preamble

The preservation of the highest standards of integrity and ethical principles is vital to the successful discharge of the professional responsibilities of all long-term health care administrators. This Code of Ethics has been promulgated by the American College of Health Care Administrators (ACHCA) in an effort to stress the fundamental rules considered essential to this basic purpose. It shall be the obligation of members to seek to avoid not only conduct specifically proscribed by the code but also conduct that is inconsistent with its spirit and purpose. Failure to specify any particular responsibility or practice in this Code of Ethics should not be construed as denial of the existence of other responsibilities or practices. Recognizing that the ultimate responsibility for applying standards and ethics falls upon the individual, the ACHCA establishes the following Code of Ethics to make clear its expectation of the membership.

Expectation I

Individuals shall hold paramount the welfare of persons for whom care is provided.

PRESCRIPTIONS: The Health Care Administrator shall:

- Strive to provide to all those entrusted to his or her care the highest quality of appropriate services possible in light of resources or other constraints.
- Operate the facility consistent with laws, regulations, and standards of practice recognized in the field of health care administration.
- Consistent with law and professional standards, protect the confidentiality of information regarding individual recipients of care.
- Perform administrative duties with the personal integrity that will earn the confidence, trust, and respect of the general public.
- Take appropriate steps to avoid discrimination on the basis of race, color, sex, religion, age, national origin, handicap, marital status, ancestry, or any other factor that is illegally discriminatory or not related to bona fide requirements of quality care.

PROSCRIPTION: The Health Care Administrator shall not:

- Disclose professional or personal information regarding recipients of service to unauthorized personnel unless required by law or to protect the public welfare.

Expectation II

Individuals shall maintain high standards of professional competence.

PRESCRIPTIONS: The Health Care Administrator shall:

- Possess and maintain the competencies necessary to effectively perform his or her responsibilities.
- Practice administration in accordance with capabilities and proficiencies and, when appropriate, seek counsel from qualified others.
- Actively strive to enhance knowledge of and expertise in long-term care administration through continuing education and professional development.

PROSCRIPTIONS: The Health Care Administrator shall not:

- Misrepresent qualifications, education, experience, or affiliations.
- Provide services other than those for which he or she is prepared and qualified to perform.

Expectation III

Individuals shall strive, in all matters relating to their professional functions, to maintain a professional posture that places paramount the interests of the facility and its residents.

PRESCRIPTIONS: The Health Care Administrator shall:

- Avoid partisanship and provide a forum for the fair resolution of any disputes which may arise in service delivery or facility management.
- Disclose to the governing body or other authority as may be appropriate, any actual or potential circumstance concerning him or her that might reasonably be thought to create a conflict of interest or have a substantial adverse impact on the facility or its residents.

PROSCRIPTION: The Health Care Administrator shall not:

- Participate in activities that reasonably may be thought to create a conflict of interest or have the potential to have a substantial adverse impact on the facility or its residents.

Expectation IV

Individuals shall honor their responsibilities to the public, their profession, and their relationships with colleagues and members of related professions.

PRESCRIPTIONS: The Health Care Administrator shall:

- Foster increased knowledge within the profession of health care administration and support research efforts toward this end.

- Participate with others in the community to plan for and provide a full range of health care services.
- Share areas of expertise with colleagues, students, and the general public to increase awareness and promote understanding of health care in general and the profession in particular.
- Inform the ACHCA Standards and Ethics Committee of actual or potential violations of this Code of Ethics, and fully cooperate with ACHCA's sanctioned inquiries into matters of professional conduct related to this Code of Ethics.

PROSCRIPTION: The Health Care Administrator shall not:

- Defend, support, or ignore unethical conduct perpetrated by colleagues, peers, or students.

From the American College of Health Care Administrators, Alexandria, Virginia. (1994). Reprinted with permission.

American Medical Association (AMA) Principles of Medical Ethics

Preamble

The medical profession has long subscribed to a body of ethical statements developed primarily for the benefit of the patient. As a member of this profession, a physician must recognize responsibility not only to patients but also to society, to other health professionals, and to self. The following Principles adopted by the American Medical Association are not laws, but standards of conduct which define the essentials of honorable behavior for the physician.

I.   A physician shall be dedicated to providing competent medical service with compassion and respect for human dignity.

II. A physician shall deal honestly with patients and colleagues, and strive to expose those physicians deficient in character or competence, or who engage in fraud or deception.

III. A physician shall respect the law and also recognize a responsibility to seek changes in those requirements which are contrary to the best interests of the patient.

IV. A physician shall respect the rights of patients, of colleagues, and of other health professionals, and shall safeguard patient confidences within the constraints of the law.

V.   A physician shall continue to study, apply and advance scientific knowledge; make relevant information available to patients, colleagues, and the public; obtain consultation; and use the talents of other health professionals when indicated.

VI. A physician shall, in the provision of appropriate patient care, except in emergencies, be free to choose whom to serve, with whom to associate, and the environment in which to provide medical services.

VII. A physician shall recognize a responsibility to participate in activities contributing to an improved community.

Source: *Code of Medical Ethics: Current Opinions with Annotations*, American Medical Association, © 1996. Reprinted with permission.

American Medical Association
Council on Ethical and Judicial Affairs

Fundamental Elements of the Patient–Physician Relationship (1994)

From ancient times, physicians have recognized that the health and well-being of patients depend upon a collaborative effort between physician and patient. Patients share with physicians the responsibility for their own health care. The patient–physician relationship is of greatest benefit to patients when they bring medical problems to the attention of their physicians in a timely fashion, provide information about their medical condition to the best of their ability, and work with their physicians in a mutually respectful alliance. Physicians can best contribute to this alliance by serving as their patients' advocates and by fostering these rights:

1. The patient has the right to receive information from physicians and to discuss the benefits, risks, and costs of appropriate treatment alternatives. Patients should receive guidance from their physicians as to the optimal course of action. Patients are also entitled to obtain copies or summaries of their medical records, to have their questions answered, to be advised of potential conflicts of interest that their physicians might have, and to receive independent professional opinions.
2. The patient has the right to make decisions regarding the health care that is recommended by his or her physician. Accordingly, patients may accept or refuse any recommended medical treatment.
3. The patient has the right to courtesy, respect, dignity, responsiveness, and timely attention to his or her needs.
4. The patient has the right to confidentiality. The physician should not reveal confidential communications or information without the consent of the patient, unless provided for by law or by the need to protect the welfare of the individual or the public interest.
5. The patient has the right to continuity of health care. The physician has an obligation to cooperate in the coordination of medically indicated care with other health care providers treating the patient. The physician may not discontinue treatment of a patient as long as further treatment is

medically indicated without giving the patient reasonable assistance and sufficient opportunity to make alternative arrangements for care.

6. The patient has a basic right to have available adequate health care. Physicians, along with the rest of society, should continue to work toward this goal. Fulfillment of this right is dependent on society providing resources so that no patient is deprived of necessary care because of an inability to pay for the care. Physicians should continue their traditional assumption of a part of the responsibility for the medical care of those who cannot afford essential health care. Physicians should advocate for patients in dealing with third parties when appropriate.

Source: *Code of Medical Ethics: Current Opinions with Annotations*, American Medical Association, copyright 1996. Reprinted with permission.

American Nurses Association (ANA) Code for Nurses

1. The nurse provides services with respect for human dignity and the uniqueness of the client, unrestricted by considerations of social or economic status, personal attributes, or the nature of health problems.
2. The nurse safeguards the client's right to privacy by judiciously protecting information of a confidential nature.
3. The nurse acts to safeguard the client and the public when health care and safety are affected by the incompetent, unethical, or illegal practice of any person.
4. The nurse assumes responsibility and accountability for individual nursing judgments and actions.
5. The nurse maintains competence in nursing.
6. The nurse exercises informed judgment and uses individual competence and qualifications as criteria in seeking consultation, accepting responsibilities, and delegating nursing activities to others.
7. The nurse participates in activities that contribute to the ongoing development of the profession's body of knowledge.
8. The nurse participates in the profession's efforts to implement and improve standards of nursing.
9. The nurse participates in the profession's efforts to establish and maintain conditions of employment conducive to high-quality nursing care.
10. The nurse participates in the profession's effort to protect the public from misinformation, and misrepresentation and to maintain the integrity of nursing.
11. The nurse collaborates with members of the health professions and other citizens in promoting community and national efforts to meet the health needs of the public.

From "Code for Nurses with Interpretive Statements," © 1985 American Nurses Association, Kansas City, MO. Reprinted with permission.

Select Bibliography

Aaron, H.J., & W.B. Schwartz. (1985, March/April). Hospital cost control: A bitter pill to swallow. *Harvard Business Review, 63,* 160–167.

Aday, L.A., & R.M. Anderson. (1981, December). Equity of access to medical care: A conceptual and empirical overview. *Medical Care, 19*(12 Suppl.), 4–27.

American College of Healthcare Executives. (1995). *Code of ethics.* Chicago: Author.

Angell, M. (1984, April). Respecting the autonomy of competent patients. *New England Journal of Medicine, 310,* 1115–1116.

Angell, M. (1985, September). Cost containment and the physician. *Journal of the American Medical Association, 254,* 1203–1207.

Annas, G.J. (1986, February). Do feeding tubes have more rights than patients? *Hastings Center Report, 11,* 26–32.

Arras, J.D. (1981, August). Health care vouchers and the rhetoric of equity. *Hastings Center Report, 11,* 29–39.

Bayer, R. (1991, May). The HIV-infected clinician: To exclude or not to exclude? *Trustee, 44,* 14, 17.

Beauchamp, T.L., & J.F. Childress. (1994). *Principles of biomedical ethics* (4th ed.). New York: Oxford University Press.

Beauchamp, T.L., & L. Walters. (1994). *Contemporary issues in bioethics* (4th ed.). Belmont, CA: Wadsworth Publishing.

Bell, N.K. (1993, April). Ethics committees: Providing moral guidance in the hospital. *Trustee, 46,* 6–8.

Blake, D.C. (1989, May/June). State interests in terminating medical treatment. *Hastings Center Report, 19,* 5–13.

Brody, B.A. (1988). *Life and death decision making.* New York: Oxford University Press.

Brody, H. (1989, September/October). Transparency: Informed consent in primary care. *Hastings Center Report, 19,* 5–9.

Brozovich, J.P. (1986, March/April). Managing change through values. *Healthcare Executive, 1,* 45–47.

Callahan, D. (1983, October). On feeding the dying. *Hastings Center Report, 13,* 22.

Callahan, D. (1986, February). How technology is reframing the abortion debate. *Hastings Center Report, 16,* 33–42.

Callahan, D. (1987, October/November). Terminating treatment: Age as a standard. *Hastings Center Report, 17,* 21–25.

Callahan, D. (1991, July–August). Medical futility, medical necessity: The-problem-without-a-name. *Hastings Center Report, 21,* 30–35.

Callahan, D. (1995, November–December). Terminating life-sustaining treatment of the demented. *Hastings Center Report, 25,* 25–31.

Caplan, A.L. (1981, Fall). Kidneys, ethics, and politics: Policy lessons of the ESRD experience. *Journal of Health, Politics and Law, 6,* 488–503.

Capron, A.M. (1995, July–August). Abandoning a waning life. *Hastings Center Report, 25,* 24–26.

Capron, A.M. (1995, November–December). Constitutionalizaing death. *Hastings Center Report, 25,* 23–24.

Childress, J.F. (1990, January/February). The place of autonomy in bioethics. *Hastings Center Report, 20,* 12–17.

Cleveland, H.C., III, & B.L. Crawford. (1988, March). When physicians refuse to treat patients with AIDS. *Trustee, 41,* 18–19.

Cohen, C.B. (Ed.). (1988, August/September). Ethics committees. *Hastings Center Report, 18,* 23–28.

Cohen, C.B. (Ed.). (1989, January/February). Ethics committees. *Hastings Center Report, 19,* 19–24.

Cohen, C.B. (Ed.). (1989, September/October). Ethics committees. *Hastings Center Report, 19,* 21–26.

Cranford, R.E., & A.E. Doudera (Eds.). (1984). *Institutional ethics committees and health care decision making.* Ann Arbor, MI: Health Administration Press.

Curtin, L.L. (1993, May). Damage control and the whistleblower. *Nursing Management, 24,* 33–34.

Curtis, J. (1984, July). Multidisciplinary input on institutional ethics committees: A nursing perspective. *Quality Review Bulletin, 10,* 199–202.

Darr, K. (1984, March/April). Administrative ethics and the health services manager. *Hospital & Health Services Administration, 29,* 120–136.

Darr, K. (1985). *Ethics for health services managers.* Vol. 4, *Case studies in health administration.* Chicago: Foundation of the American College of Hospital Administrators.

Darr, K., B. Longest, Jr., & J.S. Rakich. (1986, March/April). The ethical imperative in health services governance and management. *Hospital & Health Services Administration, 31,* 53–66.

DeGeorge, R.T. (1990). *Business ethics* (3rd ed.). New York: Macmillan.

Dine, D.D. (1988, October). Ethics. *Modern Healthcare, 18,* 22–30.

Do ethics committees work? (1994, July). *Trustee, 47,* 17.

Dolenc, D.A., & C.J. Dougherty. (1985, June). DRGs: The counterrevolution in financing health care. *Hastings Center Report, 15,* 19–29.

Dougherty, C.J. (1989, January/February). Cost containment, DRGs, and the ethics of health care. *Hastings Center Report, 19,* 5–11.

Ebell, M.H. (1994, November 1). Practical guidelines for do-not-resuscitate orders. *American Family Physician, 50*(6), 1293–1299.

Emanuel, L.L. (1996, January 15). A professional response to demands for accountability: Practical recommendations regarding ethical aspects of patient care. *Annals of Internal Medicine, 124,* 240–249.

Emanuel, L.L. (1995, July–August). Reexamining death: The asymptotic model and a bounded zone definition. *Hastings Center Report, 25,* 27–35.

Emery, D.D., & L.J. Schneiderman. (1989, July/August). Cost-effectiveness analysis in health care. *Hastings Center Report, 19,* 8–13.

Engelhardt, H.T. (1984, July). Allocating scarce medical resources and the availability of organ transplantation. *New England Journal of Medicine, 311,* 66–71.

Engelhardt, H.T., Jr. (1986). *The foundations of bioethics.* New York: Oxford University Press.

Ertel, P.Y., & R.V. Harrison. (1984, March). Ethical and operational issues concerning DRGs and the prospective payment system. *Topics in Health Care Management*, 4, 10–31.

Ethics committees: How are they doing? (1986, June). *Hastings Center Report*, 16, 9–24.

Evans, A., & B. Brody. (1985, April). The do-not-resuscitate order in teaching hospitals. *Journal of the American Medical Association*, 293, 2236–2239.

Fletcher, J.C., N. Quist, & A.R. Johnson. (1989). *Ethics consultation in health care*. Ann Arbor, MI: Health Administration Press.

Fost, N., & R.E. Cranford. (1985, May). Hospital ethics committees, administrative aspects. *Journal of the American Medical Association*, 253, 2687–2692.

Frankena, W.K. (1973). *Ethics* (2nd ed.). Englewood Cliffs, NJ: Prentice Hall.

Glazer, M. (1983, December). Ten whistleblowers and how they fared. *Hastings Center Report*, 13, 33–41.

Gostin, L. (1989, January/February). HIV-infected physicians and the practice of seriously invasive procedures. *Hastings Center Report*, 19, 32–39.

Gregory, C.L. (1984, March/April). Ethics: A management tool? *Hospital & Health Services Administration*, 29, 102–119.

Grodin, M.A., & B. Zaharoff. (1986, March). A 12-year audit of IRB decisions. *Quality Review Bulletin*, 12, 82–86.

Heitman, E. (1995). Institutional ethics committees: Local perspectives on ethical issues in medicine. In R.E. Bulger, E. Meyer Bobby, & H.V. Fineberg (Eds.), *Society's choices: Social and ethical decision making in medicine* (pp. 409–431). Washington, DC: National Academy Press.

Hofmann, P.B. (1987, September/October). Business ethics: Not an oxymoron. *Healthcare Executive*, 2, 22–24.

Holleman, W.L., D.C. Edwards, & C.C. Matson. (1994, Summer). Obligations of physicians to patients and third-party payers. *Journal of Clinical Ethics*, 5(2), 113–120.

Hudson, T. (1994, February 20). Are futile-care policies the answer? *Hospitals & Health Networks*, 68, 26–32.

Hudson, T. (1994, March 20). Advance directives: Still problematic for providers. *Hospitals & Health Networks*, 68, 46, 48, 50.

Jonsen, A.R. (1986). Casuistry and clinical ethics. *Theoretical Medicine*, 7, 65–74.

Jonsen, A.R., & S. Toulmin. (1988). *The abuse of casuistry: A history of moral reasoning*. Berkeley, CA: University of California Press.

Kapp, M.B. (1984, December). Legal and ethical implications of health care reimbursement by diagnosis-related groups. *Law, Medicine and Health Care*, 12, 245–253.

Lipton, H. (1987, July). Do-not-resuscitate decisions in a community hospital: Implications for quality care. *Quality Review Bulletin*, 13, 226–231.

Lo, B., T.A. Raffin, & N.H. Cohen. (1987, November/December). Ethical dilemmas about intensive care for patients with AIDS. *Reviews of Infectious Diseases*, 9, 1163–1167.

Longo, D., M. Warren, & J.S. Roberts. (1988, June). Extent of DNR policies varies across healthcare settings. *Health Progress*, 69, 66–73.

Lynn, J., & J.F. Childress. (1983, October). Must patients always be given food and water? *Hastings Center Report*, 13, 17–21.

Macklin, R. (1985, Autumn). Are we in the lifeboat yet? Allocation and rationing of medical resources. *Social Research*, 52, 607–623.

Macrae, N. (1993, September 11). Some moral dilemmas, 1993–2143. *Economist, 302,* 83–84, 87.

May, L. (1995, January–February). Challenging medical authority: The refusal of treatment by Christian Scientists. *Hastings Center Report, 25,* 15–21.

McCullough, L.B. (1985, September/October). Moral dilemmas and economic realities. *Hospital & Health Services Administration, 30,* 63–75.

Medical Consultants on the Diagnosis of Death to the President's Commission for the Study of Ethical Problems in Medicine and Biomedical and Behavioral Research. (1981, November). Guidelines for the determination of death. *Journal of the American Medical Association, 246,* 2184–2186.

Monagle, J.F., & D.C. Thomasma. (1994). *Health care ethics: Critical issues.* Frederick, MD: Aspen Publishers.

Mooney, G.H. (1980, December). Cost-benefit analysis and medical ethics. *Journal of Medical Ethics, 6,* 177–179.

Morreim, E.H. (1985, June). The MD and the DRG. *Hastings Center Report, 15,* 30–38.

Morreim, E.H. (1994, January–February). Profoundly diminished life: The casualties of coercion. *Hastings Center Report, 24,* 33–42.

Morreim, E.H. (1995, November–December). Lifestyles of the risky and infamous: From managed care to managed lives. *Hastings Center Report, 25,* 5–12.

Moskowitz, E.H., & J.L. Nelson. (Eds.). (1995, November–December). The best laid plans. *Hastings Center Report, 25*(Spec. Supp.), S1–S36.

Murray, T.H. (1985, June). The final, anticlimactic rule on Baby Doe. *Hastings Center Report, 15,* 5–9.

Nelson, L.J., H.W. Clark, R.L. Goldman, & J.E. Schore. (1989, September/October). Taking the train to a world of strangers: Health care marketing and ethics. *Hastings Center Report, 19,* 36–43.

Nolan, K. (1987, October/November). In death's shadow: The meanings of withholding resuscitation. *Hastings Center Report, 17,* 9–14.

Pellegrino, E.D. (1994, Fall). Managed care and managed competition: Some ethical reflections. *Calyx, 4*(4), 1–5.

Pellegrino, E.D., & D.C. Thomasma. (1988). *For the patient's good: The restoration of beneficence in health care.* New York: Oxford University Press.

Pendola, C.J. (1992, Winter). Administrative ethics in health care resource allocation. *Review of Business, 14,* 20–22.

Perry, C.B. (1994, April). Conflicts of interest and the physician's duty to inform. *American Journal of Medicine, 96,* 375–379.

Powderly, K.E., & E. Smith. (1989, January/February). The impact of DRGs on health care workers and their clients. *Hastings Center Report, 19,* 16–18.

President's Commission for the Study of Ethical Problems in Medicine and Biomedical and Behavioral Research. (1980–1983). *Summing up; Compensating for research injuries,* 2 vol.; *Deciding to forego life-sustaining treatment; Defining death; Implementing human research regulations; Making health care decisions,* 2 vol.; *Protecting human subjects; Screening and counseling for genetic conditions; Securing access to health care,* 3 vol.; *Splicing life;* and *Whistleblowing in biomedical research.* Washington, DC: U.S. Government Printing Office.

Rasinski, D.C. (1984, March). Ethics committees in hospitals: Alternative structures and responsibilities. *Quality Review Bulletin, 10,* 62–64.

Reiser, S.J. (1994, November/December). The ethical life of health care organizations. *Hastings Center Report, 24,* 29–35.

Relman, A.S. (1985, August). AIDS: The emerging ethical dilemma. *Hastings Center Report, 15*, 1–7.

Relman, A.S. (1985, September). Dealing with conflicts of interest. *New England Journal of Medicine, 313*, 749–751.

Rhoden, N.K. (1989, July/August). A compromise on abortion? *Hastings Center Report, 19*, 32–37.

Robertson, J.A. (1984, January). Ethics committees in hospitals: Alternative structures and responsibilities. *Quality Review Bulletin, 10*, 6–10.

Rosner, F. (1985, May). Hospital medical ethics committees: A review of their development. *Journal of the American Medical Association, 253*, 2693–2697.

Ross, J.W., & D. Pugh. (1988, January). Limited cardiopulmonary resuscitation: The ethics of partial codes. *Quality Review Bulletin, 14*, 4–8.

Sabatino, F. (1992, August). How collaboration is influencing boards' strategic plans. *Trustee, 45*, 8–9, 27.

Sandrick, K.M. (1993, March). Ethical misconduct in healthcare financial management. *Healthcare Financial Management*, pp. 35–41.

Schneiderman, L.J., N.S. Jecker, & A. Jonsen. (1990, June 15). Medical futility: Its meaning and ethical implications. *Annals of Internal Medicine, 112*(12), 949–954.

Seiden, D.J. (1983, March/April). Ethics for hospital administrators. *Hospital & Health Services Administration, 28*, 81–89.

Solomon, M.Z., L. O'Donnell, B. Jennings, V. Guilfoy, S.M. Wolf, K. Nolan, R. Jackson, D. Koch-Weser, & S. Donnelley. (1993, January). Decisions near the end of life: Professional views on life-sustaining treatments. *American Journal of Public Health, 83*(1), 14–21.

Stein, K. (1987, September). Last rights. *Omni, 9*, 59.

Steinbock, B. (1989, July/August). Recovery from persistent vegetative state? The case of Carrie Coons. *Hastings Center Report, 19*, 14–15.

Teisberg, E.O., M.E. Porter, & G.B. Brown. (1994, July–August). Making competition in health care work. *Harvard Business Review, 72*(4), 131–141.

ten Have, H.A.M.J. (1995, September–October). Medical technology assessment and ethics: Ambivalent relations. *Hastings Center Report, 25*(5), 13–19.

Thomasma, D.C. (1988, August). The range of euthanasia. *American College of Surgeons Bulletin, 73*, 4–13.

Tomlinson, T., & H. Brody. (1988, January). Ethics and communication in do-not-resuscitate orders. *New England Journal of Medicine, 318*, 43–46.

Tomlinson, T., & D. Czlonka. (1995, May/June). Futility and hospital policy. *Hastings Center Report, 25*, 28–35.

U.S. Department of Health and Human Services. Basic HHS Policy for Protection of Human Research Subjects. 46 C.F.R. § 98 *et seq.* (1981, as modified).

U.S. Department of Health and Human Services, Office of Human Development Services. Child Abuse and Neglect Prevention and Treatment Program (Final Rule); and Model Guidelines for Health Care Providers to Establish Infant Care Review Committees (Notice). 45 C.F.R. § 1340 (April 15, 1985).

Veatch, R.M. (1980, June). Professional ethics: New principles for physicians? *Hastings Center Report, 10*, 16–19.

Veatch, R.M. (1981). *A theory of medical ethics.* New York: Basic Books.

Veatch, R.M. (1981, June). Protecting human subjects: The federal government steps back. *Hastings Center Report, 11*, 9–14.

Veatch, R.M. (1986, June). DRGs and the ethical allocation of resources. *Hastings Center Report*, 16, 32–40.

Veatch, R.M. (1991, Fall). Allocating health resources ethically: New roles for administrators and clinicians. *Frontiers of Health Services Management*, 7, 3–29.

Vinten, G. (1994). *Whistleblowing: Subversion or corporate citizenship?* New York: St. Martin's Press.

Waisel, D.B., & R.D. Truong. (1995, February 15). The cardiopulmonary resuscitation-not-indicated order: Futility revisited. *Annals of Internal Medicine*, 122(4), 304–309.

Weiss, R. (1988, November). Forbidding fruits of fetal-cell research. *Science News*, 134, 296–298.

Weitz, R. (1987, June). The interview as legacy: A social scientist confronts AIDS. *Hastings Center Report*, 17, 21–23.

Wigodsky, H.S. (1981, June). New regulations, new responsibilities for institutions. *Hastings Center Report*, 11, 12–14.

Wing, K.R. (1990). *The law and the public's health* (3rd ed.). Ann Arbor, MI: Health Administration Press.

Wolf, S.M. (Ed.). (1988, February/March). The persistent problem of PVS. *Hastings Center Report*, 18, 26–47.

Younger, S.J. (1987, February). Do-not-resuscitate orders: No longer secret, but still a problem. *Hastings Center Report*, 17, 24–33.

Zimmerman, J.E., W.A. Knaus, & S.M. Sharpe. (1986, January). The use and implications of do-not-resuscitate orders in intensive care units. *Journal of the American Medical Association*, 255, 351–356.

Index

Page numbers followed by "*f*" indicate figures; page numbers followed by "*t*" indicate tables.